BASIC AND CLINICAL SCIENCE COURSE

Glaucoma

Section 10
2011–2012
(Last major revision 2008–2009)

LIFELONG
EDUCATION FOR THE
OPHTHALMOLOGIST®

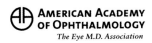

AMERICAN ACADEMY
OF OPHTHALMOLOGY
The Eye M.D. Association

The Basic and Clinical Science Course is one component of the Lifelong Education for the Ophthalmologist (LEO) framework, which assists members in planning their continuing medical education. LEO includes an array of clinical education products that members may select to form individualized, self-directed learning plans for updating their clinical knowledge. Active members or fellows who use LEO components may accumulate sufficient CME credits to earn the LEO Award. Contact the Academy's Clinical Education Division for further information on LEO.

The American Academy of Ophthalmology is accredited by the Accreditation Council for Continuing Medical Education to provide continuing medical education for physicians.

The American Academy of Ophthalmology designates this enduring material for a maximum of 10 *AMA PRA Category 1 Credits*™. Physicians should claim only credit commensurate with the extent of their participation in the activity.

The Academy provides this material for educational purposes only. It is not intended to represent the only or best method or procedure in every case, nor to replace a physician's own judgment or give specific advice for case management. Including all indications, contraindications, side effects, and alternative agents for each drug or treatment is beyond the scope of this material. All information and recommendations should be verified, prior to use, with current information included in the manufacturers' package inserts or other independent sources, and considered in light of the patient's condition and history. Reference to certain drugs, instruments, and other products in this course is made for illustrative purposes only and is not intended to constitute an endorsement of such. Some material may include information on applications that are not considered community standard, that reflect indications not included in approved FDA labeling, or that are approved for use only in restricted research settings. **The FDA has stated that it is the responsibility of the physician to determine the FDA status of each drug or device he or she wishes to use, and to use them with appropriate, informed patient consent in compliance with applicable law.** The Academy specifically disclaims any and all liability for injury or other damages of any kind, from negligence or otherwise, for any and all claims that may arise from the use of any recommendations or other information contained herein.

Cover image courtesy of M. Roy Wilson, MD.

Basic and Clinical Science Course

Gregory L. Skuta, MD, Oklahoma City, Oklahoma, *Senior Secretary for Clinical Education*

Louis B. Cantor, MD, Indianapolis, Indiana, *Secretary for Ophthalmic Knowledge*

Jayne S. Weiss, MD, Detroit, Michigan, *BCSC Course Chair*

Section 10

Faculty Responsible for This Edition

George A. Cioffi, MD, *Chair,* Portland, Oregon
F. Jane Durcan, MD, Spokane, Washington
Christopher A. Girkin, MD, Birmingham, Alabama
Ronald L. Gross, MD, Houston, Texas
Peter A. Netland, MD, Memphis, Tennessee
John R. Samples, MD, Portland, Oregon
Thomas W. Samuelson, MD, Minneapolis, Minnesota
Keith Barton, MD, *Consultant,* London, United Kingdom
Sara S. O'Connell, MD, Overland Park, Kansas
    Practicing Ophthalmologists Advisory Committee for Education

Financial Disclosures

The authors state the following financial relationships:

Dr Barton: Alcon, consultant, grant and lecture honoraria recipient; Allergan, consultant, lecture honoraria recipient; Merck US Human Health, consultant, lecture honoraria recipient; New World Medical, grant recipient; Pfizer Ophthalmics, consultant, grant and lecture honoraria recipient; Santen, grant recipient

Dr Girkin: Alcon, consultant, grant recipient; Allergan, consultant, lecture honoraria recipient; Carl Zeiss Meditec, consultant, grant recipient; Heidelberg Engineering, consultant; Merck US Human Health, lecture honoraria recipient; Pfizer Ophthalmics, consultant

Dr Gross: Alcon, consultant, grant and lecture honoraria recipient; Allergan, consultant, grant and lecture honoraria recipient; Cambridge Antibody Technology, grant recipient; ISTA Pharmaceuticals, consultant; Merck US Human Health, lecture honoraria recipient; Pfizer Ophthalmics, consultant, grant and lecture honoraria recipient

Dr Samples: Alcon, consultant, lecture honoraria recipient; Allergan, grant recipient; Cascade Biologicals, equity/stock options; IRIDEX, lecture honoraria recipient; ISTA

Pharmaceuticals, consultant, lecture honoraria recipient; Merck US Human Health, consultant, lecture honoraria recipient; Refocus Group, consultant

Dr Samuelson: Alcon, Allergan, Carl Zeiss Meditec, Glaukos Corporation, Heidelberg Engineering, iScience, Pfizer Ophthalmics, and SOLX, lecture honoraria recipient; Advanced Medical Optics, Denali Medical, and Medtronic Ophthalmics, consultant

The other authors state that they have no significant financial interest or other relationship with the manufacturer of any commercial product discussed in the chapters that they contributed to this course or with the manufacturer of any competing commercial product.

Recent Past Faculty

Jonathan S. Myers, MD
Steven T. Simmons, MD
Martha M. Wright, MD

In addition, the Academy gratefully acknowledges the contributions of numerous past faculty and advisory committee members who have played an important role in the development of previous editions of the Basic and Clinical Science Course.

American Academy of Ophthalmology Staff

Richard A. Zorab, *Vice President, Ophthalmic Knowledge*
Hal Straus, *Director, Publications Department*
Christine Arturo, *Acquisitions Manager*
Stephanie Tanaka, *Publications Manager*
D. Jean Ray, *Production Manager*
Brian Veen, *Medical Editor*
Steven Huebner, *Administrative Coordinator*

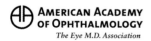

**AMERICAN ACADEMY
OF OPHTHALMOLOGY**
The Eye M.D. Association

655 Beach Street
Box 7424
San Francisco, CA 94120-7424

Contents

8 Surgical Therapy for Glaucoma 187

General Introduction

The Basic and Clinical Science Course (BCSC) is designed to meet the needs of residents and practitioners for a comprehensive yet concise curriculum of the field of ophthalmology. The BCSC has developed from its original brief outline format, which relied heavily on outside readings, to a more convenient and educationally useful self-contained text. The Academy updates and revises the course annually, with the goals of integrating the basic science and clinical practice of ophthalmology and of keeping ophthalmologists current with new developments in the various subspecialties.

The BCSC incorporates the effort and expertise of more than 80 ophthalmologists, organized into 13 Section faculties, working with Academy editorial staff. In addition, the course continues to benefit from many lasting contributions made by the faculties of previous editions. Members of the Academy's Practicing Ophthalmologists Advisory Committee for Education serve on each faculty and, as a group, review every volume before and after major revisions.

Organization of the Course

The Basic and Clinical Science Course comprises 13 volumes, incorporating fundamental ophthalmic knowledge, subspecialty areas, and special topics:

1 Update on General Medicine
2 Fundamentals and Principles of Ophthalmology
3 Clinical Optics
4 Ophthalmic Pathology and Intraocular Tumors
5 Neuro-Ophthalmology
6 Pediatric Ophthalmology and Strabismus
7 Orbit, Eyelids, and Lacrimal System
8 External Disease and Cornea
9 Intraocular Inflammation and Uveitis
10 Glaucoma
11 Lens and Cataract
12 Retina and Vitreous
13 Refractive Surgery

In addition, a comprehensive Master Index allows the reader to easily locate subjects throughout the entire series.

References

Readers who wish to explore specific topics in greater detail may consult the references cited within each chapter and listed in the Basic Texts section at the back of the book.

These references are intended to be selective rather than exhaustive, chosen by the BCSC faculty as being important, current, and readily available to residents and practitioners.

Related Academy educational materials are also listed in the appropriate sections. They include books, online and audiovisual materials, self-assessment programs, clinical modules, and interactive programs.

Study Questions and CME Credit

Each volume of the BCSC is designed as an independent study activity for ophthalmology residents and practitioners. The learning objectives for this volume are given on page 1. The text, illustrations, and references provide the information necessary to achieve the objectives; the study questions allow readers to test their understanding of the material and their mastery of the objectives. Physicians who wish to claim CME credit for this educational activity may do so by mail, by fax, or online. The necessary forms and instructions are given at the end of the book.

Conclusion

The Basic and Clinical Science Course has expanded greatly over the years, with the addition of much new text and numerous illustrations. Recent editions have sought to place a greater emphasis on clinical applicability while maintaining a solid foundation in basic science. As with any educational program, it reflects the experience of its authors. As its faculties change and as medicine progresses, new viewpoints are always emerging on controversial subjects and techniques. Not all alternate approaches can be included in this series; as with any educational endeavor, the learner should seek additional sources, including such carefully balanced opinions as the Academy's Preferred Practice Patterns.

The BCSC faculty and staff are continuously striving to improve the educational usefulness of the course; you, the reader, can contribute to this ongoing process. If you have any suggestions or questions about the series, please do not hesitate to contact the faculty or the editors.

The authors, editors, and reviewers hope that your study of the BCSC will be of lasting value and that each Section will serve as a practical resource for quality patient care.

Objectives

Upon completion of BCSC Section 10, *Glaucoma,* the reader should be able to

- identify the epidemiologic features of glaucoma, including the social and economic impacts of the disease

- summarize recent advances in the understanding of hereditary and genetic factors in glaucoma

- outline the physiology of aqueous humor dynamics and the control of intraocular pressure (IOP)

- review the clinical evaluation of the glaucoma patient, including history and general examination, gonioscopy, optic nerve examination, and visual field

- describe the clinical features of the patient considered a "glaucoma suspect"

- summarize the clinical features, evaluation, and treatment of primary open-angle glaucoma and normal-tension glaucoma

- list the various clinical features of and therapeutic approaches for the primary and secondary open-angle glaucomas

- explain the underlying causes of the increased IOP in various forms of secondary open-angle glaucoma and the impact these underlying causes have on management

- review the mechanisms and pathophysiology of primary angle-closure glaucoma

- review the pathophysiology of secondary angle-closure glaucoma, both with and without pupillary block

- outline the pathophysiology of and therapy for primary congenital and juvenile-onset glaucomas

- differentiate among the various classes of medical therapy for glaucoma, including efficacy, mechanism of action, and safety

- compare the indications for and techniques of various laser and incisional surgical procedures for glaucoma

- describe cyclodestructive therapy for refractory glaucoma

CHAPTER 1

Introduction to Glaucoma: Terminology, Epidemiology, and Heredity

Definitions

The term *glaucoma* refers to a group of diseases that have in common a characteristic *optic neuropathy* with associated *visual function loss*. Although elevated *intraocular pressure (IOP)* is one of the primary risk factors, its presence or absence does not have a role in the definition of the disease. Three factors determine the IOP (Fig 1-1):

- the rate of aqueous humor production by the ciliary body
- resistance to aqueous outflow across the trabecular meshwork–Schlemm's canal system; the specific site of resistance is generally thought to be in the juxtacanalicular meshwork
- the level of episcleral venous pressure

Generally, increased IOP is caused by increased resistance to aqueous humor outflow.

In most individuals, the optic nerve and visual field changes seen in glaucoma are determined by both the level of the IOP and the resistance of the optic nerve axons to pressure damage. Other biological factors may predispose the optic nerve axons to damage. Although progressive changes in the visual field and optic nerve are usually related to increased IOP and cupping, in cases of normal-tension glaucoma, the IOP remains within statistically normal range (see Chapter 4). However, when considering whether glaucomatous damage is truly occurring at a "normal" IOP, the clinician needs to take into account the artifact in IOP measurements that is caused by variation in central corneal thickness and that occurs with the diurnal variation in IOP. In most cases of glaucoma, it is presumed that the IOP is too high for proper functioning of the optic nerve axons and that lowering the IOP will stabilize the damage. In cases involving other pathophysiologic mechanisms that may affect the optic nerve, however, progression of optic nerve damage may continue despite lowering of IOP.

Regardless of the IOP, the presence of glaucoma is defined by a characteristic optic neuropathy consistent with excavation and undermining of the neural and connective tissue elements of the optic disc and by the eventual development of characteristic visual field defects. *Preperimetric glaucoma* is a term that is sometimes used to denote glaucomatous

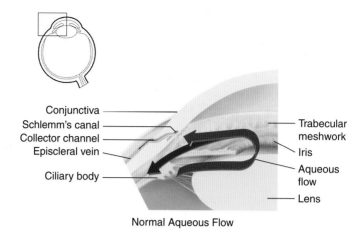

Conjunctiva
Schlemm's canal
Collector channel
Episcleral vein
Ciliary body

Trabecular meshwork
Iris
Aqueous flow
Lens

Normal Aqueous Flow

Figure 1-1 Diagrammatic cross section of the anterior segment of the normal eye, showing the site of aqueous production (ciliary body), sites of conventional aqueous outflow (trabecular meshwork–Schlemm's canal system and episcleral venous plexus), and the uveoscleral outflow pathway. Small white arrow shows normal path of outflow and indicates that resistance in this illustration is relative, not total. *(Illustration by Cyndie C. H. Wooley.)*

changes in the optic disc in patients with normal visual fields, as determined by white-on-white perimetry. Since the correct application of this term depends on the sensitivity of the visual function test used, the development of new, more sensitive tests may allow earlier confirmation of this type of glaucoma, while the patient is within this preperimetric phase.

Classification

The terms *primary* and *secondary* have been helpful in current definitions of glaucoma, and they are still in widespread use. There are separate anatomic, gonioscopic, biochemical, molecular, and genetic views of the classification of the glaucomas, among others, each with its own merit. For instance, glaucoma can be defined on the basis of genetic terms related to a specific mutation. In the future, knowing the mutation an individual with glaucoma harbors may be the most definitive method by which to understand the disease; however, it is unlikely that all glaucomas will be understood in genetic terms. By definition, the *primary glaucomas* are not associated with known ocular or systemic disorders that cause increased resistance to aqueous outflow or angle closure. The primary glaucomas usually affect both eyes. Conversely, the *secondary glaucomas* are associated with ocular or systemic disorders responsible for decreased aqueous outflow. The diseases that cause secondary glaucoma are often asymmetric or unilateral.

Open-Angle, Angle-Closure, Primary, and Secondary Glaucomas

Traditionally, glaucoma has been classified as open angle or closed angle and as primary or secondary (Table 1-1). Differentiation of open-angle glaucoma from closed-angle glaucoma is essential from a therapeutic standpoint (Figs 1-2, 1-3; see Chapters 4 and 5). The concept

Table 1-1 Classification of Glaucoma

Type	Characteristics
Open-angle glaucoma (Fig 1-2)	
Primary open-angle glaucoma (POAG)	Not associated with known ocular or systemic disorders that cause increased resistance to aqueous outflow or damage to optic nerve; usually associated with elevated IOP
Normal-tension glaucoma	Considered in continuum of POAG; terminology often used when IOP is not elevated
Juvenile open-angle glaucoma	Terminology often used when open-angle glaucoma diagnosed at young age (typically 10–30 years of age)
Glaucoma suspect	Normal optic disc and visual field associated with elevated IOP Suspicious optic disc and/or visual field with normal IOP
Secondary open-angle glaucoma	Increased resistance to trabecular meshwork outflow associated with other conditions (eg, pigmentary glaucoma, phacolytic glaucoma, steroid-induced glaucoma, exfoliation, angle-recession glaucoma) Increased posttrabecular resistance to outflow secondary to elevated episcleral venous pressure (eg, carotid cavernous sinus fistula)
Angle-closure glaucoma (Fig 1-3)	
Primary angle-closure glaucoma with relative pupillary block	Movement of aqueous humor from posterior chamber to anterior chamber restricted; peripheral iris in contact with trabecular meshwork
Acute angle closure	Occurs when IOP rises rapidly as a result of relatively sudden blockage of the trabecular meshwork
Subacute angle closure (intermittent angle closure)	Repeated, brief episodes of angle closure with mild symptoms and elevated IOP, often a prelude to acute angle closure
Chronic angle closure	IOP elevation caused by variable portions of anterior chamber angle being permanently closed by peripheral anterior synechiae
Secondary angle-closure glaucoma with pupillary block	(For example, swollen lens, secluded pupil)
Secondary angle-closure glaucoma without pupillary block	Posterior pushing mechanism: lens–iris diaphragm pushed forward (eg, posterior segment tumor, scleral buckling procedure, uveal effusion) Anterior pulling mechanism: anterior segment process pulling iris forward to form peripheral anterior synechiae (eg, iridocorneal endothelial syndrome, neovascular glaucoma, inflammation)
Plateau iris syndrome	An anatomic variation in the iris root in which narrowing of the angle occurs independent of pupillary block
Childhood glaucoma	
Primary congenital glaucoma	Primary glaucoma present from birth to first few years of life
Glaucoma associated with congenital anomalies	Associated with ocular disorders (eg, anterior segment dysgenesis, aniridia) Associated with systemic disorders (eg, rubella, Lowe syndrome)
Secondary glaucoma in infants and children	(For example, glaucoma secondary to retinoblastoma or trauma)

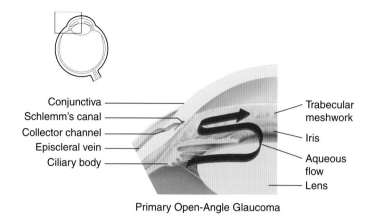

Conjunctiva
Schlemm's canal
Collector channel
Episcleral vein
Ciliary body

Trabecular meshwork
Iris
Aqueous flow
Lens

Primary Open-Angle Glaucoma

Figure 1-2 Schematic of open-angle glaucoma with resistance to aqueous outflow through the trabecular meshwork–Schlemm's canal system in the absence of gross anatomic obstruction. *(Illustration by Cyndie C. H. Wooley.)*

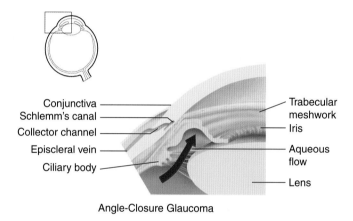

Conjunctiva
Schlemm's canal
Collector channel
Episcleral vein
Ciliary body

Trabecular meshwork
Iris
Aqueous flow
Lens

Angle-Closure Glaucoma

Figure 1-3 Schematic of angle-closure glaucoma with pupillary block leading to peripheral iris obstruction of the trabecular meshwork. *(Illustration by Cyndie C. H. Wooley.)*

of primary and secondary glaucomas is also useful, but it reflects our lack of understanding of the pathophysiologic mechanisms underlying the glaucomatous process. Open-angle glaucoma is classified as primary when no anatomically identifiable underlying cause of the events that led to outflow obstruction and IOP elevation can be found. The etiology is generally regarded as an abnormality in the trabecular meshwork extracellular matrix and in trabecular cells in the juxtacanalicular region, although other views exist. Trabecular cells and their surrounding extracellular matrix are understood in fairly specific terms, and the basic scientific understanding of the outflow structures is constantly increasing. Glaucoma has been classified as secondary when an abnormality is identified and a putative role in the pathogenesis can be ascribed to this abnormality. With the development of a specific understanding of the genetic and biochemical abnormalities in the outflow pathway, the classic division of glaucoma as either primary or secondary breaks down, and it has been recognized that all glaucomas are secondary to some abnormality, whether currently identified or not. As knowledge of the mechanisms underlying the causes of glaucoma continues to expand, the primary/secondary classification has become increasingly artificial.

Other schemes for classifying glaucoma have been proposed. Classification of the glaucomas based on initial events and on mechanisms of outflow obstruction are 2 schemes that have gained increasing popularity (Table 1-2).

Ritch R, Shields MB, Krupin T, eds. *The Glaucomas.* 2nd ed. St Louis: Mosby; 1996:722.

Combined-Mechanism Glaucoma

Combined-mechanism glaucoma can appear in a patient with open-angle glaucoma who develops secondary angle closure from other causes. Examples include a patient with open-angle glaucoma who develops angle closure as a result of miotic therapy, when the miotic causes a forward shift of the lens–iris diaphragm, or a patient with pseudophakic open-angle glaucoma who develops peripheral anterior synechiae (PAS) after an episode of pupillary block. Perhaps more often, combined mechanism glaucoma occurs in a patient who has been successfully treated for a narrow angle but who continues to demonstrate reduced outflow facility and elevated IOP.

IOP elevation in these cases can occur as a result of either or both of the following:

- the intrinsic resistance of the trabecular meshwork to aqueous outflow in open-angle glaucoma
- the direct anatomic obstruction of the filtering meshwork by synechiae in angle-closure glaucoma

Treatment is modified based on the proportion of open angle to closed angle and the etiology of the angle-closure component, as well as the status and vulnerability of the optic nerve.

Epidemiologic Aspects of Glaucoma

Primary Open-Angle Glaucoma

Magnitude of the problem

Primary open-angle glaucoma (POAG) represents a significant public health problem. The estimated prevalence of POAG in the United States in individuals older than 40 years is 1.86% (95% confidence interval, 1.75%–1.96%), based on a meta-analysis of population-based studies. Applied to data from the 2000 US census, this percentage translates to nearly 2.22 million Americans affected. Estimates based on the available data indicate that between 84,000 and 116,000 of them have become bilaterally blind (best-corrected visual acuity ≤20/200 or visual field <20°). With the rapidly aging US population, the number of POAG patients is estimated to increase by 50% to 3.36 million in 2020. This staggering number may be an underestimate, since visual field loss is required in the definition of POAG, and many individuals have glaucoma without documented visual field loss. POAG is thus an important cause of blindness in the United States and the most frequent cause of nonreversible blindness in blacks.

Table 1-2 Classification of the Glaucomas Based on Mechanisms of Outflow Obstruction*

Pretrabecular (Membrane Overgrowth)	Open-Angle Glaucoma Mechanisms		Angle-Closure Glaucoma Mechanisms		Developmental Anomalies of Anterior Chamber Angle
	Trabecular	Posttrabecular	Anterior ("Pulling")	Posterior ("Pushing")	
Fibrovascular membrane (neovascular glaucoma)	Idiopathic	Obstruction of Schlemm's canal, eg. collapse at canal	Contracture of membranes	With pupillary block	Incomplete development of trabecular meshwork–Schlemm's canal
Endothelial layer, often with	Chronic open-angle glaucoma	Elevated episcleral venous pressure	Neovascular glaucoma	Pupillary-block glaucoma	Congenital (infantile) glaucoma
Descemet-like membrane	Juvenile open-angle glaucoma	Carotid cavernous fistula	Iridocorneal endothelial syndrome	Lens-induced mechanisms	Axenfeld-Rieger syndrome
Iridocorneal endothelial syndrome	"Clogging" of trabecular meshwork	Cavernous sinus thrombosis	Posterior polymorphous dystrophy	Phacomorphic lens	Peters anomaly
Posterior polymorphous dystrophy	Red blood cells	Retrobulbar tumors	Penetrating and nonpenetrating trauma	Ectopia lentis	Glaucomas associated with other developmental anomalies
Penetrating and non-penetrating trauma	Hemorrhagic glaucoma	Thyroid ophthalmopathy	Consolidation of inflammatory products	Posterior synechiae	Iridocorneal adhesions
Epithelial downgrowth	Ghost cell glaucoma	Superior vena cava obstruction		Iris–vitreous block	Broad strands (Axenfeld-Rieger syndrome)
Fibrous ingrowth	Sickled red blood cells	Mediastinal tumors		Pseudophakia	Fine strands that contract to close angle (aniridia)
Inflammatory membrane	Macrophages	Sturge-Weber syndrome		Uveitis	
Fuchs heterochromic iridocyclitis	Hemolytic glaucoma	Familial episcleral venous pressure elevation		Without pupillary block	
Luetic interstitial keratitis	Phacolytic glaucoma			Ciliary block (malignant) glaucoma	
	Melanomalytic glaucoma			Lens-induced mechanisms	
	Neoplastic cells			Phacomorphic lens	
	Primary ocular tumors			Ectopia lentis	
	Neoplastic tumors			Following lens extraction (forward vitreous shift)	
	Juvenile xanthogranuloma			Anterior rotation of ciliary body	
	Pigment particles			Following scleral buckling	
	Pigmentary glaucoma			Following panretinal photocoagulation	
	Exfoliation syndrome (glaucoma capsulare)			Central retinal vein occlusion	
	Malignant melanoma			Intraocular tumors	
	Protein			Malignant melanoma	
	Uveitis			Retinoblastoma	
	Lens-induced glaucoma			Cysts of the iris and ciliary body	
	Viscoelastic agents			Retrolenticular tissue contracture	
	α-Chymotrypsin–induced glaucoma			Retinopathy of prematurity (retrolental fibroplasia)	
	Alterations of the trabecular meshwork			Persistent hyperplastic primary vitreous	
	Steroid-induced glaucoma				
	Edema				
	Uveitis (trabeculitis)				
	Scleritis and episcleritis				
	Alkali burns				
	Trauma (angle recession)				
	Intraocular foreign bodies (hemosiderosis, chalcosis)				

Plateau Iris Syndrome

* Clinical examples cited in this table do not represent an inclusive list of the glaucomas.

Modified with permission from Ritch R, Shields MB, Krupin T, eds. *The Glaucomas.* 2nd ed. St Louis: Mosby; 1996:722.

The World Health Organization (WHO) undertook an analysis of the literature to esti-mate the prevalence, incidence, and severity of the different types of glaucoma on a world-wide basis. Using data collected predominantly in the late 1980s and early 1990s, WHO estimated the global population of people with high IOP (>21 mm Hg) at 104.5 million. The incidence (newly identified cases) of POAG was estimated at 2.4 million people per year. Blindness prevalence for all types of glaucoma was estimated at more than 8 million people, with 4 million cases caused by POAG. The different types of glaucoma were theo-retically calculated to be responsible for 15% of blindness, placing glaucoma as the third leading cause of blindness worldwide, following cataract and river blindness.

Despite these staggering statistics, the impact of glaucoma from a public health per-spective has not been fully appreciated. Relatively little information is currently avail-able regarding the individual burden associated with the psychological effects of having a potentially blinding chronic disease, the debilitating side effects of treatment, and the qualitative functional loss associated with diminished visual fields. Nor does reliable in-formation exist on the societal costs associated with the detection, treatment, and reha-bilitation of this disease.

Prevalence

The estimated prevalence (the proportion of individuals with a disease) varies widely across population-based samples, with the Rotterdam Study showing a prevalence of 0.8% and the Barbados Eye Study showing a prevalence of 7% in individuals older than 40 years. But in all of these studies there is a significant increase in the prevalence of glaucoma in older individuals, with estimates for persons in their 70s being generally 3 to 8 times higher than those for persons in their 40s. In addition, multiple population-based surveys have demonstrated a higher prevalence of glaucoma in specific ethnic groups. Among whites aged 40 years and older, a prevalence of between 1.1% and 2.1% has been reported based on population-based studies performed throughout the world. The prevalence among blacks is 3 to 4 times higher, with at least 4 times the likelihood of blindness. This racial disparity increases with age, with the likelihood of blindness from POAG increasing to 15 times higher for blacks in the age group 46–65 years.

Friedman DS, Wolfs RC, O'Colmain BJ, et al. Prevalence of open-angle glaucoma among adults in the United States. *Arch Ophthalmol.* 2004;122(4):532–538.

Javitt JC, McBean AM, Nicholson GA, Babish JD, Warren JL, Krakauer H. Undertreatment of glaucoma among black Americans. *N Engl J Med.* 1991;325:1418–1422.

Incidence

While several studies have provided estimates of the prevalence of POAG, there are few direct measurements of the incidence of POAG in population-based studies. The Barba-dos Eye Study demonstrated an overall incidence of 2.2% in subjects older than 40 years in a predominantly black population. A much lower incidence was recently demonstrated in the Visual Impairment Project, based in Melbourne, Australia (1.1% for definite and probable POAG), and in the Rotterdam Study (5-year risk of 1.8% for definite and prob-able POAG). In both studies the incidence increased significantly with age. Several other studies attempted to statistically estimate glaucoma incidence based on prevalence data.

Although the validity of these estimates has been questioned, the nonlogistic approach, when recently compared against the observed incidence, increased the similarity between observed and predicted incidence.

Risk factors

Identifying risk factors is important because this information may lead to the development of strategies for disease screening and prevention and may be useful in identifying persons for whom close medical supervision is indicated. Strictly defined, a factor can be considered a risk factor only if it predates disease occurrence. From a clinical perspective, it is often difficult to differentiate very early disease from normal. Because evolving technologies are aimed at detecting glaucoma in increasingly earlier stages, the definition of *early glaucoma* has become dependent on the sensitivity of the methods used to assess optic nerve function and structural integrity, as discussed in Chapter 3.

Glaucoma is best defined by the presence of acquired loss of retinal ganglion cells and axons. This loss is evident at the level of the retinal nerve fiber layer and/or the optic disc and eventually leads to characteristic visual field defects. How often this diagnosis is made in marginal cases is influenced by the sensitivity of available diagnostic tests and the variability in the normal appearance of the optic disc. Thus, it may be difficult to determine whether abnormalities in certain parameters—for example, optic nerve parameters such as thinner nerve fiber layer—are indicative of increased susceptibility to developing glaucoma or are signs of early disease. Individuals manifesting such abnormalities must be closely monitored for signs of clinically significant disease development or progression.

Several risk factors—and not all risk factors are known—increase the likelihood of the development of POAG. Besides increased IOP, factors known to be associated with an increased risk for the development of glaucoma include advanced age, decreased corneal thickness, racial background, and a positive family history. Although variation in central corneal thickness creates an artifact with IOP measurement, patients with thinner corneas have a greater risk of developing glaucoma independent of the relationship with IOP. It has been hypothesized that thinner corneas may be a biologic marker for increased biomechanical susceptibility of the lamina cribrosa and peripapillary sclera, although no conclusive evidence has been demonstrated.

> Dueker DK, Singh K, Lin SC, et al. Corneal thickness measurement in the management of primary open-angle glaucoma: a report by the American Academy of Ophthalmology. *Ophthalmology*. 2007;114(9):1779–1787.

In terms of the assessment of risk factors, the importance of the diurnal variation in IOP has been increasingly recognized. It has been suggested by a number of authors that fluctuation in the pressure per se is a risk factor for optic nerve damage. Clinicians should record the time of day that IOP is checked because variations occur throughout the day and medications have an impact on them. The relative degree to which peak pressures constitute a risk factor versus overall elevation of pressure and range of pressure elevation is not known. Current evidence obtained in sleep laboratory conditions suggests that in most subjects, the peak IOP occurs during the night and is therefore, unfortunately, not ascertained in the routine clinical setting. Much of this nocturnal rise may be due to variations in body position, and it has been suggested that measurement of supine IOP during office visits may approximate this nocturnal peak. The significance of nocturnal pressure elevation is not known.

The quality of available data regarding potential risk factors for the development of POAG varies greatly. Evidence that elevated IOP, advanced age, race, and positive family history are risk factors for POAG is considerable and reliable. Data also support diabetes mellitus and myopia as risk factors, but these data are generally less convincing. The relevance of gender and of various systemic factors, such as systemic hypertension and atherosclerotic and ischemic vascular diseases, to glaucoma risk has been widely debated, and currently available data are inconclusive.

Demographic risk factors for POAG include advanced age. It is clear that as an individual gets older, the risk of POAG increases. In the Baltimore Eye Survey, the prevalence of glaucoma among whites was 3.5 times higher for individuals in their 70s than for those in their 40s. Among blacks, the ratio was 7.4. The demographic view on gender is mixed. In the Framingham and Barbados eye studies, males had a higher rate of POAG, whereas the Sweden, St Lucia, and Blue Mountains studies reported higher numbers in females. In the Wales, Baltimore, Beaver Dam, and Melbourne studies, no statistical associations were found. As a result of these mixed findings, gender is not usually regarded as a risk factor for POAG.

Racial studies have generally shown that blacks are at increased risk of developing POAG. In the Baltimore Eye Survey, blacks were 3–4 times more likely than whites to have glaucoma. Independent studies have demonstrated that the risk among Hispanic individuals appears to be intermediate between the reported values for whites and blacks. The cause of the higher prevalence of glaucoma among blacks is not known. The eyes of black persons do have larger discs and more nerve fibers, in addition to thinner central corneas, which may be an independent predictor of progression. These eyes also possibly have deeper cups. It has been hypothesized that the increased disc size is associated with increased mechanical strain in the region of the optic nerve.

Type 2 diabetes mellitus has been demonstrated to be associated with POAG, although debate persists. People with diabetes undergo frequent detailed eye examinations to rule out diabetic retinopathy, and this may mean that there is a greater opportunity to diagnose POAG.

Primary Angle-Closure Glaucoma

Race

The prevalence of primary angle-closure glaucoma (PACG) varies among different racial and ethnic groups. Among white populations in the United States and Europe, it is estimated at 0.1%. Inuit populations from Arctic regions have the highest-known prevalence of PACG—20–40 times higher than that for whites. The relative prevalence of PACG and POAG among Inuits is also the reverse of what is noted in white populations, with POAG being uncommon.

Estimates of the prevalence of PACG in Asian populations have varied considerably. Some of this variability may be the result of differences in the definition used and in the design of the studies from which the estimates were derived. Another factor, however, is that Asian populations are not one homogeneous group. Available data suggest that most Asian population groups have a prevalence rate of PACG between that of whites and Inuits.

Acute angle-closure glaucoma is relatively uncommon among blacks. However, chronic angle-closure glaucoma is much more common than initially believed. Some studies have suggested that the prevalence of PACG among blacks is similar to that among whites, with most cases among blacks being of the chronic variety. Although most attention in the field of glaucoma genetics has gone to POAG and congenital glaucoma, a positive family history is also a risk factor for PACG. For example, among Eskimos, the prevalence of PACG in first-degree relatives of patients with this disorder may be 3.5 times higher than in the general population. A population-based survey in China suggested that a family history of glaucoma increased by sixfold the risk of PACG.

Gender

Acute angle-closure glaucoma has been reported more often in women than in men, and several population surveys demonstrate that women are at increased risk of angle-closure glaucoma. Studies of normal eyes have shown that women have shallower anterior chambers than men.

Age

The anterior chamber decreases in depth and volume with age. These changes predispose to pupillary block, and the prevalence of pupillary-block–induced angle-closure glaucoma thus increases with age. Acute angle-closure glaucoma is most common between the ages of 55 and 65 years, but it can occur in young adults and has been reported in children.

Refraction

The anterior chamber depth and volume are smaller in hyperopic eyes. Although PACG may occur in eyes with any type of refractive error, it is thus typically associated with hyperopia.

Inheritance

Some of the anatomic features of the eye that predispose to pupillary block, such as more forward position of the lens and greater than average lens thickness, are inherited. Thus, relatives of subjects with angle-closure glaucoma are at greater risk of developing angle closure than is the general population. However, estimates of the exact risk vary greatly.

Epstein DL, Allingham RR, Schuman JS, eds. *Chandler and Grant's Glaucoma.* 4th ed. Baltimore: Williams & Wilkins; 1997:641–646.

Ritch RM, Shields MB, Krupin T, eds. *The Glaucomas.* 2nd ed. St Louis: Mosby; 1996: 753–765.

Hereditary and Genetic Factors

The recent explosion of knowledge regarding the genetic basis for many diseases has had a profound impact, including in the field of glaucoma. In glaucoma mapping techniques, the localization of several genes and the understanding of the mutations within the genes have significantly changed our knowledge of the disease. In the future, early diagnosis of specific forms of glaucoma may have a genetic basis. Eventually, this information will lead to the development of new drugs or specific types of gene therapy, with replacement of DNA, modification of messenger ribonucleic acid (mRNA), or replacement of the defective proteins providing long-term lowering of IOP or improving optic neuropathy.

Kass and Becker were among the first to observe a strong correlation between family history and glaucoma, particularly in terms of elevated pressure, cup–disc ratio, and the glucocorticoid response. Based on their observations, the researchers suggested that the most effective method of glaucoma detection would be to check family members. However, in the early study of glaucoma, the disease seemed to defy the simple classification as either autosomal dominant or autosomal recessive. Becker, and later Armaly, found that glucocorticoid treatment elevated IOP more often in glaucoma patients than in individuals without glaucoma. Testing of family members showed that this response was usually inherited as an autosomal recessive trait. Subsequently, Polansky hypothesized that mutations of the trabecular meshwork glucocorticoid genes could cause elevated IOP. He identified a specific protein, the TIGR protein (also termed *myocilin*) produced by trabecular meshwork cells. Initially, the TIGR protein was identified in juvenile glaucoma families; later it was reported to affect up to 3% of the general open-angle glaucoma population. In the mid-1990s, *GLC1A*, the gene responsible for mutations in the TIGR protein, was mapped to chromosome 1. Since then, several additional open-angle glaucoma genes have been mapped, and many more potential genes are being explored. Although major gene defects cause glaucoma in specific individuals, the proportion of all glaucoma patients affected by 1 or several major genes is unknown. This is likely due to the complex nature of glaucoma and to complex interactions between genetic and environmental factors. The relative contributions of environmental factors versus genetic factors remain unknown for glaucoma. Known genes account for only a small percentage of glaucoma (Table 1-3). Researchers have started to apply genome-wide scanning techniques to large cohorts of glaucoma subjects. These techniques may be useful in determining which regions of the genome are associated with the disease. In addition, use of genome-wide scanning techniques may lead to the identification of future genetic markers.

The prevalence of glaucoma, enlarged cup–disc ratio, and elevated IOP are all much higher in siblings and offspring of patients with glaucoma than in the general population. A positive family history is a risk factor for the development of POAG. The prevalence of glaucoma among siblings of patients is approximately 10%. However, in prospective studies, a family history of POAG has not been consistently demonstrated to be a risk factor for the progression of existing POAG or for the development of POAG in patients with ocular hypertension.

The precise mechanism of inheritance is not always clear. Complicated genetic interactions may involve the presence of both causal and susceptibility genes. To date, many of the glaucomas appear to have an autosomal dominant inheritance that may involve more than 1 gene (polygenic); have a late or variable age of onset; demonstrate incomplete penetrance (the disease may not develop even when the causative gene has been inherited); and may be substantially influenced by environmental factors. See also BCSC Section 2, *Fundamentals and Principles of Ophthalmology*, Part III, Genetics.

Kass MA, Becker B. Genetics of primary open-angle glaucoma. *Sight Sav Rev.* 1978;48:21–28.

Wolfs RC, Klaver CC, Ramrattan RS, et al. Genetic risk of primary open-angle glaucoma: population-based familial aggregation study. *Arch Ophthalmol.* 1998;116:1640–1645.

Table 1-3 Currently Mapped Glaucoma Genes

Locus	Chromosome Location	Phenotype	Inheritance	Gene
GLC1A	1q23	Early and adult POAG	Dominant	TIGR/MYOC
GLC1B	2cen-q13	NTG, adult POAG	Dominant	—
GLC1C	3q21-24	Adult POAG	Dominant	—
GLC1D	8q23	Adult POAG	Dominant	—
GLC1E	10P15-14	NTG, adult POAG	Dominant	OPTN
GLC1F	7q35	Adult POAG	Dominant	—
GLC1G	5q22	Adult POAG	Dominant, complex	WDR36
GLC1I	15q11-q13	Adult POAG	Complex	—
GLC1J	9q22	Early POAG	Dominant	—
GLC1K	20p12	Early POAG	Dominant	—
GPDS1	7q35-q36	PDS	Dominant	—
GLC3A	2p21	Congenital	Recessive	CYP1B1
GLC3B	1p36	Congenital	Recessive	—
GLC3C	14q24.3	Congenital	Recessive	—
NNO1	11p	Nanophthalmos	Dominant	—
VMD2	11q12	Nanophthalmos	Dominant	—
MFRP	11q23	Nanophthalmos	Recessive	—
RIEG1	4q25	Rieger syndrome	Dominant	PITX2
RIEG2	13q14	Rieger syndrome	Dominant	—
IRID1	6p25	Iridogoniodysgenesis	Dominant	FOXC1
	7q35	PDS	Dominant	—
NPS	9q34	Nail-patella syndrome	Dominant	LMX1B
	15q24	PXE		LOXL1

POAG = primary open-angle glaucoma; NTG = normal-tension glaucoma; PDS = pigment dispersion syndrome; PXE = pseudoexfoliation

Adapted from Wiggs JL. Genetic etiologies of glaucoma. *Arch Ophthalmol.* 2007;125(1):30–37.

Open-Angle Glaucoma Genes

GLC1A, the first open-angle glaucoma gene, was initially mapped in a large juvenile glaucoma family and localized to chromosome 1. The mutations in this gene, which are suspected to be responsible for open-angle glaucoma, produce a protein, myocilin, that is also induced in trabecular meshwork cells by treatment with dexamethasone (TIGR). Because of this protein, the *TIGR/myocilin* gene has been given the gene symbol *TIGR/MYOC*. The mutations in *TIGR/MYOC* are not limited to juvenile glaucoma and have been reported in 3% of individuals with adult-onset POAG. Although use of corticosteroids may increase IOP in a high percentage of glaucoma patients, it is hypothesized that a *TIGR/MYOC*-related protein could be responsible. However, the TIGR/MYOC protein is also expressed in the retina, especially in retinoblastomas, skeletal muscle, and fetal heart.

Other researchers have identified 2 loci for the normal-tension forms of open-angle glaucoma: *GLC1B* maps to chromosome 2 and *GLC1E* maps to chromosome 10. Because most individuals with the *GLC1B* and *GLC1E* genes appear to develop a type of glaucoma with lower pressure, these mutations may render the optic nerve abnormally sensitive to IOP or otherwise facilitate optic nerve damage independent of IOP. Mutations in *OPTN*, the gene that encodes the optineurin protein, have been identified in patients with the *GLC1E* gene. The characterization of the protein(s) governed by these genes may potentially lead to greater insight.

A recent genomewide scan found multiple single-nucleotide polymorphisms (SNPs) in the 15q24.1 region associated with exfoliation syndrome. These polymorphisms are associated with the *LOXL1* gene, which produces a protein that catalyzes the formation of elastin fibers, the major component of exfoliative material.

In contrast to *GLC1A* and *GLC1B*, *GLC1C*, located on chromosome 3, appears to produce a glaucoma characterized by high pressure, late onset, and moderate response to glaucoma medications. Although *GLC1C* is relatively rare, its phenotypic similarity to POAG suggests that this gene may provide valuable insight into the mechanism of many other types of adult-onset open-angle glaucoma. The glaucoma associated with *GLC1D* also resembles high-pressure POAG and may provide further insights into POAG. *GLC1D* has been mapped to band 23 on the long arm of chromosome 8.

GLC1F and *GLC1G*, additional loci for POAG, have been mapped. Linkage studies with another family have been used to map pigment dispersion syndrome to a chromosome distal to *GLC1F*.

Each of these gene locations represents only a small fraction of the total open-angle glaucoma population. Their identification indicates the diversity of glaucoma genetics. Given this diversity and the many families that do not map to any of these regions, it is likely that many other regions exist.

Angle-Closure Glaucoma Genes

Two autosomal dominant genes and one recessive gene have been associated with nan-ophthalmos (see Table 1-3), which is associated with angle-closure glaucoma due to the distortion of the anterior segment. These 3 loci map to chromosome 11.

Primary Congenital Glaucoma Genes

Three primary congenital glaucoma genes have been mapped. The majority of congenital glaucoma families map to *GLC3A* on band 2p21. In addition, several *GLC3A* genes appear to be associated with a mutation of the cytochrome P450 gene *(CYP1B1)*. In most patients with *CYP1B1* mutations, the disease is more severe. However, there is significant phenotypic variation and variable penetrance. As a second locus for congenital glaucoma, *GLC3B*, which probably affects fewer cases, has been mapped to band 1p36. An autosomal dominant form of congenital glaucoma has also been identified.

Other Identified Glaucoma Genes

Other genetic discoveries are directly relevant to glaucoma. For instance, *PITX2*, a ho-meobox gene, is associated with Rieger anomaly and forkhead transcription factor (con-genital glaucoma, Rieger anomaly, Axenfeld anomaly, and iris hypoplasia). Patients with abnormalities of the *PAX6* gene develop aniridia with associated glaucoma.

Environmental Factors

Evidence that environmental factors can also affect glaucoma arises from studies of twins, analysis of the season of birth of patients with glaucoma, and light exposure in animal models. Theoretically, if glaucoma is genetically determined, identical twins should share this trait more often than fraternal twins. In the Finnish Twin Cohort Study, 3 of 29 monozygotic twin pairs were concordant for POAG compared with 1 of 79 dizygotic twin pairs. Although a higher percentage of monozygotic twins were concordant for glaucoma, most were not. These data suggest that although genetic factors contribute to the etiology of glaucoma, other factors such as environmental influences are important.

Genetic Testing

In the future, glaucoma management in some individuals will involve testing of multiple, and potentially interacting, genetic loci. While there have been rapid advances in genetic techniques that will allow this type of testing, advances in the study of genetic diseases require accurate categorization of individuals and families with specific phenotypes. By appropriately identifying families with strong histories of glaucoma, the practicing clinical ophthalmologist has the opportunity to provide important information to researchers in genetics. Thus, the cooperation of the clinician is critical to the advancement of this crucial area of research.

Thorleifsson G, Magnusson KP, Sulem P, et al. Common sequence variants in the *LOXL1* gene confer susceptibility to exfoliation glaucoma. *Science.* 2007;317(5843):1397–1400.

CHAPTER 2

Intraocular Pressure and Aqueous Humor Dynamics

An understanding of *aqueous humor dynamics* is essential for the evaluation and management of glaucoma. As noted in Figure 1-1, aqueous humor is produced in the posterior chamber and flows through the pupil into the anterior chamber. Aqueous humor exits the eye by passing through the *trabecular meshwork* and into *Schlemm's canal* before draining into the venous system through a plexus of collector channels, as well as through the uveoscleral pathway, which is proposed to exit through the root of the iris and the ciliary muscle, into the suprachoroidal spaces and through the sclera. The *Goldmann equation* summarizes the relationship between many of these factors and the intraocular pressure (IOP) in the undisturbed eye:

$$P_0 = (F/C) + P_v$$

where P_0 is the IOP in millimeters of mercury (mm Hg), F is the rate of aqueous formation in microliters per minute (μL/min), C is the facility of outflow in microliters per minute per millimeter of mercury (μL/min/mm Hg), and P_v is the episcleral venous pressure in millimeters of mercury. Resistance to outflow (R) is the inverse of facility (C).

Table 2-1 illustrates the impact of reduced outflow facility (C value) of aqueous humor through the trabecular meshwork both in an open angle and in various amounts of angle closure.

Aqueous Humor Formation

Aqueous humor formation is a biological process that is subject to circadian rhythms. Aqueous humor is formed by the *ciliary processes,* each of which is composed of a double layer of epithelium over a core of stroma and a rich supply of fenestrated capillaries (Fig 2-1). Each of the 80 or so processes contains a large number of capillaries, which are supplied mainly by branches of the major arterial circle of the iris. The apical surfaces of both the outer pigmented and the inner nonpigmented layers of epithelium face each other and are joined by tight junctions, which are an important component of the blood–aqueous barrier. The inner nonpigmented epithelial cells, which protrude into the posterior chamber, contain numerous mitochondria and microvilli; these cells are thought to

Table 2-1 Theoretical Examples of Difference in the Degree to Which the Intraocular Pressure (P) Is Calculated to Be Affected by Changes in Flow (F) and Facility of Outflow (C) in Different Types of Eyes, Assuming Constant Episcleral Venous Pressure (P_e [or P_v])

	(mm Hg) P_e	+	(μL/min) (F	÷	(μL/min/mm Hg) C)	=	(mm Hg) P
Normal =	9		1.5		0.22		15
	9		1 to 2		0.22		13 to 17
	9		1.5		0.30		14
Glaucoma =	9		1.5		0.05		39
	9		1 to 2		0.05		29 to 49
	9		1.5		0.10		24
Good normal =	9		1.5		0.30		14
½ angle closed =	9		1.5		0.15		19
¾ angle closed =	9		1.5		0.075		29
Poor normal =	9		1.5		0.15		19
½ angle closed =	9		1.5		0.075		29
¾ angle closed =	9		1.5		0.0375		49

Modified with permission from Epstein DL, Allingham RR, Schuman JS. *Chandler and Grant's Glaucoma.* 4th ed. Baltimore: Williams & Wilkins; 1997:21.

be the actual site of aqueous production. The ciliary processes provide a large surface area for secretion.

Aqueous humor formation and secretion into the posterior chamber result from

- active secretion, which takes place in the double-layered ciliary epithelium
- ultrafiltration
- simple diffusion

Active secretion, or *transport,* consumes energy to move substances against an electrochemical gradient and is independent of pressure. The identity of the precise ion or ions transported is not known, but sodium, chloride, and bicarbonate are involved. Active secretion accounts for the majority of aqueous production and involves, at least in part, activity of the enzyme carbonic anhydrase II. *Ultrafiltration* refers to a pressure-dependent movement along a pressure gradient. In the ciliary processes, the hydrostatic pressure difference between capillary pressure and IOP favors fluid movement into the eye, whereas the oncotic gradient between the two resists fluid movement. The relationship between secretion and ultrafiltration is not known. *Diffusion* is the passive movement of ions across a membrane related to charge and concentration.

In humans, aqueous humor has an excess of hydrogen and chloride ions, an excess of ascorbate, and a deficit of bicarbonate relative to plasma. Aqueous humor is essentially protein free (1/200–1/500 of the protein found in plasma), which allows for optical clarity and reflects the integrity of the blood–aqueous barrier of the normal eye. Albumin accounts for about half of the total protein. Other components include growth factors; several enzymes, such as carbonic anhydrase, lysozyme, diamine oxidase, plasminogen activator, dopamine β-hydroxylase, and phospholipase A_2; and prostaglandins, cyclic adenosine monophosphate (cAMP), catecholamines, steroid hormones, and hyaluronic acid. Aqueous humor is

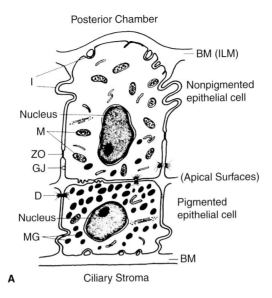

Posterior Chamber

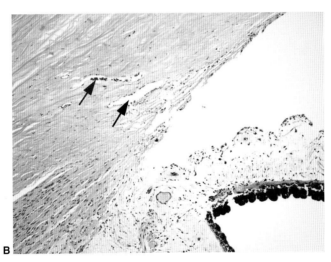

Figure 2-1 **A,** The 2 layers of the ciliary epithelium showing apical surfaces in apposition to each other. Basement membrane *(BM)* lines the double layer and constitutes the internal limiting membrane *(ILM)* on the inner surface. The nonpigmented epithelium is characterized by large numbers of mitochondria *(M)*, zonula occludens *(ZO)*, and lateral and surface interdigitations *(I)*. The pigmented epithelium contains numerous melanin granules *(MG)*. Additional intercellular junctions include desmosomes *(D)* and gap junctions *(GJ)*. **B,** Light micrograph of the anterior chamber angle demonstrates Schlemm's canal *(black arrow)* to the trabecular meshwork in the sclera. One of the external collector vessels can be seen adjacent to Schlemm's canal *(red arrow)*. *(Part A reproduced with permission from Shields MB. Textbook of Glaucoma. 3rd ed. Baltimore: Williams & Wilkins; 1992. Part B courtesy of Nasreen A. Syed, MD.)*

produced at an average rate of 2.0–2.5 µL/min, and its composition is altered as it flows from the posterior chamber, through the pupil, and into the anterior chamber. This alteration occurs across the hyaloid face of the vitreous, the surface of the lens, the blood vessels of the iris, and the corneal endothelium and is secondary to other dilutional exchanges and active processes. BCSC Section 2, *Fundamentals and Principles of Ophthalmology,* discusses aqueous humor composition and production in detail in Part IV, Biochemistry and Metabolism.

Suppression of Aqueous Formation

The mechanisms of action of the various classes of drugs that suppress aqueous formation—the *carbonic anhydrase inhibitors, β-adrenergic antagonists (beta-blockers),* and *α₂-agonists*—are not precisely understood. The role of the enzyme carbonic anhydrase has been debated vigorously. Evidence suggests that the bicarbonate ion is actively secreted in human eyes; thus, the function of the enzyme may be to provide this ion. Carbonic anhydrase may also provide bicarbonate or hydrogen ions for an intracellular buffering system.

Current evidence indicates that β_2-receptors are the most prevalent adrenergic receptors in the ciliary epithelium. The significance of this finding is unclear, but β-adrenergic antagonists may affect active transport by causing a decrease either in the efficiency of the Na^+/K^+ pump or in the number of pump sites. For a detailed discussion and illustration of the sodium pump and pump–leak mechanism, see BCSC Section 2, *Fundamentals and Principles of Ophthalmology.*

Rate of Aqueous Formation

The most common method used to measure the rate of aqueous formation is *fluorophotometry.* Fluorescein is administered systemically or topically, and the subsequent decline in its anterior chamber concentration is measured optically and used to calculate aqueous flow. As previously noted, the normal flow is approximately 2.0–2.5 µL/min, and the aqueous volume is turned over at a rate of 1% per minute.

Aqueous formation varies diurnally and drops during sleep. It also decreases with age, as does outflow facility. The rate of aqueous formation is affected by a variety of factors, including

- integrity of the blood–aqueous barrier
- blood flow to the ciliary body
- neurohumoral regulation of vascular tissue and the ciliary epithelium

Aqueous humor production may decrease following trauma or intraocular inflammation and following the administration of certain drugs, such as general anesthetics and some systemic hypotensive agents. Carotid occlusive disease may also decrease aqueous humor production.

Aqueous Humor Outflow

Aqueous humor outflow occurs by 2 major mechanisms: pressure-dependent outflow and pressure-independent outflow. The facility of outflow (*C* in the Goldmann equation; see the beginning of the chapter) varies widely in normal eyes. The mean value reported ranges from 0.22 to 0.30 μL/min/mm Hg. Outflow facility decreases with age and is affected by surgery, trauma, medications, and endocrine factors. Patients with glaucoma and elevated IOP have decreased outflow facility.

Trabecular Outflow

Traditional thought contended that most of the aqueous humor exits the eye by way of the trabecular meshwork–Schlemm's canal–venous system. However, recent evidence questions the exact ratio of trabecular to uveoscleral outflow. As with outflow facility, this ratio is affected by age and by ocular health. The meshwork is classically divided into 3 parts (Fig 2-2). The uveal part is adjacent to the anterior chamber and is arranged in bands that extend from the iris root and the ciliary body to the peripheral cornea. The corneoscleral meshwork consists of sheets of trabeculum that extend from the scleral spur to the lateral wall of the scleral sulcus. The juxtacanalicular meshwork, which is thought to be the major site of outflow resistance, is adjacent to, and actually forms the inner wall of, Schlemm's canal. Aqueous moves both across and between the endothelial cells lining the inner wall of Schlemm's canal.

The trabecular meshwork is composed of multiple layers, each of which consists of a collagenous connective tissue core covered by a continuous endothelial layer covering. It is the site of pressure-dependent outflow. The trabecular meshwork functions as a 1-way valve that permits aqueous to leave the eye by bulk flow but limits flow in the other direction, independent of energy. Its cells are phagocytic, a function they may exhibit in the presence of inflammation and after laser treatment.

In most older eyes, trabecular cells contain a large number of pigment granules within their cytoplasm that give the entire meshwork a brown or muddy appearance. In addition, the number of trabecular cells decreases with age, and the basement membrane beneath them thickens. There are relatively few trabecular cells—approximately 200,000–300,000 cells per eye. An interesting effect of all types of laser trabeculoplasty is to induce trabecular cell division and cause a change in the production of cytokines and other structurally important elements of the extracellular matrix. The extracellular matrix material is found through the dense portions of the trabecular meshwork.

Schlemm's canal is completely lined with an endothelial layer that does not rest on a continuous basement membrane. The canal is a single channel, with an average diameter of approximately 370 μm, and is transversed by tubules. The inner wall of Schlemm's canal contains giant vacuoles that have direct communication with the intertrabecular spaces. The outer wall is actually a single layer of endothelial cells that do not contain pores. A complex system of vessels connects Schlemm's canal to the episcleral veins, which subsequently drain into the anterior ciliary and superior ophthalmic veins. These, in turn, ultimately drain into the cavernous sinus.

When IOP is low, the trabecular meshwork may collapse, or blood may reflux into Schlemm's canal and be visible on gonioscopy.

Uveoscleral Outflow

In the normal eye, any nontrabecular outflow is termed *uveoscleral outflow*. Uveoscleral outflow is also termed *pressure-independent outflow*. A variety of mechanisms are likely

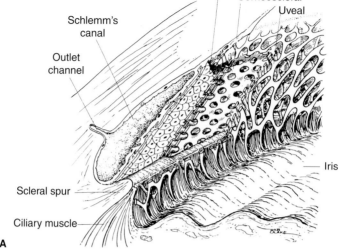

Trabecular Meshwork

Figure 2-2 **A,** Three layers of trabecular meshwork (shown in cutaway views): uveal, corneoscleral, and juxtacanalicular. **B,** Pars plicata of the ciliary body showing the 2 epithelial layers in the eye of an older person. The unpigmented epithelial cells measure approximately 20 μm high by 12 μm wide. The cuboidal pigmented epithelial cells are approximately 10 μm high. The thickened internal limiting membrane *(a)* is laminated and vesicular; such thickened membranes are a characteristic of older eyes. The cytoplasm of the unpigmented epithelium is characterized by its numerous mitochondria *(b)* and the cisternae of the rough-surfaced endoplasmic reticulum *(c).* A poorly developed Golgi apparatus *(d)* and several lysosomes and residual bodies *(e)* are shown. The pigmented epithelium contains many melanin granules, measuring about 1 μm in diameter and located mainly in the apical portion. The basal surface is rather irregular, having many fingerlike processes *(f).* The basement membrane of the pigmented epithelium *(g)* and a smooth granular material containing vesicles *(i)* and coarse granular particles are seen at the bottom of the figure. The appearance of the basement membrane is typical of older eyes and can be discerned with the light microscope (×5700). *(Part A reproduced with permission from Shields MB. Textbook of Glaucoma. 3rd ed. Baltimore: Williams & Wilkins; 1992. Part B reproduced with permission from Hogan MJ, Alvarado JA, Weddell JE. Histology of the Human Eye. Philadelphia: Saunders; 1971:283.)* *(continued)*

involved, predominantly aqueous passage from the anterior chamber into the ciliary muscle and then into the supraciliary and suprachoroidal spaces. The fluid then exits the eye through the intact sclera or along the nerves and the vessels that penetrate it. As noted, uveoscleral outflow is largely pressure-independent and is believed to be influenced by age. There is evidence that humans, like nonhuman primates, have significant outflow via the uveoscleral pathway. Uveoscleral outflow has been estimated to account for 5%–15% of total aqueous outflow, but recent studies indicate it may be a higher percentage of total outflow, especially in normal eyes of young people. It is increased by cycloplegia, adrenergic agents, prostaglandin analogs, and certain complications of surgery (eg, cyclodialysis) and is decreased by miotics.

Tonography

Tonography is a method used to measure the facility of aqueous outflow. The clinician can take the measurement by using a Schiøtz tonometer of known weight. The tonometer

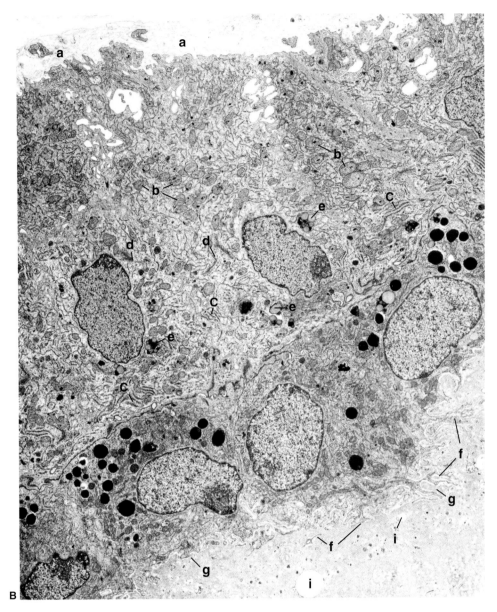

Figure 2-2 *(continued from previous page)*

is placed on the cornea, acutely elevating the IOP. The rate at which the pressure declines with time is related to the ease with which the aqueous leaves the eye. The decline in IOP over time can be used to determine outflow facility in μL/min/mm Hg through a series of mathematical calculations.

Unfortunately, tonography depends on a number of assumptions (eg, the elastic properties of the eye, stability of aqueous formation, and constancy of ocular blood volume) and is subject to many sources of error, such as calibration problems, patient fixation, and eyelid squeezing. These problems reduce the accuracy and reproducibility of tonography for an individual patient. In general, tonography is best used as a research tool for the investigation of pharmacokinetics and is rarely used clinically.

Episcleral Venous Pressure

Episcleral venous pressure is relatively stable, except with alterations in body position and with certain diseases of the orbit, the head, and the neck that obstruct venous return to the heart or shunt blood from the arterial to the venous system. The usual range of values is 8–10 mm Hg. The pressure in the episcleral veins can be measured with specialized equipment. In acute conditions, according to the Goldmann equation, IOP rises approximately 1 mm Hg for every 1 mm Hg increase in episcleral venous pressure. The relationship is more complex and less well understood, however, in chronic conditions. Chronic elevations of episcleral venous pressure may be accompanied by changes in IOP that are of greater or less magnitude than predicted by the Goldmann equation. In addition, these changes may not vary directly with the episcleral venous pressure. Abnormal elevated episcleral venous pressure can cause the collapse of Schlemm's canal and an increase in aqueous humor outflow resistance. Episcleral venous pressure is often increased in syndromes with facial hemangiomas (eg, Sturge-Weber) and in thyroid-associated orbitopathy and is partially responsible for the elevated IOP seen in thyroid eye disease.

Intraocular Pressure

Distribution in the Population and Relation to Glaucoma

Pooled data from large western epidemiologic studies indicate that the mean IOP is approximately 16 mm Hg, with a standard deviation of 3 mm Hg. However, IOP has a non-Gaussian distribution with a skew toward higher pressures, especially in individuals older than age 40 (Fig 2-3). The value 22 mm Hg (greater than 2 standard deviations above the mean) has been used in the past both to separate normal and abnormal pressures and to define which patients required ocular hypotensive therapy. This division was based on the erroneous clinical assumptions that glaucomatous damage is caused exclusively by pressures that are higher than normal and that normal pressures do not cause damage. An example of the shortcomings created by these assumptions is that screening for glaucoma based solely on IOP >21 mm Hg misses up to half of the people with glaucoma and optic nerve damage in the screened population.

General agreement has been reached that, for the population as a whole, there is no clear IOP level below which IOP can be considered "normal" or safe and above which IOP can be considered "elevated" or unsafe: some eyes undergo damage at IOPs of 18 mm Hg or less, whereas others tolerate IOPs in the 30s. However, elevation of IOP is still seen as a very important risk factor for the development of glaucomatous optic nerve damage. Although other risk factors affect an individual's susceptibility to glaucomatous damage, IOP is the only one that can be effectively altered at this time.

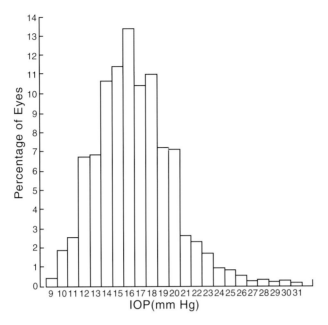

Figure 2-3 Frequency distribution of intraocular pressure: 5220 eyes in the Framingham Eye Study. *(Reproduced from Colton T, Ederer F. The distribution of intraocular pressures in the general population.* Surv Ophthalmol. *1980;25:123–129.)*

Factors Influencing Intraocular Pressure

IOP varies with a number of factors, including the following (Table 2-2):

- time of day
- heartbeat
- respiration
- exercise
- fluid intake
- systemic medications
- topical medications

Alcohol consumption results in a transient decrease in IOP. In most studies, caffeine has not shown an appreciable effect on IOP. Cannabis decreases IOP but has not been proven clinically useful because of its short duration of action and poor side effect profile. IOP is higher when an individual is recumbent rather than upright, predominantly because of an increase in the episcleral venous pressure. Some people have an exaggerated rise in IOP when they lie down, and this tendency may be important in the pathogenesis of some forms of glaucoma. IOP usually increases with age and is genetically influenced: higher pressures are more common in relatives of patients with POAG than in the general population.

Table 2-2 Factors That Affect Intraocular Pressure

Factors that may increase intraocular pressure
  Elevated episcleral venous pressure
    Valsalva maneuver
    Breath holding
    Playing a wind instrument
    Wearing a tight collar or tight necktie
    Bending over or being in a supine position
    Elevated central venous pressure
    Orbital venous outflow obstruction
    Intubation
  Pressure on the eye
    Blepharospasm
    Squeezing and crying, especially in young children
  Elevated body temperature: associated with increased aqueous humor production
  Hormonal influences
    Hypothyroidism
    Thyroid ophthalmitis
  Drugs unrelated to therapy
    Lysergic acid diethylamide (LSD)
    Topiramate (Topamax)
    Corticosteroids
    Anticholinergics: may precipitate angle closure
    Ketamine

Factors that may decrease intraocular pressure
  Aerobic exercise
  Anesthetic drugs
    Depolarizing muscle relaxants such as succinylcholine
  Metabolic or respiratory acidosis: decreases aqueous humor production
  Hormonal influences
    Pregnancy
  Drugs unrelated to therapy
    Alcohol consumption
    Heroin
    Marijuana (cannabis)

Diurnal Variation

In normal individuals, IOP varies 2–6 mm Hg over a 24-hour period, as aqueous humor production and outflow change. Higher IOP is associated with greater fluctuation, and a diurnal fluctuation of greater than 10 mm Hg is suggestive of glaucoma. The time at which peak IOPs occur in any individual is quite variable; however, many people reach their peak daytime pressures in the morning hours. Such fluctuations can be detected through measurement of ocular pressure at multiple times around the clock. Recent evidence suggests that with around-the-clock IOP measurement performed in individuals in habitual body positions (standing or sitting during the daytime and lying down at night), many individuals, those with glaucoma and those without, will show peak pressures in the early morning hours while they are still in bed. Measurement of IOP during nonoffice hours may be useful for determining why optic nerve damage occurs despite apparently adequately controlled pressure. However, the impact of IOP fluctuations on the optic nerve remains unknown. The relationship between blood pressure and IOP may be important in optic nerve damage: systemic hypotension, especially during sleep, has been suggested as a possible cause of decreased optic nerve perfusion resulting in damage.

Clinical Measurement of Intraocular Pressure

Measurement of IOP in a clinical setting requires a force that indents or flattens the eye. *Applanation tonometry* is the method used most widely. It is based on the Imbert-Fick principle, which states that the pressure inside an ideal dry, thin-walled sphere equals the force necessary to flatten its surface divided by the area of the flattening:

$P = F/A$

where P = pressure, F = force, and A = area. In applanation tonometry, the cornea is flattened, and IOP is determined by measuring the applanating force and the area flattened (Fig 2-4).

The *Goldmann applanation tonometer* measures the force necessary to flatten an area of the cornea of 3.06 mm diameter. At this diameter, the resistance of the cornea to flattening is counterbalanced by the capillary attraction of the tear film meniscus for the tonometer head. Furthermore, the IOP (in mm Hg) equals the flattening force (in grams) multiplied by 10. A split-image prism allows the examiner to determine the flattened area with great accuracy. Fluorescein in the tear film is used to outline

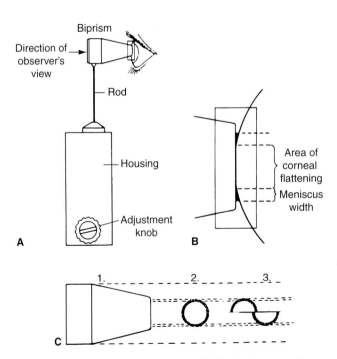

Figure 2-4   Goldmann-type applanation tonometry. **A,** Basic features of tonometer, shown in contact with patient's cornea. **B,** Enlargement shows tear film meniscus created by contact of biprism and cornea. **C,** View through biprism *(1)* reveals circular meniscus *(2),* which is converted into semicircle *(3)* by prisms. *(Reproduced with permission from Shields MB. Textbook of Glaucoma. 3rd ed. Baltimore: Williams & Wilkins; 1992.)*

the area of flattening. The semicircles move with the ocular pulse, and the endpoint is reached when the inner edges of the semicircles touch each other at the midpoint of their excursion (Fig 2-5).

Applanation measurements are safe, easy to perform, and relatively accurate in most clinical situations. Of the currently available devices, the Goldmann applanation tonometer is the most valid and reliable. Because applanation does not displace much fluid (approximately 0.5 µL) or substantially increase the pressure in the eye, this method is relatively unaffected by ocular rigidity. Table 2-3 lists possible sources of error in tonometry.

An excessive amount of fluorescein results in wide mires and an inaccurately high reading, whereas an inadequate amount of fluorescein leads to artificially low readings.

Marked corneal astigmatism causes an elliptical fluorescein pattern. To obtain an accurate reading, the clinician should rotate the prism so the red mark on the prism holder

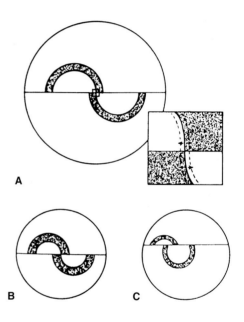

Figure 2-5 Semicircles of Goldmann-type applanation tonometer. **A,** Proper width and position. Enlargement depicts excursions of semicircles caused by ocular pulsations. **B,** Semicircles are too wide. **C,** Improper vertical and horizontal alignment. *(Reproduced with permission from Shields MB.* Textbook of Glaucoma. *3rd ed. Baltimore: Williams & Wilkins; 1992.)*

Table 2-3 Possible Sources of Error in Tonometry

Squeezing of the eyelids
Breath holding or Valsalva maneuver
Pressure on the globe
Extraocular muscle force applied to a restricted globe
Tight collar or tight necktie
Obesity or straining to reach slit lamp
An inaccurately calibrated tonometer
Excessive or inadequate amount of fluorescein
High corneal astigmatism
Corneal thickness greater or less than normal
Corneal biomechanical properties (eg, rigidity)
Corneal scarring or band keratopathy
Corneal irregularity
Technician errors

is set at the least curved meridian of the cornea (along the negative axis). Alternatively, 2 pressure readings taken 90° apart can be averaged.

The accuracy of applanation tonometry is reduced in certain situations. Corneal edema predisposes to inaccurate low readings, whereas pressure measurements taken over a corneal scar will be falsely high. Tonometry performed over a soft contact lens gives falsely low values. Alterations in scleral rigidity may compromise the accuracy of measurements; for example, applanation readings that follow scleral buckling procedures may be inaccurately low.

Applanation tonometry measurements are also affected by the central corneal thickness (CCT). Recently, the importance of CCT and its effect on the accuracy of IOP measurement has become better understood. The Goldmann tonometer is most accurate, with a CCT of 520 µm; however, population studies have shown a wide range of normal, with mean CCT between 537 and 554 µm.

Increased CCT may give an artificially high IOP measurement; decreased CCT, an artificially low reading. IOP measured after photorefractive keratectomy (PRK) and laser in situ keratomileusis (LASIK) may be reduced because of changes in the corneal thickness induced by these and other refractive procedures. As a rough guide, using an overview of published studies, it can be estimated that for every 10-µm difference in CCT from the population mean (approximately 542 µm), there is a 0.5 mm Hg difference between actual IOP and the IOP measured with a Goldmann tonometer. However, because the relationship of measured IOP and CCT is not linear, it is important to remember that such correction factors as this are only estimates at best. In addition, the biomechanical properties of an individual cornea may vary, resulting in changes of the relative stiffness or rigidity of the cornea and altering the measurement. The Goldmann tonometer, Perkins tonometer, pneumatonometer, noncontact tonometer, and Tono-Pen are all affected by CCT. Currently, there is no validated correction factor for the effect of CCT on applanation tonometers; therefore, clinical application of any of the proposed correction methods should be avoided.

The Ocular Hypertension Treatment Study (OHTS) found that a thinner central cornea was a strong predictive factor for the development of glaucoma in subjects with ocular hypertension. Subjects with a corneal thickness of 555 µm or less had a threefold greater risk of developing POAG compared with participants who had a corneal thickness of more than 588 µm. Whether this increased risk of glaucoma is due to underestimating actual IOP in patients with thinner corneas or whether thin corneas are a risk factor independent of IOP measurement has not been completely determined, but the OHTS found CCT to be a risk factor for progression independent of IOP level.

The *Perkins tonometer* is a counterbalanced applanation tonometer that is portable and can be used with the patient either upright or supine. It is similar to the Goldmann tonometer in using a split-image device and fluorescein staining of the tears.

Methods other than Goldmann-type applanation tonometry

The recognition that the accuracy of applanation tonometry is dependent on many uncontrollable factors has led to a renewed interest in the development of novel tonometric methodologies. In particular, new tonometers aim to lessen the potential inaccuracy secondary to differences in corneal thickness and rigidity. One such technology is the *dynamic contour tonometer (DCT)*, a nonapplanation contact tonometer that may be more independent of corneal biomechanical properties and thickness than are older tonometers.

Noncontact (air-puff) tonometers measure IOP without touching the eye, by measuring the time necessary for a given force of air to flatten a given area of the cornea. Readings obtained with these instruments vary widely, and IOP is often overestimated with these instruments. The instruments are often used in large-scale glaucoma-screening programs or by nonmedical health care providers.

The group of *portable electronic applanation* devices (eg, Tono-Pen) that applanate a very small area of the cornea are particularly useful in the presence of corneal scars or edema. The *pneumatic tonometer,* or *pneumatonometer,* has a pressure-sensing device that consists of a gas-filled chamber covered by a Silastic diaphragm. The gas in the chamber escapes through an exhaust vent. As the diaphragm touches the cornea, the gas vent decreases in size and the pressure in the chamber rises. Because this instrument, too, applanates only a small area of the cornea, it is especially useful in the presence of corneal scars or edema.

Schiøtz tonometry determines IOP by measuring the indentation of the cornea produced by a known weight. The indentation is read on a linear scale on the instrument and is converted to millimeters of mercury by a calibration table. Because of a number of practical and theoretical problems, however, Schiøtz tonometry is now rarely used.

It is possible to estimate IOP by *digital pressure* on the globe. This test may be used with uncooperative patients, but it may be inaccurate even in very experienced hands. In general, tactile tensions are only useful for detecting large differences between 2 eyes.

Infection Control in Clinical Tonometry

Many infectious agents, including the viruses responsible for acquired immunodeficiency syndrome (AIDS), hepatitis, and epidemic keratoconjunctivitis, can be recovered from tears. Tonometers must be cleaned after each use so that transfer of such agents can be prevented:

- The prism head of both Goldmann-type tonometers and the Perkins tonometer should be cleaned immediately after use. The prisms should either be soaked in a 1:10 sodium hypochlorite solution (household bleach), in 3% hydrogen peroxide, or in 70% isopropyl alcohol for 5 minutes, or be thoroughly wiped with an alcohol sponge. If a soaking solution is used, the prism should be rinsed and dried before reuse. If alcohol is employed, it should be allowed to evaporate, or the prism head should be dried before reuse, to prevent damage to the epithelium.
- The front surface of the air-puff tonometer should be wiped with alcohol between uses because the instrument may be contaminated by tears from the patient.
- Portable electronic applanation devices employ a disposable cover, which should be replaced immediately after each use.
- The Schiøtz tonometer requires disassembly to clean both the plunger and the footplate. Unless the plunger is clean (as opposed to sterile), the measurements may be falsely elevated because of increased friction between the plunger and the footplate.

A pipe cleaner can be used to clean the inside of the footplate, removing tears and any tear film debris. The same solutions used for cleaning prism heads may then be employed to sterilize the instrument.

For other tonometers, consult the manufacturer's recommendations.

Brandt JD. The influence of corneal thickness on the diagnosis and management of glaucoma. *J Glaucoma.* 2001;10(5 Suppl 1):S65–S67.

Brubaker RF. Measurement of uveoscleral outflow in humans. *J Glaucoma.* 2001;10(5 Suppl 1): S45–S48.

Doherty MJ, Zaman ML. Human corneal thickness and its impact on intraocular pressure measures: a review and meta-analysis approach. *Surv Ophthalmol.* 2000;44:367–408.

Gordon MA, Beiser JA, Brandt JA, et al. The Ocular Hypertension Treatment Study: baseline factors that predict the onset of primary open-angle glaucoma. *Arch Ophthalmol.* 2002;120(6):714–720.

Mills RP. If intraocular pressure measurement is only an estimate—then what? *Ophthalmology.* 2000;107:1807–1808.

Shah S. Accurate intraocular pressure measurement—the myth of modern ophthalmology? *Ophthalmology.* 2000;107:1805–1807.

Sommer A, Tielsch JM, Katz J, et al. Relationship between intraocular pressure and primary open angle glaucoma among white and black Americans. The Baltimore Eye Survey. *Arch Ophthalmol.* 1991;109:(8)1090–1095.

CHAPTER 3

Clinical Evaluation

History and General Examination

Appropriate management of glaucoma depends on the clinician's ability to diagnose the specific form of glaucoma in a given patient, to determine the severity of the condition, and to detect progression in that patient's disease status. The most important aspects of the clinical evaluation of a glaucoma patient are presented in the following discussion.

History

The history should include the following:

- patient's current complaint
- symptoms, onset, duration, severity, location
- ocular history
- history of present illness
- past ocular, medical, and surgical history
- general medical history
- past systemic medical history (including medications and allergies)
- review of systems
- social history
- history of alcohol and tobacco use
- occupation, avocation, interests
- family history

It is often useful to question the patient specifically about symptoms and conditions associated with glaucoma, such as pain, redness, colored halos around lights, alteration of vision, and loss of vision. Similarly, the general medical history should include specific inquiry about diseases that may have ocular manifestations or that may affect the patient's ability to tolerate medications. Such conditions include diabetes, cardiac and pulmonary disease, hypertension, hemodynamic shock, systemic hypotension, sleep apnea, Raynaud phenomenon, migraine and other neurologic diseases, and renal stones. In addition to identifying present medications and medication allergies, the clinician should take note of a history of corticosteroid use. See also BCSC Section 1, *Update on General Medicine,* for further discussion of these conditions and medications.

Refraction

Neutralizing any refractive error is crucial for accurate perimetry with most perimeters, and the clinician should understand how the patient's refractive state affects the diagnosis. Hyperopic eyes are at increased risk of angle-closure glaucoma and generally have smaller discs. Myopia is associated with disc morphologies that can be clinically confused with glaucoma, and myopic eyes are at increased risk of pigment dispersion. Whether myopic eyes have increased risk of open-angle glaucoma remains a controversial issue.

External Adnexae

Examination and assessment of the external ocular adnexae is useful for determining the presence of a variety of conditions associated with secondary glaucomas as well as external ocular manifestations of glaucoma therapy. The entities described in this section are discussed in greater depth and illustrated in other volumes of the BCSC series; consult the *Master Index.*

An example of an association between adnexal changes and systemic disease is *tuberous sclerosis (Bourneville syndrome),* in which glaucoma may occur secondary to vitreous hemorrhage, anterior segment neovascularization, or retinal detachment. Typical external and cutaneous signs of tuberous sclerosis include a hypopigmented lesion termed the "ash-leaf sign" and a red-brown papular rash (adenoma sebaceum) that is often found on the face and chin.

Glaucoma is commonly associated with *neurofibromatosis (von Recklinghausen disease),* likely secondary to developmental abnormalities of the anterior chamber angle. Subcutaneous plexiform neuromas are a hallmark of the type 1 variant of neurofibromatosis. When found in the upper eyelid, the plexiform neuroma can produce a classic S-shaped upper eyelid deformity strongly associated with risk of glaucoma.

In *juvenile xanthogranuloma,* yellow and/or orange papules are commonly found on the skin of the head and neck. Secondary glaucoma may cause acute pain and photophobia and ultimately significant visual loss. *Oculodermal melanocytosis (nevus of Ota)* presents with the key finding of hyperpigmentation of periocular skin. Intraocular pigmentation is also increased, which contributes to a higher incidence of glaucoma and may possibly increase the risk of malignant melanoma. *Axenfeld-Rieger syndrome,* an autosomal dominant disorder with variable penetrance, is associated with microdontia (small, peglike incisors), hypodontia (decreased number of teeth), and anodontia (focal absence of teeth). Maxillary hypoplasia may also be present. Glaucoma occurs in 50% of cases in late childhood or adulthood.

A number of entities are associated with signs of increased episcleral venous pressure. The presence of a facial cutaneous angioma (nevus flammeus, or port-wine stain) can indicate *encephalofacial angiomatosis (Sturge-Weber syndrome).* Hemifacial hypertrophy may also be observed. The cutaneous hemangiomas of the *Klippel-Trénaunay-Weber syndrome* extend over an affected, secondarily hypertrophied limb and may also involve the face.

Orbital varices are associated with secondary glaucoma. Intermittent unilateral proptosis and dilated eyelid veins are key external signs of orbital varices. Carotid cavernous, dural cavernous, and other *arteriovenous fistulae* can produce orbital bruits, restricted ocular motility, proptosis, and pulsating exophthalmos. *Superior vena cava syndrome* can cause proptosis and facial and eyelid edema, as well as conjunctival chemosis. *Thyroid-associated orbitopathy* and its associated glaucoma are associated with exophthalmos, eyelid retraction, and motility disorders.

Use of prostaglandin analogs may result in trichiasis, hypertrichosis, distichiasis, and growth of facial hair around the eyes, as well as increased skin pigmentation involving the eyelids. Use of glaucoma hypotensive agents may also result in an allergic contact dermatitis. Chapter 7, Medical Management of Glaucoma, discusses these agents in detail.

Pupils

Pupil size may be affected by glaucoma therapy, and pupillary responses are one measure of compliance in patients who are on miotic therapy. Testing for a relative afferent pupillary defect may detect asymmetric optic nerve damage, a common and important finding in glaucoma. Corectopia, ectropion uveae, and pupillary abnormalities may also be observed in some forms of secondary open-angle glaucoma and angle-closure glaucoma. In some clinical situations, it is not possible to assess the pupils objectively for the presence of a relative afferent defect. Under those circumstances, it can be useful to ask the patient to make a subjective comparison between the eyes of the perceived brightness of a test light.

Biomicroscopy

Biomicroscopy of the anterior segment is performed for signs of underlying or associated ocular disease. BCSC Section 8, *External Disease and Cornea,* discusses slit-lamp technique and the examination of the external eye in greater depth.

Conjunctiva

Eyes with acutely elevated IOP may show conjunctival hyperemia. The chronic elevation of IOP that can occur with arteriovenous fistulae may produce massive episcleral venous dilation. Long-term use of sympathomimetics and prostaglandin analogs may also cause conjunctival injection, and long-term use of epinephrine derivatives may result in black adrenochrome deposits in the conjunctiva. The use of topical antiglaucoma medication can also cause decreased tear production, allergic and hypersensitivity reactions (papillary and follicular conjunctivitis), foreshortening of the conjunctival fornices, and scarring. Prior to filtering surgery, the presence or absence of subconjunctival scarring or other conjunctival abnormalities should be assessed. The presence or absence of any filtering bleb should be noted. If a bleb is present, its size, height, degree of vascularization, and integrity should be noted, and in the situation of postoperative hypotony, a Seidel test performed.

Episclera and sclera

Dilation of the episcleral vessels may indicate elevated episcleral venous pressure, a finding that can be seen in the secondary glaucomas associated with Sturge-Weber syndrome, arteriovenous fistulae, or thyroid-associated orbitopathy. Sentinel vessels may be seen in eyes harboring an intraocular tumor. Any thinning or staphylomatous areas should be noted.

Cornea

Enlargement of the cornea associated with breaks in Descemet's membrane (Haab striae) is commonly found in developmental glaucoma patients. Glaucomas associated with other anterior segment anomalies are described in the following discussions. Punctate epithelial defects, especially in the inferonasal interpalpebral region, are often indicative of medication toxicity. Microcystic epithelial edema is commonly associated with elevated IOP, particularly when the IOP rise is acute. Corneal endothelial abnormalities, such as the following, can be important clues to the presence of an underlying associated secondary glaucoma:

- Krukenberg spindle in pigmentary glaucoma
- deposition of exfoliation material in exfoliation syndrome
- keratic precipitates in uveitic glaucoma
- guttae in Fuchs endothelial dystrophy
- irregular and vesicular lesions in posterior polymorphous dystrophy
- a "beaten bronze" appearance in the iridocorneal endothelial syndrome

An anteriorly displaced Schwalbe line is found in Axenfeld-Rieger syndrome. The presence of traumatic or surgical corneal scars should be noted. The central corneal thickness (CCT) of all patients suspected of glaucoma should be assessed by corneal pachymetry because of the effect of CCT on the accuracy of applanation tonometry and its possible implication as a risk factor in some types of glaucomas. (See Chapters 2 and 4.)

Anterior chamber

To estimate the width of the chamber angle, the examiner directs a narrow slit beam at an angle of 60° onto the cornea just anterior to the limbus (Van Herick method). If the distance from the anterior iris surface to the posterior surface of the cornea is less than one-fourth the thickness of the cornea, the angle may be narrow. This test should alert the examiner to narrow angles, but it is not a substitute for gonioscopy, which is discussed in detail in the following major section (Figs 3-1, 3-2, Table 3-1).

The uniformity of depth of the anterior chamber should be noted. Iris bombé can result in an anterior chamber that is deep centrally and shallow or flat peripherally. Iris masses, choroidal effusions, or trauma can produce an irregular iris surface contour and nonuniformity or asymmetry in anterior chamber depth. In many circumstances, especially in the assessment of narrow-angle glaucoma, comparison of chamber depth between eyes is of substantial value. The presence of inflammatory cells, red blood cells, ghost cells, fibrin, vitreous, or other findings should be noted. The degree of inflammation (flare and cell) should be determined prior to instillation of eyedrops.

Iris

Examination should be performed prior to dilation. Heterochromia, iris atrophy, transillumination defects, ectropion uveae, corectopia, nevi, nodules, and exfoliative material should be noted. Early stages of neovascularization of the anterior segment may appear as either fine tufts around the pupillary margin or a fine network of vessels on the surface of the iris. Visualization of neovascular tufts with biomicroscopy may require increased

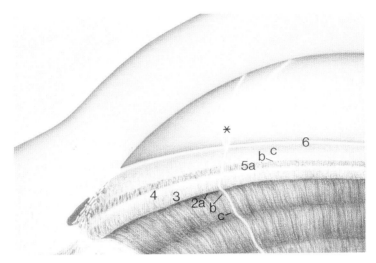

Figure 3-1 Gonioscopic appearance of a normal anterior chamber angle. *2,* Peripheral iris: *a,* insertion; *b,* curvature; *c,* angular approach. *3,* Ciliary body band. *4,* Scleral spur. *5,* Trabecular meshwork: *a,* posterior; *b,* mid; *c,* anterior. *6,* Schwalbe line. *Asterisk,* Corneal optical wedge.

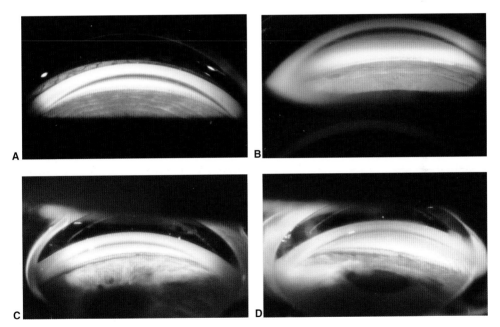

Figure 3-2 **A,** Normal open angle. Gonioscopic photograph shows trace pigmentation of the posterior trabecular meshwork and normal insertion of the iris into a narrow ciliary body band. The Goldmann lens was used. **B,** Normal open angle. This gonioscopic view using the Goldmann lens shows mild pigmentation of the posterior trabecular meshwork. A wide ciliary body band with posterior insertion of the iris can also be seen. **C,** Narrow angle. This gonioscopic view using the Zeiss lens without indentation shows pigment in the inferior angle but poor visualization of angle anatomy. **D,** Narrow angle. Gonioscopy with a Zeiss lens with indentation shows peripheral anterior synechiae in the posterior trabecular meshwork. Pigment deposits on the Schwalbe line can also be seen. This is the same angle as shown in **C.** *(Courtesy of Elizabeth A. Hodapp, MD.)*

Table 3-1 Gonioscopic Examination

Tissue	Features
Posterior cornea	Pigmentation, guttae, corneal endothelium
Schwalbe line	Thickening, anterior displacement
Trabecular meshwork	Pigmentation, peripheral anterior synechiae (PAS), inflammatory or neovascular membranes, keratic precipitates
Scleral spur	Iris processes, presence or absence
Ciliary body band	Width, regularity, cyclodialysis cleft
Iris	Contour, rubeosis, atrophy, cysts, iridodonesis
Pupil and lens	Exfoliation syndrome, posterior synechiae, position and regularity, sphincter rupture, ectropion uveae
Zonular fibers	Pigmentation, rupture

magnification. The iris should also be examined for evidence of trauma, such as sphincter tears or iridodonesis. The degree of baseline iris pigmentation should be noted, especially in patients being considered for treatment with a prostaglandin analog.

Lens

The lens is generally best examined after dilation. However, if phacodonesis is suspected in traumatic glaucoma, this should be evaluated prior to dilation because the increased tension on the zonules following cycloplegia will reduce lens movement. Material associated with pseudoexfoliation, phacodonesis, subluxation, and dislocation should be noted, along with lens size, shape, and clarity. A posterior subcapsular cataract may be indicative of long-term corticosteroid use. An intraocular foreign body with siderosis and glaucoma may also result in characteristic lens changes. The presence, type, and position of an intraocular lens should be recorded, along with the status of the posterior capsule.

Fundus

Careful assessment of the optic disc is an essential part of the clinical examination for glaucoma, and this is covered in detail later in the chapter. In addition, fundus examination may reveal posterior segment pathology such as hemorrhages, effusions, masses, inflammatory lesions, retinovascular occlusions, diabetic retinopathy, or retinal detachments that can be associated with the glaucomas. Funduscopy is best performed with a dilated pupil.

Gonioscopy

Gonioscopy is an essential diagnostic tool and examination technique used to visualize the structures of the anterior chamber angle. Mastering the various techniques of gonioscopy is crucial in the evaluation of glaucoma patients. Figures 3-1 and 3-2 give schematic and clinical views of the angle as seen with gonioscopy. Gonioscopy is required to visualize the chamber angle because under normal conditions light reflected from the angle structures undergoes total internal reflection at the tear–air interface. At the tear–air interface, the critical angle (approximately 46°) is reached and light is totally reflected back into the corneal stroma. This prevents direct visualization of the angle structures.

All gonioscopy lenses eliminate the tear–air interface by placing a plastic or glass surface adjacent to the front surface of the eye. The small space between the lens and cornea is filled by the patient's tears, saline solution, or a clear viscous substance. Depending on the type of lens employed, the angle can be examined with a direct (eg, Koeppe) system or a mirrored indirect (eg, Goldmann or Zeiss) system (Fig 3-3).

Direct and Indirect Gonioscopy

Gonioscopy techniques fall into 1 of 2 broad categories: direct and indirect (see Fig 3-3). To diagnose the various types of outflow obstruction, the clinician must master several gonioscopic techniques. Direct gonioscopy is performed with a binocular microscope, a fiberoptic illuminator or slit-pen light, and a direct goniolens, such as the Koeppe, Barkan, Wurst, Swan-Jacob, or Richardson lens. The lens is placed on the eye, and saline solution is used to fill the space between the cornea and the lens. The saline acts as an optical coupler between the 2 surfaces. The lens provides direct visualization of the chamber angle (ie, light reflected directly from the chamber angle is visualized). With direct gonioscopy lenses, the physician has an erect view of the angle structures, which is essential when performing goniotomies. Direct gonioscopy is most easily performed with the patient in a supine position and is commonly used in the operating room for examination of the eyes of infants under anesthesia.

Direct gonioscopy

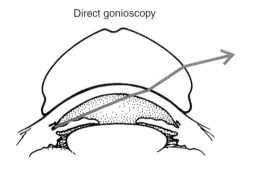

Indirect

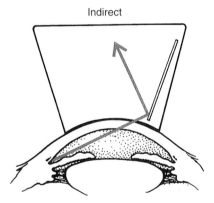

Dynamic

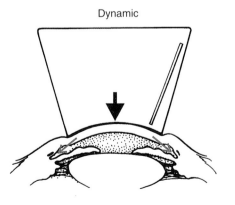

Figure 3-3 Direct and indirect gonioscopy. Gonioscopic lenses eliminate the tear–air interface and total internal reflection. With a direct lens, the light ray reflected from the anterior chamber angle is observed directly, whereas with an indirect lens the light ray is reflected by a mirror within the lens. Posterior pressure with an indirect lens forces open an appositionally closed or narrow anterior chamber angle (dynamic gonioscopy). *(Reprinted with permission from Wright KW, ed.* Textbook of Ophthalmology. *Baltimore: Williams & Wilkins; 1997.)*

Koeppe-type lenses are also quite useful for performing funduscopy. When used with a direct ophthalmoscope and a high-plus-power lens, they can provide a good view of the fundus, even through a very small pupil. These lenses are especially helpful in individuals with nystagmus or irregular corneas. Inconvenience is the major disadvantage of the direct gonioscopy systems.

Indirect gonioscopy is more frequently used in the clinician's office. Indirect gonioscopy also eliminates the total internal reflection at the surface of the cornea. Light reflected from the chamber angle passes into the indirect gonioscopy lens and is reflected by a mirror within the lens. Indirect gonioscopy may be used with the patient in an upright position, with illumination and magnification provided by a slit lamp. A *goniolens,* which contains a mirror or mirrors, yields an inverted and slightly foreshortened image of the opposite angle. Although the image is inverted with an indirect goniolens, the right–left orientation of a horizontal mirror and the up–down orientation of a vertical mirror remain unchanged. The foreshortening, combined with the upright position of the patient, makes the angle appear a little shallower than it does with direct gonioscopy systems. A large variety of lenses have been developed for indirect gonioscopy.

The Goldmann-type goniolens requires a viscous fluid such as methylcellulose for optical coupling with the cornea. In lenses with only 1 mirror, the lens must be rotated to view the entire angle. Posterior pressure on the lens, especially if it is tilted, indents the sclera and may falsely narrow the angle. The combination of the lens manipulation and the use of viscous fluid often temporarily reduces the clarity of the cornea and may make subsequent fundus examination, visual field testing, and photography more difficult. These lenses provide the clearest visualization of the anterior chamber angle structures and may be modified with antireflective coatings for use during laser procedures.

The Posner, Sussman, and Zeiss 4-mirror goniolenses allow all 4 quadrants of the chamber angle to be visualized without rotation of the lens during examination. They have a smaller area of contact than the Goldmann-type lens and about the same radius of curvature as the cornea, thus they are optically coupled by the patient's tears. Pressure on the cornea may distort the chamber angle. The examiner can detect this pressure by noting the induced Descemet's membrane folds. Although pressure may falsely open the angle, the technique of dynamic gonioscopy is sometimes essential for distinguishing iridocorneal apposition from synechial closure. Many clinicians prefer these lenses because of their ease of use, as well as their ability to perform dynamic gonioscopy.

With dynamic gonioscopy (compression or indentation gonioscopy), gentle pressure is placed on the cornea, and aqueous humor is forced into the chamber angle (see Fig 3-3). The posterior diameter of these goniolenses is smaller than the corneal diameter, and posterior pressure can be used to force open a narrowed angle. In inexperienced hands, dynamic gonioscopy may be misleading, as undue pressure on the anterior surface of the cornea may distort the chamber angle or may give the observer the false impression of an open angle. The examiner can detect this pressure by noting the induced folds in Descemet's membrane. With all indirect gonioscopy techniques, the observer may manipulate the chamber angle by repositioning the patient's eye (having the patient look toward the mirror) or by applying pressure with the posterior surface of the lens to provide more complete evaluation of the chamber angle. However, caution must be used not to induce artificial opening or closing of the anterior chamber angle with these techniques.

Gonioscopic Assessment and Documentation

In performing both direct and indirect gonioscopy, the clinician must recognize the angle landmarks. It is important to perform gonioscopy with dim room light and a thin, short light beam in order to minimize the light entering the pupil that could result in increased pupillary constriction and a change in the peripheral angle appearance that could falsely open the angle and prevent the proper identification of a narrow or occluded angle. The scleral spur and the Schwalbe line are the most consistent; a convenient gonioscopic technique to determine the exact position of the Schwalbe line is the parallelopiped technique. The parallelopiped, or corneal light wedge, technique allows the observer to determine the exact junction of the cornea and the trabecular meshwork. Using a narrow slit beam and sharp focus, the examiner sees 2 linear reflections, one from the external surface of the cornea and its junction with the sclera and the other from the internal surface of the cornea. The 2 reflections meet at the Schwalbe line (see Fig 3-1). The scleral spur is a thin, pale stripe between the ciliary face and the pigmented zone of the trabecular meshwork. The inferior portion of the angle is generally wider and is the easiest place in which to locate the landmarks. After verifying the landmarks, the clinician should examine the entire angle in an orderly manner (see Table 3-1).

Proper management of glaucoma requires that the clinician determine not only whether the angle is open or closed, but also whether other pathologic findings, such as angle recession or low PAS, are present. In angle closure, the peripheral iris obstructs the trabecular meshwork—that is, the meshwork is not visible on gonioscopy. The width of the angle is determined by the site of insertion of the iris on the ciliary face, the convexity of the iris, and the prominence of the peripheral iris roll. In many cases, the angle appears to be open but very narrow. It is often difficult to distinguish a narrow but open angle from an angle with partial closure; dynamic gonioscopy is useful in this situation (see Figs 3-2 and 3-3).

The best method for describing the angle is to use a standardized grading system or draw the iris contour, the location of the iris insertion, and the angle between the iris and the trabecular meshwork. A variety of gonioscopic grading systems have been developed. All grading systems facilitate standardized description of angle structures and abbreviate that description. Keep in mind that, with abbreviated descriptions, some details of the angle structure will be eliminated. The most commonly used gonioscopic grading systems are the Shaffer and Spaeth systems. A quadrant-by-quadrant narrative description of the chamber angle noting localized findings such as neovascular tufts, angle recession, or PAS may also be used to document serial gonioscopic findings. If a grading system is used, the clinician should specify which system is being used.

The *Shaffer system* describes the angle between the trabecular meshwork and the iris as follows:

- *Grade 4:* The angle between the iris and the surface of the trabecular meshwork is 45°.
- *Grade 3:* The angle between the iris and the surface of the trabecular meshwork is greater than 20° but less than 45°.
- *Grade 2:* The angle between the iris and the surface of the trabecular meshwork is 20°. Angle closure is possible.

- *Grade 1:* The angle between the iris and the surface of the trabecular meshwork is 10°. Angle closure is probable in time.
- *Slit:* The angle between the iris and the surface of the trabecular meshwork is less than 10°. Angle closure is very likely.
- *0:* The iris is against the trabecular meshwork. Angle closure is present.

The *Spaeth gonioscopic grading system* expands this system to include a description of the peripheral iris contour, the insertion of the iris root, and the effects of dynamic gonioscopy on the angle configuration (Fig 3-4).

Ordinarily, Schlemm's canal is invisible by gonioscopy. Occasionally during gonioscopy, at times in normal eyes, blood refluxes into Schlemm's canal, where it is seen as a faint red line in the posterior portion of the trabecular meshwork (Fig 3-5). Blood enters Schlemm's canal when episcleral venous pressure exceeds IOP, most commonly because of compression of the episcleral veins by the lip of the goniolens. Pathologic causes include hypotony and elevated episcleral venous pressure, as in carotid cavernous fistula or Sturge-Weber syndrome.

Normal blood vessels in the angle include radial iris vessels, portions of the arterial circle of the ciliary body, and vertical branches of the anterior ciliary arteries. Normal

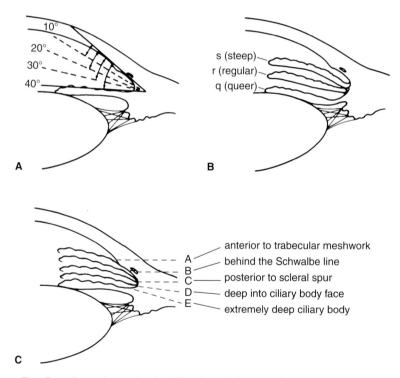

Figure 3-4   The Spaeth gonioscopic classification of the anterior chamber angle, based on 3 variables: **A,** angular width of the angle recess; **B,** configuration of the peripheral iris; and **C,** apparent insertion of the iris root. *(Reproduced with permission from Shields MB. Textbook of Glaucoma. 3rd ed. Baltimore: Williams & Wilkins; 1992.)*

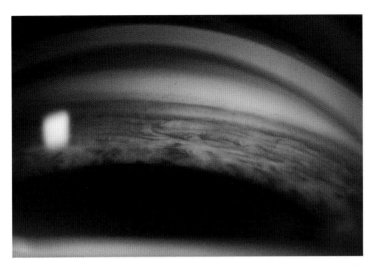

Figure 3-5 Blood in Schlemm's canal. Note the red line posterior to the trabecular meshwork in this patient with elevated episcleral venous pressure resulting in blood reflux into Schlemm's canal. *(Courtesy of G. A. Cioffi, MD.)*

vessels are oriented either radially along the iris or circumferentially (in a serpentine manner) in the ciliary body face. Vessels that cross the scleral spur to reach the trabecular meshwork are usually abnormal (Fig 3-6). The vessels seen in Fuchs heterochromic iridocyclitis are fine, branching, unsheathed, and meandering. Patients with neovascular glaucoma have trunklike vessels crossing the ciliary body and scleral spur and arborizing over the trabecular meshwork. Contraction of the myofibroblasts accompanying these vessels leads to PAS formation.

It is important to distinguish PAS from iris processes (the uveal meshwork), which are open and lacy and follow the normal curve of the angle. The angle structures are visible in the open spaces between the processes. Synechiae are more solid or sheetlike (Fig 3-7). They are composed of iris stroma and obliterate the angle recess.

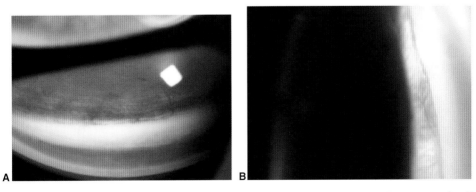

Figure 3-6 Goniophotos of neovascularization of the angle. **A,** Anatomically open angle. **B,** Closed angle. *(Part A courtesy of Keith Barton, MD; part B courtesy of Ronald L. Gross, MD.)*

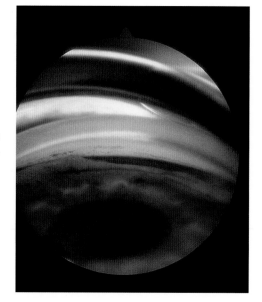

Figure 3-7 Goniophoto showing both an area of sheetlike PAS *(left)* and an open angle *(right)*. *(Courtesy of Louis B. Cantor, MD.)*

Pigmentation of the trabecular meshwork increases with age and tends to be more marked in individuals with darkly pigmented irides. Pigmentation can be segmental and is usually most marked in the inferior angle. The pigmentation pattern of an individual angle is dynamic over time, especially in conditions such as pigment dispersion syndrome. Heavy pigmentation of the trabecular meshwork should suggest pigment dispersion or exfoliation syndrome. Exfoliation syndrome may appear clinically similar to pigment dispersion syndrome, with pigment granules on the anterior surface of the iris, increased pigment in the anterior chamber angle, and secondary open-angle glaucoma. Pigmentation of the angle structures is usually patchy in exfoliation syndrome, as compared with the more uniform pigment distribution seen in pigment dispersion syndrome. In addition, a line of pigment deposition anterior to the Schwalbe line is often present in exfoliation syndrome (Sampaolesi line). Other conditions that cause increased anterior chamber angle pigmentation include malignant melanoma, trauma, surgery, inflammation, angle closure, and hyphema.

Posttraumatic angle recession may be associated with monocular open-angle glaucoma. The gonioscopic criteria for diagnosing angle recession include

- an abnormally wide ciliary body band (Fig 3-8)
- increased prominence of the scleral spur
- torn iris processes
- marked variation of ciliary face width and angle depth in different quadrants of the same eye

In evaluating for angle recession, it is helpful to compare one part of the angle to other areas in the same eye or to the same area in the fellow eye.

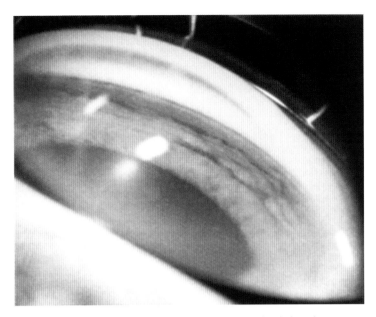

Figure 3-8 Angle recession. Note the widening of the ciliary body band. *(Reprinted with permission from Wright KW, ed.* Textbook of Ophthalmology. *Baltimore: Williams & Wilkins; 1997.)*

Figure 3-9 illustrates the variety of gonioscopic findings caused by blunt trauma. If the ciliary body separates from the scleral spur (cyclodialysis), it will appear gonioscopically as a deep angle recess with a gap between the scleral spur and the ciliary body. Detection of a very small cleft may require ultrasound biomicroscopy.

Other findings that may be visible by gonioscopy are

- microhyphema or hypopyon
- retained anterior chamber foreign body
- iridodialysis
- angle precipitates suggestive of glaucomatocyclitic crisis
- pigmentation of the lens equator
- other peripheral lens abnormalities
- intraocular lens haptics
- ciliary body tumors

Alward WLM. *Color Atlas of Gonioscopy.* San Francisco: Foundation of the American Academy of Ophthalmology; 2001.

Campbell DG. A comparison of diagnostic techniques in angle-closure glaucoma. *Am J Ophthalmol.* 1979;88:197–204.

Fellman RL, Spaeth GL, Starita RJ. Gonioscopy: key to successful management of glaucoma. *Focal Points: Clinical Modules for Ophthalmologists.* San Francisco: American Academy of Ophthalmology; 1984, module 7.

Savage JA. Gonioscopy in the management of glaucoma. *Focal Points: Clinical Modules for Ophthalmologists.* San Francisco: American Academy of Ophthalmology; 2006, module 3.

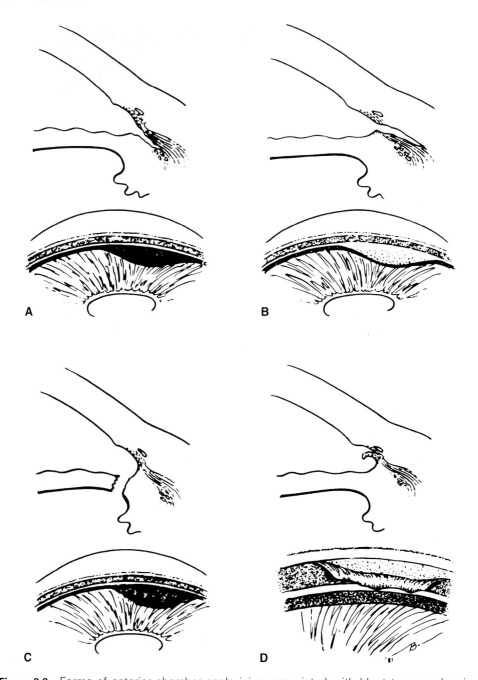

Figure 3-9 Forms of anterior chamber angle injury associated with blunt trauma, showing cross-sectional and corresponding gonioscopic appearance. **A,** Angle recession (tear between longitudinal and circular muscles of ciliary body). **B,** Cyclodialysis (separation of ciliary body from scleral spur) with widening of suprachoroidal space. **C,** Iridodialysis (tear in root of iris). **D,** Trabecular damage (tear in anterior portion of meshwork, creating a flap that is hinged at the scleral spur). *(Reproduced with permission from Shields MB.* Textbook of Glaucoma. *3rd ed. Baltimore: Williams & Wilkins; 1992.)*

The Optic Nerve

The entire visual pathway is described and illustrated in BCSC Section 5, *Neuro-Ophthalmology*. For further discussion of retinal involvement in the visual process, see Section 12, *Retina and Vitreous*.

Anatomy and Pathology

The optic nerve is the neural connection between the neurosensory retina and the lateral geniculate body. An understanding of the normal and pathologic appearance of the optic nerve allows the clinician to detect glaucoma, as well as to follow glaucoma patients. The optic nerve is composed of neural tissue, glial tissue, extracellular matrix, and blood vessels. The human optic nerve consists of approximately 1.2–1.5 million axons of retinal ganglion cells (RGCs), although there is significant individual variability. The cell bodies of the RGCs lie in the ganglion cell layer of the retina. The intraorbital optic nerve is divided into 2 components: the anterior optic nerve and the posterior optic nerve. The anterior optic nerve extends from the retinal surface to the retrolaminar region, just where the nerve exits the posterior aspect of the globe. The diameter of the optic nerve head and the intraocular portion of the optic nerve is approximately 1.5 mm; it expands to approximately 3–4 mm immediately upon exiting the globe. The increase in size is accounted for by axonal myelination, glial tissue, and the beginning of the leptomeninges (optic nerve sheath). The axons are separated into fascicles within the optic nerve, with the intervening spaces occupied by astrocytes.

In primates there are 3 major RGC types involved in conscious visual perception: magnocellular neurons (M cells), parvocellular neurons (P cells), and koniocellular neurons (bistratified cells). M cells have large-diameter axons, synapse in the magnocellular layer of the lateral geniculate body, are sensitive to luminance changes in dim illumination (scotopic conditions), have the largest dendritic field, primarily process information related to motion perception, and are not responsive to color. In comparison to the M cells, the P cells account for approximately 80% of all ganglion cells and are concentrated in the central retina, and they have smaller-diameter axons, smaller receptive fields, and slower conduction velocity. They synapse in the parvocellular layers of the lateral geniculate body. P cells subserve color vision, are most active under higher luminance conditions, and discriminate fine detail. The cells are motion-insensitive and process information of high spatial frequency (high resolution). The more recently described bistratified cells (koniocellular neurons) process information concerned with blue-yellow color opponency. This system, which is likely preferentially activated by short-wavelength perimetry, is inhibited when red and green cones (yellow) are activated and stimulated when blue cones are activated. Bistratified and large M cells each account for approximately 10% of RGCs.

The distribution of nerve fibers as they enter the optic nerve head is shown in Figure 3-10. The arcuate nerve fibers entering the superior and inferior poles of the disc seem to be more susceptible to glaucomatous damage. This susceptibility explains the frequent occurrence of arcuate nerve fiber bundle visual field defects in glaucoma. The arrangement of the axons in the optic nerve head and their differential susceptibility to

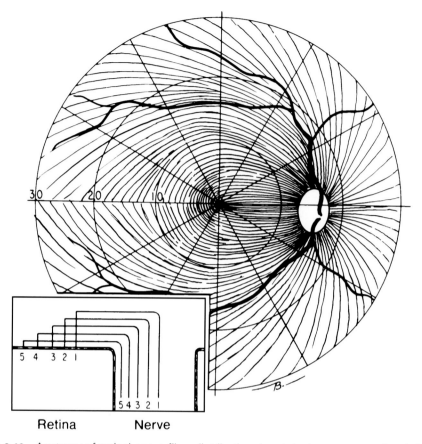

Retina   Nerve

Figure 3-10 Anatomy of retinal nerve fiber distribution. Inset depicts cross-sectional view of axonal arrangement. Peripheral fibers run closer to the choroid and exit in the periphery of the optic nerve, while fibers originating closer to the nerve head are situated closer to the vitreous and occupy a more central portion of the nerve. *(Reproduced with permission from Shields MB. Textbook of Glaucoma. 3rd ed. Baltimore: Williams & Wilkins; 1992.)*

damage determine the patterns of visual field loss seen in glaucoma, which are described and illustrated later in this chapter.

The anterior optic nerve can be divided into 4 layers (Fig 3-11):

- nerve fiber
- prelaminar
- laminar
- retrolaminar

The most anterior zone is the superficial nerve fiber layer region, which is continuous with the *nerve fiber layer* of the retina. This region is primarily composed of the axons of the RGCs in transition from the superficial retina to the neuronal component of the optic nerve. The nerve fiber layer can be viewed with the ophthalmoscope when the red-free (green) filter is used. Immediately posterior to the nerve fiber layer is the *prelaminar region,* which lies adjacent to the peripapillary choroid. More posteriorly, the *laminar region* is continuous with the sclera and is composed of the lamina cribrosa, a structure consist-

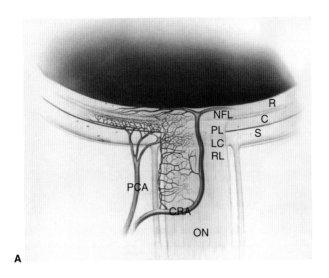

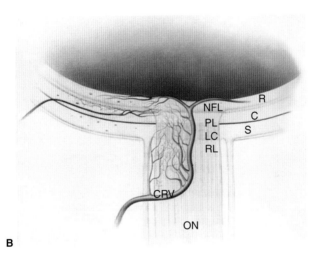

Figure 3-11 Anterior optic nerve vasculature. **A,** Arterial supply to the anterior optic nerve and peripapillary choroid. Lamina cribrosa *(LC)*, superficial nerve fiber layer *(NFL)*, prelamina *(PL)*, retrolamina *(RL)*, cranial retinal artery *(CRA)*, optic nerve *(ON)*, choroid *(C)*, posterior ciliary artery *(PCA)*, retina *(R)*, sclera *(S)*. **B,** Venous drainage of the anterior optic nerve and peripapillary choroid. Lamina cribrosa *(LC)*, nerve fiber layer *(NFL)*, prelamina *(PL)*, retrolamina *(RL)*, choroid *(C)*, optic nerve *(ON)*, central retinal vein *(CRV)*. *(Reprinted with permission from Wright KW, ed.* Textbook of Ophthalmology. *Baltimore: Williams & Wilkins; 1997:592, Figs 44-2, 44-3. Originally from Ritch R, Shields MB, Krupin T, eds.* The Glaucomas. *2nd ed. St Louis: Mosby; 1996:178.)*

ing of fenestrated connective tissue lamellae that allow the transit of neural fibers through the scleral coat. Finally, the *retrolaminar region* lies posterior to the lamina cribrosa, is marked by the beginning of axonal myelination, and is surrounded by the leptomeninges of the central nervous system.

The lamina cribrosa is composed of a series of fenestrated sheets of connective tissue and elastic fibers. The lamina cribrosa provides the main support for the optic nerve as it exits the eye, penetrating the scleral coat. The beams of connective tissue are composed primarily of collagen; other extracellular matrix components include elastin, laminin, and fibronectin. These connective tissue beams are perforated by various-sized fenestrations through which the neural component of the optic nerve passes. In addition, larger, central fenestrations allow transit of the central retinal artery and central retinal vein. The fenestrations within the lamina have been described histologically as larger superiorly and inferiorly as compared with the temporal and nasal aspects of the optic nerve. It has been suggested that these differences play a role in the development of glaucomatous optic neuropathy. The fenestrations of the lamina cribrosa (laminar dots) may often be seen by ophthalmoscopy at the base of the optic nerve head cup. Between the optic nerve and the adjacent choroidal and scleral tissue lies a rim of connective tissue, the ring of Elschnig. The connective tissue beams of the lamina cribrosa extend from this surrounding connective tissue border and are arranged in a series of parallel, stacked plates.

The vascular anatomy of the anterior optic nerve and peripapillary region has been extensively studied (see Fig 3-11). The arterial supply of the anterior optic nerve is derived entirely from branches of the ophthalmic artery via 1 to 5 posterior ciliary arteries. Typically, between 2 and 4 posterior ciliary arteries course anteriorly before dividing into approximately 10–20 short posterior ciliary arteries prior to entering the posterior globe. Often, the posterior ciliary arteries separate into a medial and a lateral group before branching into the short posterior ciliary arteries. The short posterior ciliary arteries penetrate the perineural sclera of the posterior globe to supply the peripapillary choroid, as well as most of the anterior optic nerve. Some short posterior ciliary arteries course, without branching, through the sclera directly into the choroid; others divide within the sclera to provide branches to both the choroid and the optic nerve. Often a noncontinuous arterial circle exists within the perineural sclera, the circle of Zinn-Haller. The central retinal artery, also a posterior orbital branch of the ophthalmic artery, penetrates the optic nerve approximately 10–15 mm behind the globe. The central retinal artery has few if any intraneural branches, the exception being an occasional small branch within the retrolaminar region, which may anastomose with the pial system. The central retinal artery courses adjacent to the central retinal vein within the central portion of the optic nerve.

The superficial nerve fiber layer is supplied principally by recurrent retinal arterioles branching from the central retinal artery. These small vessels, originating in the peripapillary nerve fiber layer, run toward the center of the optic nerve head and have been referred to as "epipapillary vessels." The capillary branches from these vessels are continuous with the retinal capillaries at the disc margin, but they also have posterior anastomoses with the prelaminar capillaries of the optic nerve. The temporal nerve fiber layer may have an arterial contribution from the cilioretinal artery, when it is present.

The prelaminar region is principally supplied by direct branches of the short posterior ciliary arteries and by branches of the circle of Zinn-Haller, when it is present. In eyes with a well-developed circle of Zinn-Haller, arterial branches emerge to supply both the prelaminar and laminar regions. The lamina cribrosa region also receives its blood supply from branches of the short posterior ciliary arteries or from branches of the circle of Zinn-Haller; this is similar to the prelaminar region. These precapillary branches perforate the outer aspects of the lamina cribrosa before branching into an intraseptal capillary network. Arterioles also branch from the short posterior ciliary arteries and the circle of Zinn-Haller and course posteriorly to supply the pial arteries. These pial arteries often contribute to the laminar region. As in the prelaminar region, the larger vessels of the peripapillary choroid may contribute occasional small arterioles to this region, although there is no connection between the peripapillary choriocapillaris and the capillaries of the optic nerve.

The retrolaminar region is also supplied by branches from the short posterior ciliary arteries, as well as by the pial arterial branches coursing adjacent to the retrolaminar optic nerve region. The pial arteries originate from both the central retinal artery, before it pierces the retrobulbar optic nerve, and branches of the short posterior ciliary arteries more anteriorly. The central retinal artery may supply several small intraneural branches in the retrolaminar region.

The rich capillary beds of each of the 4 anatomic regions within the anterior optic nerve are anatomically confluent. The venous drainage of the anterior optic nerve is almost exclusively via a single vein, the central retinal vein. In the nerve fiber layer, blood is drained directly into the retinal veins, which then join to form the central retinal vein. In the prelaminar, laminar, and retrolaminar regions, venous drainage also occurs via the central retinal vein or axial tributaries to the central retinal vein.

Glaucomatous Optic Neuropathy

Glaucomatous optic neuropathy is the sine qua non of all forms of glaucoma (Fig 3-12). On a histologic level, early glaucomatous cupping consists of loss of axons, blood vessels, and glial cells. The loss of tissue seems to start at the level of the lamina cribrosa and is associated with compaction and fusion of the laminar plates. It is most pronounced at the superior and inferior poles of the disc. Structural optic nerve changes may precede detectable functional loss. Tissue destruction in more advanced glaucoma extends behind the cribriform plate, and the lamina bows backward. The optic nerve head takes on an excavated and undermined appearance that has been likened to a bean pot.

Glaucomatous cupping in infants and children is accompanied by an expansion of the entire scleral ring, which may explain why cupping seems to occur earlier in children and why reversibility of cupping is more prominent with successful treatment in these cases. Cupping may be reversed in adults as well, but such reversal is less frequent and more subtle.

Theories of Glaucomatous Optic Nerve Damage

The development of glaucomatous optic neuropathy likely results from a variety of factors, both intrinsic and extrinsic to the optic nerve. Elevated IOP plays a major role in the development of glaucomatous optic neuropathy in most individuals and is considered the most significant risk factor. Unilateral secondary glaucoma, experimental models of glaucoma, and observations of the effect of lowering IOP in patients all point to this conclusion. But it is also clear that factors other than IOP contribute to a given individual's susceptibility to glaucomatous damage.

Two hypotheses have emerged to explain the development of glaucomatous optic neuropathy, the mechanical and ischemic theories. The *mechanical theory* stresses the importance of direct compression of the axonal fibers and support structures of the

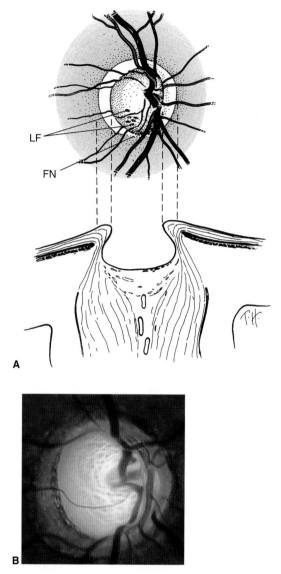

LF

FN

A

B

Figure 3-12   A, Glaucomatous optic nerve (anterior optic nerve head and transverse view, right eye). Note thinning and undermining and focal notching *(FN)* of inferior neuroretinal rim, enlarged central cup with visible laminar fenestrations *(LF),* nasal shift of retinal vessels, and peripapillary atrophy. **B,** Clinical view of glaucomatous optic nerve head demonstrating extensive loss of the neuroretinal rim. *(Part A reprinted with permission from Wright KW, ed.* Textbook of Ophthalmology. *Baltimore: Williams & Wilkins; 1997. Part B courtesy of Ronald L. Gross, MD.)*

anterior optic nerve, with distortion of the lamina cribrosa plates and interruption of axoplasmic flow, resulting in the death of the RGCs. The *ischemic theory* focuses on the potential development of intraneural ischemia resulting from decreased optic nerve perfusion. This perfusion may result from the stress of IOP on the blood supply to the nerve or from processes intrinsic to the optic nerve.

Disturbance of vascular *autoregulation* may contribute to decreased perfusion and thus to nerve damage. The optic nerve vessels normally increase or decrease their tone to maintain a constant blood flow independent of IOP and blood pressure variations. A disturbance in vascular autoregulation may result in decreased optic nerve blood flow from increased IOP. Alternatively, changes in systemic hemodynamics may result in perfusion deficits, even at normal IOP. Such hypothetical derangement could be related to abnormal vessels or to circulating vasoactive substances, for example.

Current thinking regarding glaucomatous optic neuropathy recognizes that both vascular and mechanical factors probably contribute to damage. The glaucomas are likely a heterogeneous family of disorders, and the ganglion cell death seen in glaucomatous optic neuropathy may be mediated by many factors. Active investigations continue to examine the potential role in glaucomatous optic neuropathy of processes such as excitotoxicity, apoptosis, neurotrophin deprivation, ischemia, and autoimmunity.

Examination of the Optic Nerve Head

The optic disc can be examined clinically with a direct ophthalmoscope, an indirect ophthalmoscope, or a slit-lamp biomicroscope using a posterior pole lens. The *direct ophthalmoscope* provides a view of the optic disc through a small pupil. In addition, when used with a red-free filter, it enhances detection of the nerve fiber layer of the posterior pole. However, the direct ophthalmoscope does not provide sufficient stereoscopic detail to detect subtle changes in optic disc topography.

The *indirect ophthalmoscope* is used for examination of the optic disc in young children, uncooperative patients, individuals with high myopia, and individuals with substantial opacities of the media. With the indirect ophthalmoscope, cupping of the optic nerve can be detected, but, in general, optic nerve cupping and pallor appear less pronounced than with slit-lamp methods, and the magnification is often inadequate for detecting subtle or localized details important in the evaluation of glaucoma. Thus, the indirect ophthalmoscope is not recommended for routine use in examining the optic disc.

The best method of examination for the diagnosis of glaucoma is the *slit lamp* combined with a Hruby lens; a posterior pole contact lens; or a 60, 78, or 90 D lens. The slit beam, rather than diffuse illumination, is useful for determining subtle changes in the contour of the nerve head. This system provides high magnification, excellent illumination, and a stereoscopic view of the disc. This also allows for quantitative measurement of the diameter of the optic disc, by adjusting the height of the slit beam. The disc is viewed through the hand-held lens until the height of the slit is the same as the vertical diameter of the disc. The disc diameter can then be calculated by taking into account the lens used. With a 60 D lens, the height of the slit equals the disc diameter in millimeters read directly from the scale. If a 78 D lens is used, the scale reading is multiplied by 1.1, and with a 90 D lens multiplication by 1.3 results in the disc diameter in millimeters. The normal-sized optic disc is approximately 1.5–2.2 mm in diameter.

Slit-lamp techniques require some patient cooperation and moderate pupil size for adequate visibility of the disc.

Clinical Evaluation of the Optic Nerve Head

The *optic nerve head,* or *optic disc,* is usually round or slightly oval in shape and contains a central *cup.* The tissue between the cup and the disc margin is called the *neural rim* or *neuroretinal rim.* In normal individuals, the rim has a relatively uniform width and a color that ranges from orange to pink. The size of the physiologic cup is developmentally determined and is related to the size of the disc. For a given number of nerve fibers, the larger the overall disc area, the larger the cup. Cup–disc ratio alone is not an adequate assessment of the optic disc for possible glaucomatous damage. For example, a 0.7 ratio in a large optic disc may be normal whereas a 0.3 ratio in a very small disc could be pathologic. This shows the importance of assessing the disc size. The size of the cup may increase slightly with age. Nonglaucomatous black individuals, on average, have larger disc areas and larger cup–disc ratios than do whites, although a substantial overlap exists. On average, people with myopia have larger eyes and larger discs and cups than do those with emmetropia and those with hyperopia.

Differentiating physiologic or normal cupping from acquired *glaucomatous cupping* of the optic disc can be difficult. The early changes of glaucomatous optic neuropathy are very subtle (Table 3-2):

- generalized enlargement of the cup
- focal enlargement of the cup
- superficial splinter hemorrhage
- loss of nerve fiber layer
- translucency of the neuroretinal rim
- development of vessel overpass
- asymmetry of cupping between the patient's eyes
- peripapillary atrophy (beta zone)

Generalized enlargement of the cup may be the earliest change detected in glaucoma. This enlargement can be difficult to appreciate unless previous photographs or diagrams are available. It is useful to compare one eye with the fellow eye because disc asymmetry is unusual in normal individuals (Fig 3-13). The vertical cup–disc ratio is normally between 0.1 and 0.4, although as many as 5% of normal individuals will have cup–disc ratios larger than 0.6. Asymmetry of the cup–disc ratio of more than 0.2 occurs in less than 1% of normal individuals. This asymmetry may be related to disc size asymmetry. Increased size of the physiologic cup may be a familial trait and it is also seen with high myopia. An oblong

Table 3-2 Ophthalmoscopic Signs of Glaucoma

Generalized	Focal	Less Specific
Large optic cup	Narrowing (notching) of the rim	Exposed lamina cribrosa
Asymmetry of the cups	Vertical elongation of the cup	Nasal displacement of vessels
Progressive enlargement of the cup	Cupping to the rim margin	Baring of circumlinear vessels
	Regional pallor	Peripapillary crescent
	Splinter hemorrhage	
	Nerve fiber layer loss	

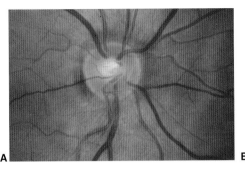
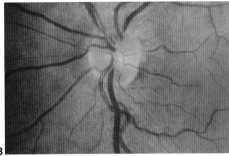

Figure 3-13 Asymmetry of optic nerve cupping. Note the generalized enlargement of the cup in the right eye **(A)** as compared with the left eye **(B).** Asymmetry of the cup–disc ratio of more than 0.2 occurs in less than 1% of normal individuals. *(Courtesy of G. A. Cioffi, MD.)*

insertion of the optic nerve into the globe of individuals with high myopia may also cause a tilted appearance to the optic nerve head. Examination of other family members may clarify whether a large cup is inherited or acquired.

Focal enlargement of the cup appears as localized notching or narrowing of the rim. Focal atrophy most typically occurs at the inferior and superior temporal poles of the optic nerve in early glaucomatous optic neuropathy. Thinning of the neuroretinal rim with development of a focal notch or extension of the cup into the neuroretinal rim may be seen. To help identify subtle thinning of the neuroretinal rim, a convention referred to as the *ISNT rule* may be useful. In general, the *I*nferior neuroretinal rim is the thickest, followed by the *S*uperior rim, the *N*asal rim, and finally the *T*emporal rim. If the rim widths do not follow this progression, there should be increased concern for the presence of focal loss of rim tissue. Deep localized notching, where the lamina cribrosa is visible at the disc margin, is sometimes termed an *acquired optic disc pit.* If notching or acquired pit formation occurs at either (or both) the superior or the inferior pole of the disc, the cup becomes vertically oval (Fig 3-14). Even in the normal eye, laminar trabeculations or pores may be seen as grayish dots in the base of the physiologic cup. With glaucomatous optic neuropathy, neural atrophy results in more extensive exposure of the underlying lamina and may reveal more laminar pores in the optic nerve cup. Nasalization of the central retinal artery and central retinal vein is often seen as the cup enlarges.

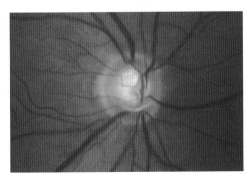

Figure 3-14 Vertical elongation of the cup with localized thinning of the inferior neuroretinal rim in the right eye of a patient with moderately advanced glaucoma. *(Courtesy of Ronald L. Gross, MD.)*

Splinter, or nerve fiber layer, hemorrhages usually appear as a linear red streak on or near the disc surface (Fig 3-15). Nerve fiber layer hemorrhages may occur in the neuro-retinal rim or in the peripapillary area in as many as one-third of glaucoma patients at some time during the course of their disease. Hemorrhages typically clear over several weeks to months but are often followed by localized notching of the rim and visual field loss. Some glaucoma patients have repeated episodes of optic disc hemorrhage; others have none. Individuals with normal-tension glaucoma are more likely to have disc hemorrhages. Optic disc hemorrhage is an important prognostic sign for the development or progression of visual field loss, and any patient with a splinter hemorrhage requires detailed evaluation and follow-up. Splinter hemorrhages may be caused by posterior vitreous detachments, diabetes mellitus, branch retinal vein occlusions, and anticoagulation therapy.

Axons in the nerve fiber layer of the normal eye may best be visualized with red-free illumination. The nerve fiber layer extending from the neuroretinal rim to the surrounding peripapillary retina appears as fine striations created by the bundles of axons. In the healthy eye, the nerve fiber layer bundles have a plush, refractile appearance. With progressive glaucomatous optic neuropathy, the nerve fiber layer thins and becomes less visible. The loss may be diffuse (generalized) or localized to specific bundles (Fig 3-16). *Focal abnormalities* can consist of slitlike grooves or wedge defects. Slitlike defects can be seen in normal retinal nerve fiber layer anatomy, although they usually do not extend to the disc margin. Early wedge defects are sometimes visible only at a distance from the optic disc margin. *Diffuse nerve fiber loss* is more common in glaucoma than focal loss but also more difficult to observe. The nerve fiber layer can be visualized clearly in high-contrast black-and-white photographs, and experienced observers can recognize even early disease if good-quality photographs are available. Direct ophthalmoscopy and slit-lamp techniques can both be successfully employed to observe the retinal nerve fiber layer. The combination of red-free filter, wide slit beam, and posterior pole lens at the slit lamp affords the best view.

In the early stages of nerve fiber loss, often before enlargement of the cup, existing neuroretinal rim tissue can be observed to become more translucent. The clinician can

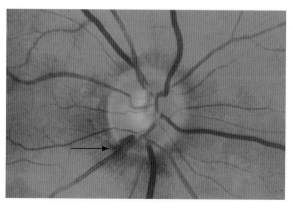

Figure 3-15 Splinter hemorrhage *(arrow)* of the right optic nerve at the 7 o'clock position in a patient with early open-angle glaucoma. *(Courtesy of G. A. Cioffi, MD.)*

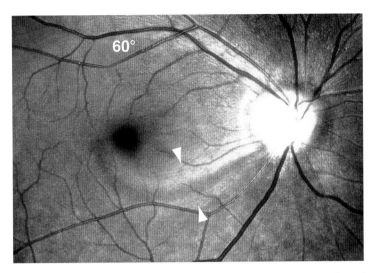

Figure 3-16 Nerve fiber layer photograph shows a nerve fiber bundle defect *(arrowheads)*. *(Courtesy of Louis B. Cantor, MD.)*

best observe this rim translucency by using a lens at the slit-lamp biomicroscope, employing a thin slit beam and confining the beam to the disc surface.

As the nerve fiber loss continues, the cup may begin to enlarge by progressive posterior collapse and compaction of the remaining viable nerve fibers. In circumstances where the neuroretinal tissue—but not the overlying nerve head vasculature—has collapsed, vessel overpass can often be observed. The blood vessels overlying the collapsed neural rim tissue look like a highway overpass suspended over—but not in contact with—the underlying tissue.

Peripapillary atrophy occurs as 2 types. Alpha-zone peripapillary atrophy is the typical temporal crescent often seen in myopia with areas of hyperpigmentation and hypopigmentation; it has no known impact on glaucoma. The second type, beta-zone peripapillary atrophy, is seen with greater frequency and is more extensive in eyes with glaucoma than in unaffected eyes. It represents loss of choriocapillaris and retinal pigment epithelium, leaving only large choroidal vessels and sclera and resulting in the characteristic white appearance adjacent to the disc margin. The location of the atrophy often correlates with the position of visual field defects. Other less specific signs of glaucomatous damage include nasal displacement of the vessels, narrowing of peripapillary retinal vessels, and baring of the circumlinear vessels. With advanced damage, the cup becomes pale and markedly excavated.

It is important to recognize that glaucomatous optic nerve damage is only one type of pathologic change of the optic nerve; other etiologies of optic nerve changes should be considered in the differential diagnosis. Optic discs where the remaining neuroretinal nerve tissue is pale may need to be evaluated for causes of nonglaucomatous optic atrophy (see BCSC Section 5, *Neuro-Ophthalmology*). Glaucoma results in increased cupping and pallor within the cup, but not pallor of the remaining rim tissue. In addition, a large cup may be physiologic in a large disc. This can best be assessed following measurement of the disc diameter. Consideration must also be given to a disc with optic disc drusen or colo-boma, which can result in visual field loss but not on the basis of glaucoma. Finally, the myopic disc represents a challenge when attempting to assess possible glaucoma damage. The size, tilting, and associated structural changes often preclude the ability to definitively determine the likelihood of glaucoma damage.

Quantitative measurement of the optic nerve head and retinal nerve fiber layer

Since the 1850s, the appearance of the optic nerve head has been recognized as critical in as-sessing the disease status of glaucoma. However, optic disc assessment can be quite subjective, and interobserver and intraobserver variation is greater than desirable, given the importance of accurate assessments. Thus, the need for reliable and objective measures of optic disc and as-sociated retinal nerve fiber layer morphology is clear. A number of sophisticated image analysis systems have been developed in recent years to evaluate the optic disc and retinal nerve fiber layer. These instruments give quantitative measurements of various anatomic parameters.

Confocal scanning laser ophthalmoscopy (Fig 3-17A) can be used to create a 3-dimen-sional image of the optic nerve head. The optical design of instruments using confocal scanning laser technology allows for a series of tomographic slices, or optical sections,

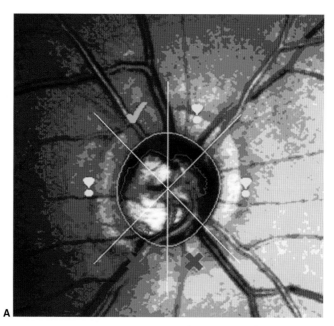

A

Figure 3-17 Commonly used instruments for optic disc and nerve fiber layer imaging in glau-coma. **A,** Optic nerve head analysis with Heidelberg Retina Tomograph (HRT) shows thin-ning of the inferior neuroretinal rim using Moorfields regression analysis (green check mark = within normal limits; yellow exclamation mark = borderline; red x = abnormal). **B,** Retinal nerve fiber layer analysis with scanning laser polarimetry. *Top,* Deviation map. *Bottom,* Generalized thinning or diffuse loss of the nerve fiber layer in the right eye. **C,** Retinal nerve fiber layer analysis with optical coherence tomography. *Top,* Thinning of the inferior bundle (blunted peak) in the right eye. *Middle,* Thinning of the inferior and nasal nerve fiber layer in the left eye. *Bot-tom,* Comparison of both eyes. *(Reproduced with permission from Salinas-Van Orman E, Bashford KP, Craven ER. Nerve fiber layer, macula, and optic disc imaging in glaucoma. Focal Points: Clinical Modules for Ophthalmologists. San Francisco: American Academy of Ophthalmology; 2006, module 8.)* *(Continued)*

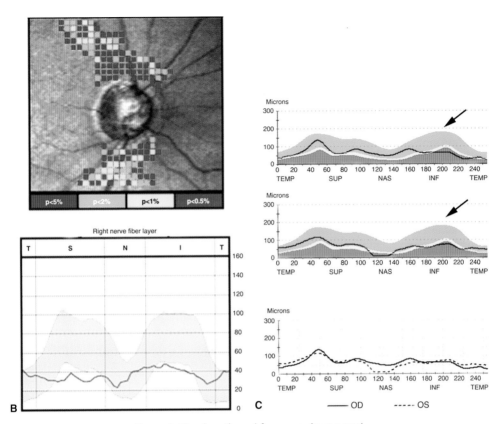

Figure 3-17 *(continued from previous page)*

of the structure being imaged. The images acquired by this method are stored as a computer data file and manipulated to reconstruct the 3-dimensional structure, display the image, and perform data analysis. Parameters such as cup area, cup volume, rim volume, cup–disc ratio, and peripapillary nerve fiber layer thickness are then calculated. Software to evaluate the images for the statistical likelihood of glaucoma damage as well as identify areas of possible progression over time are available.

Techniques such as scanning laser polarimetry and optical coherence tomography have been used to acquire images of the retinal nerve fiber layer. The *scanning laser polarimeter* (Fig 3-17B) is basically a scanning laser ophthalmoscope outfitted with a polarization modulator and detector to take advantage of the birefringent properties of the retinal nerve fiber layer arising from the predominantly parallel nature of its microtubule substructure. As light passes through the nerve fiber layer, the polarization state changes. The deeper layers of retinal tissue reflect the light back to the detector, where the degree to which the polarization has been changed is recorded. The acquired data can then be stored, displayed, and manipulated by computer programs, just as with the unmodified confocal scanning laser ophthalmoscope. The fundamental parameter being measured with this instrumentation is *relative* (not absolute) retinal nerve fiber layer thickness. The addition of a variable corneal compensator (VCC) to include analysis of potential anterior segment birefringence has improved the quality of the information available by this technique.

Optical coherence tomography (OCT) (Fig 3-17C) uses interferometry and low-coherence light to obtain a high-resolution cross section of biological structures. The resolution of OCT instrumentation in the eye is approximately 10 µm, and OCT has the potential to yield an absolute measurement of nerve fiber layer thickness. In vivo OCT measurements appear to correlate with histologic measurements of the same tissues.

Quantitative measurement of the optic disc and retinal nerve fiber layer is a promising nascent science. The instrumentation and techniques used to acquire quantitative imaging and analysis of nerve head and nerve fiber layer anatomic parameters are rapidly evolving. Both for single measurements directed at detecting the presence of glaucoma and, especially, for serial measurements necessary to determine clinical progression of glaucoma, these technologies have great potential. The clinician must remember that no system of measurement and observation is currently more useful or has proven more reliable than good-quality stereophotographs combined with detailed and careful clinical examination.

Chen YY, Chen PP, Xu L, Ernst PK, Wang L, Mills RP. Correlation of peripapillary nerve fiber layer thickness by scanning laser polarimetry with visual field defects in patients with glaucoma. *J Glaucoma.* 1998;7:312–316.

Wollstein G, Garway-Heath DF, Hitchings RA. Identification of early glaucoma cases with the scanning laser ophthalmoscope. *Ophthalmology.* 1998;105:1557–1563.

Recording of optic nerve findings

It is common practice to grade an optic disc by comparing the diameter of the cup with the diameter of the disc. This ratio is usually expressed as a decimal, for example, 0.2, but such a description poorly conveys the appearance of the nerve head. To avoid confusion, the examiner must specify whether the cup is being defined by the change in *color* or in *contour* between the central area of the disc and the surrounding rim. Furthermore, the examiner must specify what is being measured: the horizontal diameter, the vertical diameter, or the longest diameter. If cup–disc ratios are to be used, the description should include the dimensions of the cup specified by both color and contour criteria in both the vertical and horizontal meridians. The rim, which contains the neural elements, should also be described in detail: color, width, focal thinning or pallor, and slope.

A detailed, annotated diagram of the optic disc topography is preferable to the recording of a simple cup–disc ratio. The diagram must be of adequate size to allow depiction of important topographic landmarks and morphologic features. With annotation, the diagram can convey the cup–disc ratio along all dimensions and serves to document the presence or absence of regions of rim thinning, notching, hemorrhage, rim translucency, vessel overpass, and other findings.

Photography, particularly simultaneous stereophotography, is an excellent method for recording the appearance of the optic nerve for detailed examination and sequential follow-up. This record allows the examiner to compare the present status of the patient with the baseline status without resorting to memory or grading systems. Moreover, photographs allow better evaluation when a patient has changed doctors. Sometimes subtle optic disc changes become apparent when the clinician compares one set of photographs to a previous set. Careful diagrams of the optic nerve head are useful when photography is not possible or available.

Computerized optic disc and/or retinal nerve fiber layer analysis is a very good alternative for documentation of these structures. The reproducibility of these techniques is reasonable and each provides a standardized method of recording and analysis. However, care must be taken because the clinical validation of each instrument has not demonstrated sufficient sensitivity or specificity to suggest that individual patient assessments can be made solely on the basis of these analyses. In addition, as these and potential novel techniques evolve, previous images may not be useful in future evaluations.

The Visual Field

The ultimate goal of glaucoma management is the preservation of the patient's visual function and quality of life. Visual function is a very complex concept that can be measured in a variety of ways. For many years, the standard measurement has been clinical perimetry, which measures differential light sensitivity, or the ability of the subject to distinguish a stimulus light from background illumination. As usually performed in glaucoma examinations, the test uses white light and measures what is conventionally referred to as the *visual field*. The classic description of the visual field given by Harry Moss Traquair (1875–1954) is "an island hill of vision in a sea of darkness." The island of vision is usually described as a 3-dimensional graphic representation of differential light sensitivity at different positions in space (Fig 3-18).

Perimetry refers to the clinical assessment of the visual field. Perimetry has traditionally served 2 major purposes in the management of glaucoma:

1. identification of abnormal fields
2. quantitative assessment of normal or abnormal fields to guide follow-up care

Quantification of visual field sensitivity enables detection of initial loss by comparison with normative data. Regular visual field testing in known cases of disease provides valuable information for helping to differentiate between stability and progressive loss. It is likely that in individual patients, different tests will show abnormalities at different times. Some methods may be better for identification than for following the progression of defects, and vice versa.

Over the last 2 decades, automated static perimetry has become the standard for assessing visual function in glaucoma. With this procedure, threshold sensitivity measurements are usually performed at a number of test locations using white stimuli on a white background; this is known as standard automated perimetry (SAP), or achromatic automated perimetry. Assessment of threshold sensitivity by SAP traditionally uses simple staircase algorithms that employ a bracketing approach to estimate threshold. Recently, other technologies have become available that may be useful in evaluating the visual field. Evidence from detailed investigations using these newer perimetric tests—such as short-wavelength automated perimetry, high-pass resolution

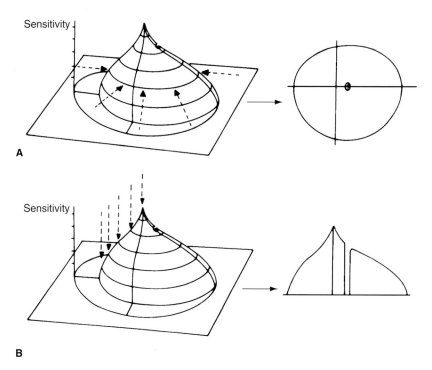

Figure 3-18   A, Isopter (kinetic) perimetry. Test object of fixed intensity is moved along several meridians toward fixation. Points where the object is first perceived are plotted in a circle. **B,** Static perimetry. Stationary test object is increased in intensity from below threshold until perceived by patient. Threshold values yield a graphic profile section. *(Reproduced with permission from Kolker AE, Hetherington J, eds.* Becker-Shaffer's Diagnosis and Therapy of the Glaucomas. *5th ed. St Louis: Mosby; 1983. Modified from Aulhorn E, Harms H. In: Leydhecker W.* Glaucoma. Tutzing Symposium. Basel: S Karger; 1967.)

perimetry, and frequency-doubling technology perimetry—strongly suggests that they may provide beneficial clinical information.

A description of these newer perimetric tests follows:

- *Short-wavelength automated perimetry (SWAP):* This is also known as blue-yellow perimetry. Standard perimeters are available that can project a blue stimulus onto a yellow background. This method is sensitive in the early identification of glaucomatous damage. Several studies suggest that the rate of development of perimetric defects in early glaucoma may be higher with blue-on-yellow (short-wavelength) testing than with conventional (achromatic) white-on-white visual fields.
- *Frequency-doubling technology (FDT) perimetry:* This visual field testing paradigm uses a low spatial frequency sinusoidal grating undergoing rapid phase-reversal flicker. Commercially available instruments employ a 0.25 cycle per degree grating, phase-reversed at a rapid 25 Hz. When a low spatial frequency grating is presented in this manner, it appears to have twice as many alternating light and dark bars than are actually present—hence the term *frequency doubling*. It is believed that the stimuli employed in this test preferentially activate the M cells and may be more sensitive in the detection of early glaucomatous loss.

- *Visually evoked cortical potentials and electroretinography:* Cortical (VECP; also VEP or VER) or retinal (ERG) electrical responses to a stimulus, such as a reversing pattern of light and dark squares or a flickering light, are recorded. The multifocal ERG and multifocal VECP may be a useful objective test for assessing RGC function. Although these tests require visual attention, they do not require a subjective response.

Other measures of visual field include contrast sensitivity, flicker sensitivity, and high-pass resolution perimetry. Several of these tests are discussed in greater detail in BCSC Section 12, *Retina and Vitreous.*

Clinical Perimetry

Two major types of perimetry are in general use today:

- automated static perimetry using a bowl perimeter or video monitor
- manual kinetic and static perimetry using a Goldmann-type bowl perimeter

In the United States, the predominant automated static perimeters are currently the Humphrey Field Analyzers (HFA) models I and II (Carl Zeiss Meditec Inc, Dublin, CA). Most of the clinical examples given in this discussion are from the Humphrey perimeters, and the descriptions apply most directly to these instruments. However, many of the principles apply to a number of other perimeters.

The following are brief definitions of some of the major perimetric terms:

- *Threshold:* The differential light sensitivity at which a stimulus of a given size and duration of presentation is seen 50% of the time—in practice, the dimmest spot detected during testing.
- *Suprathreshold:* Above the threshold; generally used to mean brighter than the threshold stimulus. A stimulus may also be made suprathreshold by increasing the size or duration of presentation. This is generally used for screening paradigms.
- *Kinetic testing:* Perimetry in which a target is moved from an area where it is not seen toward an area where it is just seen. This is usually performed manually by a perimetrist who chooses the target, moves it, and records the results.
- *Static testing:* A stationary stimulus is presented at various locations. In theory, the brightness, size, and duration of the stimulus can be varied at each location to determine the threshold. In practice, in a given automated test session, only the brightness is varied. Although static perimetry may be done manually—and is often combined with manual kinetic perimetry—in current practice the term usually refers to automated perimetry.
- *Isopter:* A line on a visual field representation—usually on a 2-dimensional sheet of paper—connecting points with the same threshold.
- *Depression:* A decrease in retinal sensitivity.
- *Scotoma:* An area of decreased retinal sensitivity within the visual field surrounded by an area of greater sensitivity.
- *Decibel (dB):* A 0.1 log unit. This is a relative term used in both kinetic and static perimetry that has no absolute value. Its value depends on the maximum illumination of the perimeter. As usually used, it refers to log units of attenuation of the maximum light intensity available in the perimeter being used.

Patterns of Glaucomatous Nerve Loss

The hallmark defect of glaucoma is the nerve fiber bundle defect that results from damage at the optic nerve head. The pattern of nerve fibers in the retinal area served by the damaged nerve fiber bundle will correspond to the specific defect. The common names for the classic visual field defects are derived from their appearance as plotted on a kinetic visual field chart. In static perimetry, however, the sample points are in a grid pattern, and the representation of visual field defects on a static perimetry chart generally lacks the smooth contours suggested by such terms as "arcuate."

Glaucomatous visual field defects include the following:

- generalized depression
- paracentral scotoma (Fig 3-19)
- arcuate or Bjerrum scotoma (Fig 3-20)

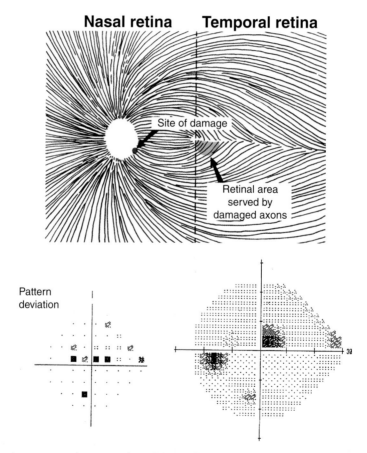

Figure 3-19   A *paracentral scotoma* is an island of relative or absolute visual loss within 10° of fixation. Loss of nerve fibers from the inferior pole, originating from the inferotemporal retina, resulted in the superonasal scotoma shown. Paracentral scotomata may be single, as in this case, or multiple, and they may occur as isolated findings or may be associated with other early defects (Humphrey 24-2 program). *(Visual field courtesy of G. A. Cioffi, MD.)*

- nasal step (Fig 3-21)
- altitudinal defect (Fig 3-22)
- temporal wedge

The superior and inferior poles of the optic nerve appear to be most susceptible to glaucomatous damage. However, damage to small, scattered bundles of optic nerve axons commonly produces a generalized decrease in sensitivity, which is harder to recognize than focal defects. Combinations of superior and inferior visual field loss, such as double arcuate scotomata, may occur, resulting in profound peripheral vision loss. Typically, the central island of vision and the inferior temporal visual field are retained until late in the course of glaucomatous optic nerve damage (Fig 3-23).

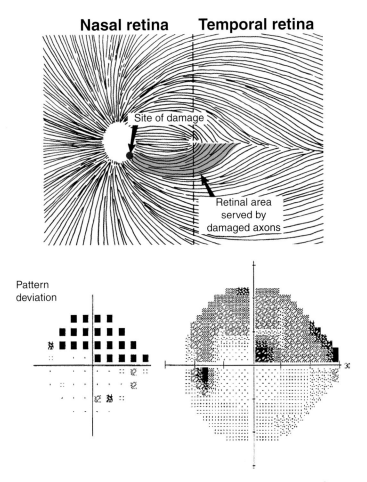

Figure 3-20 An *arcuate scotoma* occurs in the area 10°–20° from fixation. Glaucomatous damage to a nerve fiber bundle that contains axons from both inferonasal and inferotemporal retina resulted in the arcuate defect shown. The scotoma often begins as a single area of relative loss, which then becomes larger, deeper, and multifocal. In its full form an arcuate scotoma arches from the blind spot and ends at the nasal raphe, becoming wider and closer to fixation on the nasal side (Humphrey 24-2 program). *(Visual field courtesy of G. A. Cioffi, MD.)*

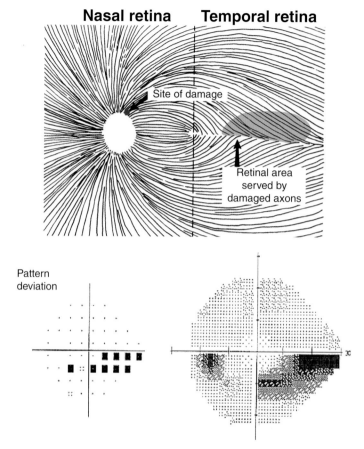

Figure 3-21 A *nasal step* is a relative depression of one horizontal hemifield compared with the other. Damage to superior nerve fibers serving the superotemporal retina beyond the paracentral area resulted in this nasal step. In kinetic perimetry the nasal step is defined as a discontinuity or depression in one or more nasal isopters near the horizontal raphe (Humphrey 24-2 program). *(Visual field courtesy of G. A. Cioffi, MD.)*

Variables in Perimetry

Whether automated or manual, perimetry is subject to many variables, including the human elements involving the patient and the perimetrist.

Patient

People vary in their attentiveness and response time from moment to moment and from day to day. Longer tests are more likely to produce fatigue and diminish the ability of the patient to maintain peak performance.

Perimetrist

The individual performing manual perimetry can administer the test slightly differently each time. Different technicians or physicians also vary from one another. Perimetrist bias is markedly diminished with automated testing. However, the perimetrist can have

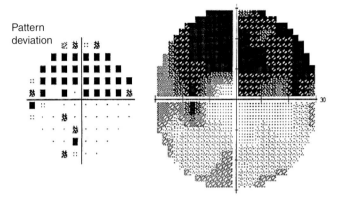

Figure 3-22 Altitudinal defect with near complete loss of the superior visual field, characteristic of moderate to advanced glaucomatous optic neuropathy (left eye). *(Visual field courtesy of G. A. Cioffi, MD.)*

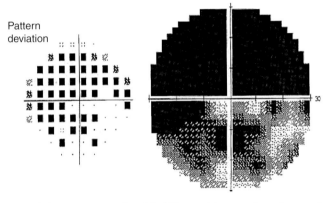

Figure 3-23 Advanced glaucomatous visual field loss with retention of a small central island of vision (foveal threshold: 33 dB) and retention of inferior temporal visual field. *(Visual field courtesy of G. A. Cioffi, MD.)*

an effect on test outcome even in automated testing, by monitoring or not monitoring the patient for proper performance and positioning. Most automated instruments can be paused during the test by perimetrist intervention, thereby allowing repositioning or other adjustments to enhance test reliability.

Other variables

Other variables of importance include the following:

- *Fixation:* If the eye is slightly cyclotorted relative to the test bowl, or if the patient's point of fixation is off center, defects may shift locations. Especially in automated static tests (because the test logic does not change), a defect may thus appear and disappear.
- *Background luminance:* The luminance of the surface onto which the perimetric stimulus is projected affects retinal sensitivity and thus the hill of vision. Clinical

perimetry is usually done with a background luminance of 4.0–31.5 apostilbs. Retinal sensitivity is greatest at fixation and falls steadily toward the periphery.

- *Stimulus luminance:* For a given stimulus size and presentation time, the brighter the stimulus, the more visible it is.
- *Size of stimulus:* For a given brightness and duration of presentation, the larger the stimulus, the more likely it is to be perceived. The sizes of standard stimuli are: 0 = 1/16 mm^2, I = 1/4 mm^2, II = 1 mm^2, III = 4 mm^2, IV = 16 mm^2, and V = 64 mm^2.
- *Presentation time:* Fixed on individual automated perimeters. Up to about 0.5 second, temporal summation occurs. In other words, the longer the presentation time, the more visible a given stimulus. Commercially available static perimeters generally employ a stimulus duration of 0.2 second or less. Comparison of perimetric thresholds between instruments is difficult because different manufacturers use different stimulus durations and background luminances.
- *Patient refraction:* Uncorrected refractive errors cause blurring on the retina and decrease the visibility of stimuli. Thus, proper neutralization of refractive errors is essential for accurate perimetry. In addition, presbyopic patients must have a refractive compensation that focuses fixation at the depth of the perimeter bowl. Care needs to be taken to center the patient close to the correcting lens to avoid a lens rim artifact (see Fig 3-28).
- *Pupil size:* Pupil size affects the amount of light entering the eye, and it should be recorded on each visual field test. Testing with pupils smaller than 3 mm in diameter may induce artifacts. Pupil size should be kept constant from test to test.
- *Wavelength of background and stimulus:* As noted, color perimetry may yield different results from white-on-white perimetry.
- *Speed of stimulus movement:* Because temporal summation occurs over a time period as long as 0.5 second, the area of retina stimulated by a test object is affected by the speed of the stimulus movement. If a kinetic target is moved quickly, by the time the patient responds, the target may have gone well beyond the location at which it was first seen. This period of time between visualization and response is termed the *latency period* or *visual reaction time*.

Automated Static Perimetry

A computerized perimeter must be able to determine threshold sensitivity at multiple points in the visual field, to perform an adequate test in a reasonable amount of time, and to present results in a comprehensible form. The objective perimeter should provide valid, reliable information describing visual sensitivity from an adequate sample of locations, obtained over a reasonable time period. The intensity of the stimulus is varied by a system of filters that attenuate the stimulus, usually allowing measurement to approximately 1 dB.

Automated static perimeters have traditionally used staircase algorithms, which produce more reliable and efficient threshold estimates compared with previous psychophysical test strategies. Any staircase strategy yields threshold estimates that are a compromise between reliability (accuracy and precision) and efficiency (test duration). Threshold estimates from strategies that cross the threshold (reversal) more often or that use smaller staircase intervals are more reliable, but at the expense of requiring a longer test time. The "standard" staircase strategy used by both the Octopus perimeters and the Humphrey Field Analyzers employs an initial 4-dB step size that decreases to 2 dB on first reversal and continues until a second reversal occurs (Fig 3-24).

Four general categories of testing strategy are currently in common use:

1. *Suprathreshold testing:* A stimulus, usually one expected to be a little brighter than threshold, is presented at various locations and recorded as seen or not seen. This type of test is designed to screen for moderate to severe defects and is only appropriate for screening; it cannot be used for follow-up of patients.

2. *Threshold-related strategy:* The threshold is determined at a few points, and a presumed hill of vision is extrapolated from these points. Then a stimulus 6 dB brighter is presented, and the results are recorded as either seen or not seen. This type of test will detect moderate to severe defects, but it may miss mild defects.

3. *Threshold:* Threshold testing is the current standard for automated perimetry in glaucoma management. As described earlier, threshold may be determined by a variety of bracketing and statistical strategies.

4. *Efficient threshold strategies:* Full-threshold testing algorithms suffer from patient fatigue, high variability, and generally poor patient acceptance. In an attempt to achieve shorter threshold testing with good accuracy and reproducibility, the *Swedish interactive thresholding algorithm (SITA)* was developed. Unlike the discrete intervals used to step toward threshold employed by staircase strategies, SITA employs a logical best guess, or forecasting, approach to threshold estimation. Briefly, the best guess intensity of SITA's initial stimulus presentation at each test location corresponds to the intensity associated with the highest probability of being seen by an age-matched individual. Depending on the patient's response to this first stimulus, the intensity of each subsequent presentation is modified. This iterative procedure is repeated until the likely threshold measurement error is reduced to below a predetermined level, with at least 1 reversal occurring at every test location. SITA also uses neighborhood comparisons to optimize the best guess procedure: if adjacent test locations show lower or higher sensitivity than expected, the initial stimulus intensity is altered. SITA monitors the timing of patient

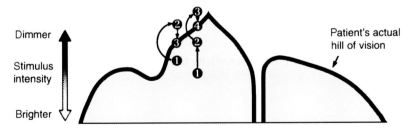

Figure 3-24 Full-threshold strategy determines retinal sensitivity at each tested point by altering the stimulus intensity in 4-dB steps until the threshold is crossed. It then recrosses the threshold, moving in 2-dB steps, in order to check and refine the accuracy of the measurement. *(Reproduced with permission from* The Field Analyzer Primer. *San Leandro, CA: Allergan Humphrey; 1989.)*

responses in order to interactively pace the test. Similar to the SITA test strategy for the HFA, the *tendency-oriented perimeter (TOP)* algorithm was developed for the Octopus perimeter as an alternative to the lengthy staircase threshold procedures. The intent of both of these strategies was to provide a faster, more efficient test procedure that maintained the same degree of accuracy and reliability as the staircase procedures.

Comparisons between SITA testing algorithms and older thresholding algorithms have suggested that the SITA Standard yields visual field results comparable to, though not exactly the same as, full-threshold testing. Both SITA (Standard and Fast) strategies yield marginally higher values for differential light sensitivity compared with other algorithms. Average test time with SITA Standard is approximately 50% the full-thresholding strategy time, and SITA Fast results in an additional reduction of approximately 30% compared with SITA Standard. The significantly reduced test time with SITA Standard appears to be achieved without significant sacrifice of accuracy or increase in variability or noise levels within the test. SITA Fast should not be used in the routine evaluation of glaucoma suspects or patients with glaucoma and should be reserved only for patients who are unable to perform SITA Standard because of mental or physical limitations.

Screening tests

These tests may or may not be threshold-related, and they cover varying areas of the visual field. Suprathreshold tests are not recommended for glaucoma suspects because they do not provide a good reference for future comparison, but they are appropriate for screening people not suspected of having glaucoma. A threshold field should be performed on glaucoma suspects unless a cause other than glaucoma is apparent on examination.

Threshold tests

The most common programs for glaucoma testing are the central 24° and 30° programs, such as the Octopus 32 and G1 and the Humphrey 24-2 and 30-2 (Fig 3-25). These programs test the central field using a 6° grid. They test points 3° above and 3° below the

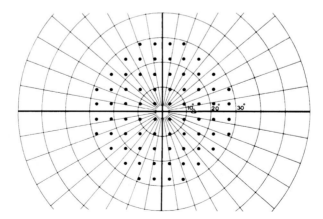

Figure 3-25 Central 30-2 threshold test pattern, right eye. *(Reproduced with permission from The Field Analyzer Primer. San Leandro, CA: Allergan Humphrey; 1989.)*

horizontal midline and facilitate diagnosis of defects that respect this line. For patients with advanced visual field loss that threatens fixation, serial 10-2 or C8 visual fields should be used. These visual fields concentrate on the central 8°–10° of the visual field and test points every 1°–2°, which enables the physician to follow many more test points within the central island and improve the detection of progression.

Although a 30°–60° program is available on most static threshold perimeters, it is rarely performed. No trend to move beyond the central program has emerged after more than 2 decades of static threshold perimetry.

Interpretation of a Single Visual Field

The clinician should exercise caution when interpreting perimetric results. Even with improved strategies, these remain subjective tests. Therefore, confirmation of a new defect or worsening of an existing defect is usually necessary to validate the clinical implication of the visual field in conjunction with all other pertinent data.

Quality

The first aspect of the field to be evaluated is its quality. The percentage of fixation losses, the false positives and false negatives, and the fluctuations of doubly determined points are assessed. Damaged areas of the field demonstrate more variability than normal areas. Glaucomatous damage may cause an increase in false-negative responses unrelated to patient reliability. In general, the average fluctuation between 2 determinations should be less than 2 dB in a normal visual field, less than 3 dB in a visual field with early damage, and less than 4 dB in a visual field with moderate damage. The clinician can evaluate patient reliability by looking at the least damaged areas in a badly damaged visual field.

Normality or abnormality

Next to be assessed is normality or abnormality. When tested under photopic conditions, the normal visual field demonstrates the greatest sensitivity centrally, with sensitivity falling steadily toward the periphery. A cluster of 2 or more points depressed ≥5 dB compared with surrounding points is suspicious. A single point depressed >10 dB is very unusual but is of less value on a single visual field than a cluster, because cluster points confirm one another. Corresponding points above and below the horizontal midline should not vary markedly; normally the superior field is depressed 1–2 dB compared with the inferior field.

To aid the clinician in interpreting the numerical data generated by threshold tests, field indices have been developed by perimeter manufacturers. In addition to the mean difference from normal and the test–retest variability, other measures of the irregularity of the visual field include Humphrey pattern standard deviation and Octopus loss variance indices. These indices highlight localized depressions in the field. When corrected for short-term fluctuation, the indices are termed *corrected pattern standard deviation* and *corrected loss variance.*

These corrected indices help distinguish between generalized field depression and localized loss. An abnormal pattern deviation has greater diagnostic specificity than a generalized loss of sensitivity. An abnormally high pattern standard deviation indicates that some points of the visual field are depressed relative to other points in the visual field after correction for the patient's moment-to-moment variability. Such a finding is suggestive of focal damage such as that occurring with glaucoma (and many other conditions). Although a normal pattern standard deviation in an eye with an abnormal visual field indicates a generalized depression of the hill of vision such as that occurring with media opacity, such generalized loss may also occur with diffuse glaucomatous damage.

The Humphrey STATPAC 2 program performs an additional calculation on a single visual field to determine the likelihood that a visual field shows glaucomatous damage. This test is designed only for glaucoma and involves comparison of corresponding points above and below the horizontal midline (Fig 3-26). This hemifield analysis is at least as accurate as other methods for the classification of single visual fields.

Comparison of various perimetric techniques

With the introduction of new perimetric techniques into the clinical arena, clinicians may be asked to derive important clinical information from several perimetric printouts. The association between glaucoma and short-wavelength (blue) color vision deficits has been known for some time. Sensitivity to blue stimuli is believed to be mediated by a small subpopulation of morphologically distinct ganglion cells, the small bistratified ganglion cells, that typically have large receptive fields, little receptive field overlap, and relatively large axon diameters. If early ganglion cell loss in open-angle glaucoma preferentially affects either sparsely represented cell groups or those with larger axons, either scenario may produce reduced short-wavelength (blue) sensitivity. If special stimuli and background illumination conditions are used, it is possible to isolate and test the sensitivity of short-wavelength mechanisms throughout the visual field with *short-wavelength automated perimetry (SWAP)*. SWAP is available on the HFA II (700 series) and the Octopus 1–2–3. A STATPAC procedure is used to analyze data, which are presented using the same layout as for standard automated perimetry. SWAP is suitable for identifying individuals likely to develop SAP visual field loss. Repeatable visual field loss on SWAP should be carefully monitored. Analyses of local loss such as glaucoma hemisphere test (GHT) and pattern threshold deviations are the best statistical tools to identify glaucomatous SWAP deficits

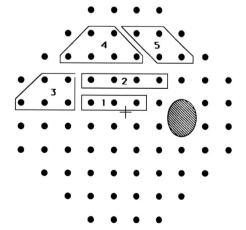

Figure 3-26 Superior visual field zones used in the glaucoma hemifield test. *(Reproduced with permission from The STATPAC User's Guide. San Leandro, CA: Allergan Humphrey; 1989.)*

and to separate them from artifacts resulting from media opacities. The availability of SWAP using the SITA testing algorithm (SITA SWAP) has decreased the testing time for SWAP testing, making it much more clinically useful.

The *frequency-doubling technology (FDT)* perimeter was developed to measure contrast detection thresholds for frequency-doubled test targets. The high temporal frequency and low spatial frequency attributes of the stimulus that causes frequency doubling mean that the stimulus is an M-cell task. Whether it is because of the isolation of specific cell populations, which are susceptible to early damage in glaucoma, or because of the reduced redundancy allowing earlier identification of defects, visual function tests that employ frequency-doubled stimuli may be useful for detection of early defects. Because of the small number of areas tested, FDT is limited in its usefulness for follow-up of glaucoma patients. The availability of the MATRIX perimeter that makes use of frequency-doubling testing with a similar number and size of testing areas as SAP 24-2 provides a potential new method to perform functional assessment in glaucoma. The greater sensitivity of both SWAP and FDT for detection of early glaucomatous damage is illustrated in Figure 3-27. Standard perimetric results reveal a small, localized region of reduced sensitivity nasally, whereas both SWAP and FDT show more extensive amounts of visual field damage.

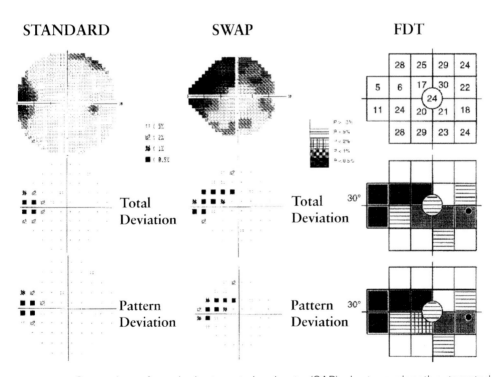

Figure 3-27 Comparison of standard automated perimetry (SAP), short-wavelength automated perimetry (SWAP), and frequency-doubling technology (FDT) in the right eye of a patient with early glaucomatous optic neuropathy. Note the more extensive superior arcuate scotoma and nasal loss detected by SWAP and FDT perimetry testing. These tests frequently detect visual field loss earlier than does SAP. *(Reproduced with permission from Johnson CA, Spry PGD. Automated perimetry. Focal Points: Clinical Modules for Ophthalmologists. San Francisco: American Academy of Ophthalmology; 2002, module 10.)*

Artifacts

Identification of artifacts is the next step in evaluation of the visual field. The following are common artifacts seen on automated perimetry:

- *Lens rim:* If the patient's corrective lens is decentered or set too far from the eye, the lens rim may project into the central 30° (Fig 3-28).
- *Incorrect corrective lens:* If an incorrect corrective lens is used, the resulting field will be generally depressed. In practice, such an error is rarely noted, but it probably accounts for the occasional inexplicably depressed field that improves on follow-up testing. This appears to be less of a problem with FDT perimetry.
- *Cloverleaf visual field:* If a patient stops paying attention and ceases to respond partway through a visual field test, a distinctive visual field pattern may develop, depending on the test logic of a given perimeter. Figure 3-29 shows a cloverleaf visual field, the result of the test logic of the Humphrey 30-2 perimeter, which begins test-

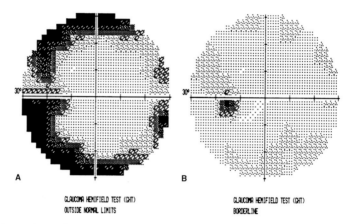

Figure 3-28 Lens rim artifact. The 2 visual fields shown were obtained 9 days apart. The visual field on the left, **A,** shows a typical lens rim artifact, whereas the corrective lens was positioned appropriately for the visual field on the right, **B** (Humphrey 30-2 program).

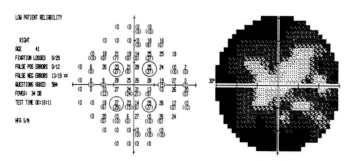

Figure 3-29 Cloverleaf visual field. The Humphrey visual field perimeter test is designed so that 4 circled points are checked initially and the testing in each quadrant proceeds outward from these points. If the patient ceases to respond after only a few points have been tested, the result is some variation of the cloverleaf visual field shown at right (Humphrey 30-2 program).

ing with the points circled and works outward. This pattern may also be seen if a patient is malingering.

- *High false-positive rate:* When a patient responds at a time when no test stimulus is being presented, a false-positive response is recorded. False-positive rates greater than 33% suggest an unreliable test that can mask or minimize an actual scotoma. A high false-positive response rate can, in extreme cases, result in a visual field with impossibly high threshold values (Fig 3-30). A high false-positive and a high fixation-loss rate will also occur if the instrument records fixation losses by presenting stimuli in the blind spot. Careful instruction of the patient may sometimes resolve this artifact.

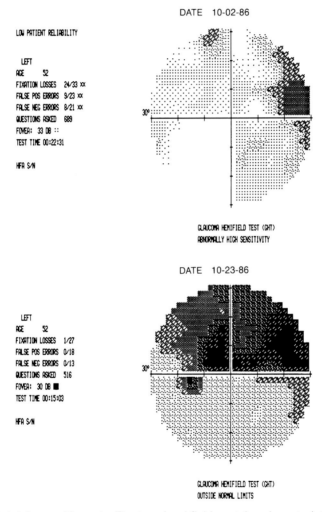

Figure 3-30 High false-positive rate. The top visual field contains characteristic "white scotomata," which represent areas of impossibly high retinal sensitivity. Upon return visit 3 weeks later, the patient was carefully instructed to respond only when she saw the light, resulting in the bottom visual field, which shows good reliability and demonstrates the patient's dense superior visual field loss (Humphrey 30-2 program).

- *High false-negative rate:* When a patient fails to respond to a stimulus presented in a location where a dimmer stimulus was previously seen, a false-negative response is recorded. False-negative rates greater than 33% suggest test unreliability. A high false-negative rate should alert the clinician to the likelihood that the patient's actual visual field might not be as depressed as suggested by the test result. However, it should also be noted that patients with significant visual field loss, including scotomata with steep edges, can demonstrate high false-negative rates that do not indicate unreliability. This effect appears to arise from presentation of stimuli at the edges of deep scotomata, where short-term threshold fluctuation can be quite variable.

Interpretation of a Series of Visual Fields

Interpretation of serial visual fields should meet 2 goals:

1. separating real change from ordinary variation
2. using the information from the visual field testing to determine the likelihood that a change is related to glaucomatous progression

A number of methods can be employed to analyze a series of visual fields for glaucomatous change. Point-by-point analysis by hand, in the absence of a statistical program package, is extremely cumbersome. The mountain of data present in a series of visual fields cannot be effectively analyzed by hand. Fortunately, statistical programs are available from the major instrument manufacturers (eg, the Humphrey STATPAC 2 or Octopus Delta programs); these are valuable aids in point-by-point series analysis. The application of each of these packages is described clearly in the owner's manual that comes with the program.

Calculation and comparison of visual field indices is another method that can be useful in visual field series analysis. Examination of visual field indices can reveal global trends that may be missed using point-by-point analysis. Raw perimetric data can also be transferred to independent software programs for change analysis. Even when computed statistical methods are employed, however, separation of true pathologic progression from normal test-to-test variability remains a difficult challenge. Moreover, the examiner interpreting a series of visual fields must keep in mind that test variability is increased as part of the pathophysiology of glaucoma.

Whatever method the clinician uses, the fundamental requirement for adequate interpretation over time is a good *baseline* visual field. Often the patient experiences a learning effect, and the second visual field may show substantial improvement over the first (Fig 3-31). At least 2 visual fields should be obtained as early in a patient's course as possible. If they are quite different, a third test should be performed. Subsequent visual fields should be compared with these baseline fields. Any follow-up visual field that appears to be quite different should be repeated for confirmation of the suspected change from baseline.

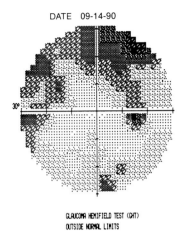

DATE   09-14-90

GLAUCOMA HEMIFIELD TEST (GHT)
OUTSIDE NORMAL LIMITS

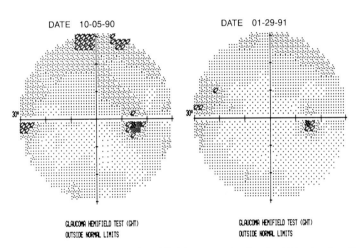

DATE   10-05-90

GLAUCOMA HEMIFIELD TEST (GHT)
OUTSIDE NORMAL LIMITS

DATE   01-29-91

GLAUCOMA HEMIFIELD TEST (GHT)
OUTSIDE NORMAL LIMITS

Figure 3-31   Learning effect. These 3 visual fields were obtained within the first 3½ months of diagnosis in a patient with very early, clinically stable glaucoma. They illustrate the learning effect between the first and the second visual field. The third visual field is similar to the second visual field, and the second and third visual fields provided a baseline for subsequent follow-up of the patient (Humphrey 30-2 program).

Progression

No hard-and-fast rules define what determines visual field progression, but the following are reasonable guidelines:

- Deepening of an existing scotoma is suggested by the reproducible depression of a point in an existing scotoma by ≥7 dB.
- Enlargement of an existing scotoma is suggested by the reproducible depression of a point adjacent to an existing scotoma by ≥9 dB.
- Development of a new scotoma is suggested by the reproducible depression of a previously normal point in the visual field by ≥11 dB, or of 2 adjacent, previously normal points by ≥5 dB.

Cases such as that shown in Figure 3-32 are easy to recognize. A general decrease in sensitivity may be secondary to glaucoma or may be related to media opacity, and clinical correlation is required, which is often difficult. Two causes of general decline in sensitivity that may confuse interpretation are variable miosis (often related to use of eyedrops) and cataract (Fig 3-33). To help avoid the problem of variable pupil size, the clinician should record pupil size at each examination; the size should remain constant from test to test if at all possible.

Suspected new defects or progression of existing defects should be reproduced on subsequent visual fields to determine their validity. Definitions of progression have varied in the numerous clinical trials; these definitions will continue to be refined with additional years of experience and further improvements in computer software.

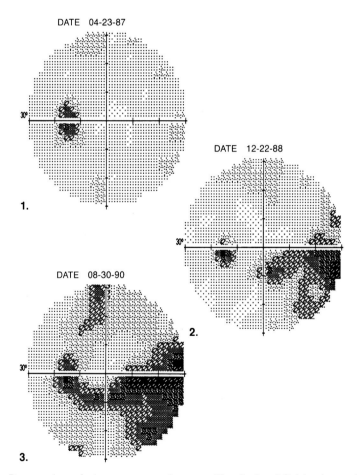

Figure 3-32 Progression of glaucomatous damage. The 3 visual fields shown illustrate the development and advancement of a visual field defect. Between the first and second visual fields, the patient developed a significant inferior nasal step. The third visual field illustrates the extension of this defect to the blind spot, as well as the development of superior visual field loss (Humphrey 30-2 program).

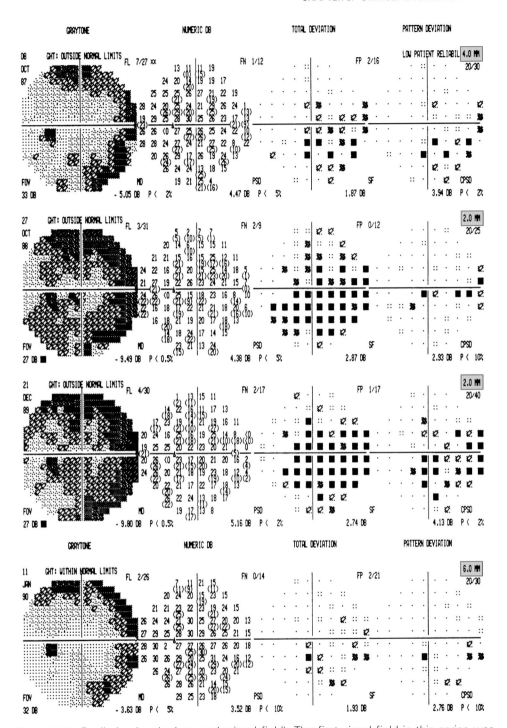

Figure 3-33 Pupil size (marked on each visual field). The first visual field in this series was obtained before the patient began pilocarpine therapy. The second and third visual fields were obtained with a miotic pupil. Before the fourth visual field was obtained, the patient's pupil was dilated (Humphrey 30-2 program).

The Glaucoma Change Probability (GCP) and the Glaucoma Probability Analysis (GPA) (Fig 3-34) currently provide a sensitive assessment of possible progression. The analysis is based on the analysis performed in the Early Manifest Glaucoma Trial (EMGT). It compares the current visual field with a baseline composed of 2 separate visual field tests. The operator must choose the 2 baseline visual fields. As a result, if progression occurs, a new baseline must be established for future analysis.

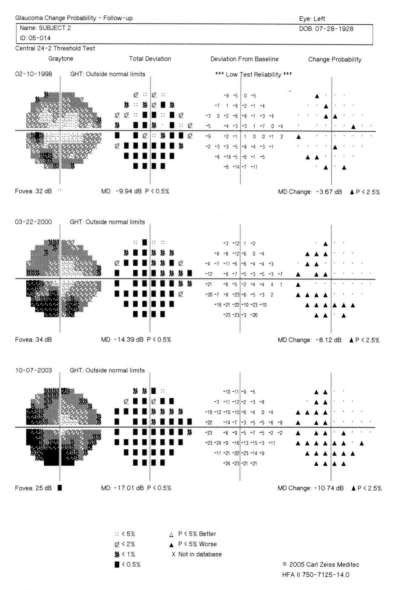

Figure 3-34 Glaucoma Change Probability. Progression of glaucomatous damage. Each of the 3 visual fields shown demonstrates progressive loss compared with the same baseline. The black triangles designate points with a probability (P < .05) that the value is worse than the baseline value. *(Courtesy of Ronald L. Gross, MD.)*

Correlation with the optic disc

It is important to correlate changes in the visual field with those of the optic disc. If such correlation is lacking, other causes of visual loss should be considered, such as ischemic optic neuropathy, demyelinating or other neurologic disease, pituitary tumor, and so forth. This consideration is especially important in the following situations:

- The patient's optic disc seems less cupped than would be expected for the degree of visual field loss.
- The pallor of the disc is more impressive than the cupping.
- The progression of the visual field loss seems excessive.
- The pattern of visual field loss is uncharacteristic for glaucoma—for example, it respects the vertical midline.
- The location of the cupping or thinning of the neural rim does not correspond to the proper location of the visual field defect.

Anderson DR, Patella VM. *Automated Static Perimetry*. 2nd ed. St Louis: Mosby; 1999.

Drake MV. A primer on automated perimetry. *Focal Points: Clinical Modules for Ophthalmologists*. San Francisco: American Academy of Ophthalmology; 1993, module 8.

Drance SM, Anderson DR, eds. *Automatic Perimetry in Glaucoma: A Practical Guide*. Orlando, FL: Grune & Stratton; 1985.

Harrington DO, Drake MV. *The Visual Fields: A Textbook and Atlas of Clinical Perimetry*. 6th ed. St Louis: Mosby; 1989.

Lieberman MF. Glaucoma and automated perimetry. *Focal Points: Clinical Modules for Ophthalmologists*. San Francisco: American Academy of Ophthalmology; 1993, module 9.

Spry PGD, Johnson CA. Advances in automated perimetry. *Focal Points: Clinical Modules for Ophthalmologists*. San Francisco: American Academy of Ophthalmology; 2002, module 10.

Walsh TJ, ed. *Visual Fields: Examination and Interpretation*. 2nd ed. Ophthalmology Monograph 3. San Francisco: American Academy of Ophthalmology; 1996.

Manual Perimetry

The 2 goals of perimetry—to identify abnormalities and to define and record visual function for comparison over time—are most commonly pursued in manual perimetry using the *Armaly-Drance screening technique*. This screening technique for the detection of early glaucomatous visual field loss was originally developed for the Goldmann perimeter but has been adapted for a number of instruments. It combines a kinetic examination of the peripheral isopters with a suprathreshold static examination of the central field.

With this technique, the kinetic perimeter—usually the Goldmann I-2e—is used to determine the stimulus that is just suprathreshold for the central 25°. The central isopter is then plotted kinetically with this stimulus to detect nasal, temporal, or vertical steps, with special attention to the 15° straddling the horizontal and vertical meridians. The blind spot is mapped with the same stimulus moving from the center of the blind spot outward in 8 directions. The same stimulus is then used in static presentations to search for paracentral and arcuate defects. A more intense stimulus, often the equivalent of a Goldmann I-4e, is used to search for both nasal step and temporal sector defects to prepare a kinetic plot of the peripheral isopter.

A different perimetric technique must be used for quantification of defects and for follow-up of patients with established glaucomatous damage. This form of perimetry quantifies visual field defects by size, shape, and depth and determines whether the disease is progressing or not. If the examiner is using a kinetic technique, targets of different size and brightness must be employed. The technique of quantifying defects with kinetic perimetry is well described in standard texts. An example of a quantified defect is shown in Figure 3-35.

Progression of glaucomatous visual field loss generally occurs in areas damaged previously. Scotomata become larger and deeper, and new scotomata appear in the same hemifield. Arcuate scotomata extend to the peripheral boundaries on the nasal side and break through to the periphery. The clinician who quantifies defects with precision can use this pattern of progression to determine a patient's ongoing stability or progression.

Because high-quality manual threshold perimetry requires a well-trained and conscientious perimetrist, and even the best perimetrist varies from day to day, automated field testing has become increasingly widespread. Computerized static perimetry has shown itself to be at least as good as the best-quality manual perimetry for the detection and quantification of glaucomatous defects. However, manual perimetry remains helpful in documenting defects outside the central 30° and in monitoring end-stage visual field loss.

Anderson DR. *Perimetry With and Without Automation.* 2nd ed. St Louis: Mosby; 1987.

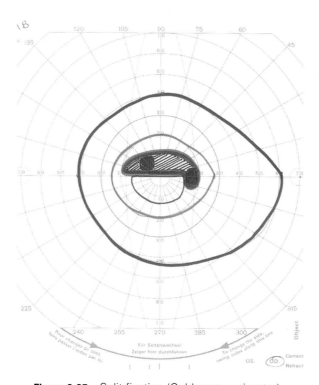

Figure 3-35   Split fixation (Goldmann perimeter).

Other Tests

Several other tests may be helpful in selected patients. Many of these tests are described elsewhere in the BCSC series, and the reader is advised to consult the *Master Index* for the following:

- fluorescein angiography
- corneal pachymetry
- measurement of episcleral venous pressure
- carotid noninvasive vascular studies
- ocular blood-flow measurements
- ultrasonography

Although it is not currently widely available, ultrasound biomicroscopy (UBM) provides valuable information about several types of glaucoma. The test employs shorter-wavelength sound waves than does conventional ocular ultrasound, limiting the penetration but increasing the resolution tenfold. The test allows detailed examination of the anterior segment, the posterior chamber, and the ciliary body (Fig 3-36).

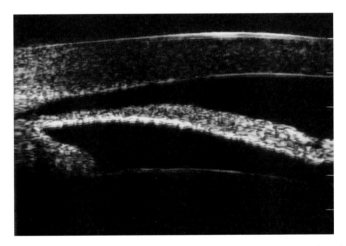

Figure 3-36 Pupillary block as shown by ultrasound biomicroscopy. Note the elevation above the lens of the peripheral iris on the left compared with the central iris on the right. *(Courtesy of Charles J. Pavlin, MD.)*

CHAPTER 4

Open-Angle Glaucoma

Primary Open-Angle Glaucoma

Primary open-angle glaucoma (POAG) is characterized as a chronic, slowly progressive, optic neuropathy with characteristic patterns of optic nerve damage and visual field loss. POAG lacks the identifiable contributing factors of the secondary open-angle glaucomas, such as pigment dispersion in pigmentary glaucoma or the exfoliative material seen in exfoliation syndrome. Elevated IOP is an important risk factor for POAG; other factors, such as race, decreased central corneal thickness (CCT), advanced age, and positive family history, also contribute to the risk of developing this disease. Reduced perfusion to the optic nerve, abnormalities of axonal or ganglion cell metabolism, and disorders of the extracellular matrix of the lamina cribrosa may be contributory factors. Unfortunately, the puzzle of the interplay of the multiple causes of POAG remains unsolved.

Clinical Features

POAG is usually insidious in onset, slowly progressive, and painless. Though usually bilateral, it can be quite asymmetric. Because central visual acuity is relatively unaffected until late in the disease, visual field loss may be significant before symptoms are noted. POAG is diagnosed by the assessment of a combination of findings, including IOP levels, optic disc appearance, and visual field loss.

Intraocular pressure

Large, population-based epidemiologic studies have revealed a mean IOP of 15.5 mm Hg, with a standard deviation of 2.6 mm Hg. This led to the definition of "normal" IOP as 2 standard deviations above and below the mean IOP, or approximately 10–21 mm Hg.

Although IOP greater than 21 mm Hg has in the past been defined as "abnormal," this definition has a number of shortcomings. It is known that IOP in the general population is not represented by a Gaussian distribution but is skewed toward higher pressures (see Fig 2-3). IOPs of 22 mm Hg and above would thus not necessarily represent abnormality from a statistical standpoint. More importantly, IOP distribution curves in glaucomatous and nonglaucomatous eyes show a great deal of overlap. An IOP screening value of 21 or 22 mm Hg, by itself, has little real clinical significance. Several studies have indicated that as many as 30%–50% of individuals in the general population who have glaucomatous optic neuropathy and/or visual field loss have initial screening IOPs below 22 mm Hg. Furthermore, because of diurnal fluctuation, elevations of IOP may occur only intermittently in some glaucomatous eyes, with as many as one-third of the measurements being normal.

The IOP in glaucoma patients may vary widely, by 10 mm Hg or more, over a 24-hour period. Most patients without glaucoma show a diurnal range of 2–6 mm Hg. Patterns of diurnal fluctuation have been broken into several types depending on time of peak pressure: morning, day, night, or flat (meaning little diurnal variation). Most individuals manifest similar patterns from day to day; however, 10%–20% of patients are "erratic," manifesting different patterns of diurnal IOP fluctuation over time. The shift from daytime upright posture to supine posture at night may be associated with increased nocturnal IOP measurements. Spontaneous asymmetric fluctuations of IOP between fellow eyes occur commonly in individuals without glaucoma and in glaucoma patients.

Thus, single office measurements of IOP do not adequately depict the degree of fluctuation of IOP. Diurnal IOP fluctuations have been associated with progression of glaucoma in some studies. Whether or not fluctuation of IOP is an independent risk factor, elevation of IOP is a strong risk factor for glaucoma progression.

Asrani S, Zeimer R, Wilensky J, Gieser D, Vitale S, Lindenmuth K. Large diurnal fluctuations in intraocular pressure are an independent risk factor in patients with glaucoma. *J Glaucoma.* 2000;9(2):134–142.

Bengtsson B, Leske MC, Hyman L, Heijl A, Early Manifest Glaucoma Trial Group. Fluctuation of intraocular pressure and glaucoma progression in the Early Manifest Glaucoma Trial. *Ophthalmology.* 2007;114(2):205–209.

Bergea B, Bodin L, Svedbergh B. Impact of intraocular pressure regulation on visual fields in open-angle glaucoma. *Ophthalmology.* 1999;106(5):997–1004.

Liu JHK, Kripke DF, Twa MD, et al. Twenty-four-hour pattern of intraocular pressure in the aging population. *Invest Ophthalmol Vis Sci.* 1999;40:2912–2917.

Realini T, Barber L, Burton D. Frequency of asymmetric intraocular pressure fluctuations among patients with and without glaucoma. *Ophthalmology.* 2002;109(7):1367–1371.

Zeimer RC. Circadian variations in intraocular pressure. In: Ritch R, Shields MB, Krupin T. *The Glaucomas.* 2nd ed. St Louis: Mosby; 1996:chap 21, pp 429–445.

Corneal thickness affects the measurement of IOP. Thicker corneas resist the indentation inherent in nearly all methods of IOP measurement, including applanation tonometry, airpuff method, and pneumotonometry. Some measurement techniques, such as dynamic contour tonometry (DCT), may be less affected by corneal thickness.

Corneal thickness may be measured (pachymetry) by optical and ultrasonic methods. Average corneal thickness, determined by optical and ultrasonic pachymetry, is approximately 530–545 μm in eyes without glaucoma. Central corneal thickness (CCT) has been found to be increased in groups of patients with the condition termed *ocular hypertension (OHT),* which is elevated IOP in the absence of identifiable optic nerve damage or visual field loss, and decreased in patients with normal-tension glaucoma. Above-average thickness tends to cause overestimation of IOP, but the relationship between corneal thickness and applanation tonometry measurements is probably not linear. Corneal curvature may also play a role in the measurement of IOP, since more sharply curved (steeper) corneas resist indentation more.

Bhan A, Browning AC, Shah S, Hamilton R, Dave D, Dua HS. Effect of corneal thickness on intraocular pressure measurements with the pneumotonometer, Goldmann applanation tonometer, and Tono-Pen. *Invest Ophthalmol Vis Sci.* 2002;43:1389–1392.

Brandt JD, Beiser JA, Kass MA, Gordon MO. Central corneal thickness in the Ocular Hypertension Treatment Study (OHTS). *Ophthalmology.* 2001;108:1779–1788.

Doughty MJ, Zaman ML. Human corneal thickness and its impact on intraocular pressure measures: a review and meta-analysis approach. *Surv Ophthalmol.* 2000;44:367–408.

Optic disc appearance and visual field loss

Although elevated IOP is still considered a key risk factor for glaucoma, it is no longer considered essential to the diagnosis. Optic nerve head appearance and visual field defects have assumed predominant roles in the diagnosis of POAG, although treatment at this time remains aimed at lowering the IOP. Table 4-1 and Clinical Trials 4-1 through 4-4 summarize clinical trials to evaluate control of IOP and POAG.

Careful periodic evaluation of the optic disc and visual field is vital in the follow-up of glaucoma patients. Stereophotographic documentation or computerized imaging of the disc enhances the clinician's ability to detect subtle changes over time. Pertinent clinical signs of glaucoma affecting the optic disc include the following:

- asymmetry of the neuroretinal rim area or cupping
- focal thinning or notching of the neuroretinal rim
- optic disc hemorrhage
- any acquired change in the disc rim appearance or the surrounding retinal nerve fiber layer

Visual field loss should correlate with the appearance of the optic disc. Significant discrepancies in the pattern of field loss and optic nerve damage warrant additional investigation, as noted in Chapter 3.

Gonioscopy should be performed in all patients evaluated for glaucoma and should be repeated periodically in patients with open-angle glaucoma to detect possible progressive angle closure caused by miotic therapy or age-related lens changes, especially in patients with hyperopia. Repeated gonioscopy is also indicated when the chamber becomes shallow, when strong miotics are prescribed, after laser trabeculoplasty or iridectomy is performed, and when IOP rises.

Jonas JB, Budde WM, Panda-Jonas S. Ophthalmoscopic evaluation of the optic nerve head. *Surv Ophthalmol.* 1999;43:293–320.

Preferred Practice Patterns Committee, Glaucoma Panel. *Primary Open-Angle Glaucoma.* San Francisco: American Academy of Ophthalmology; 2005.

Risk Factors for POAG Other Than IOP

Advanced age is an important risk factor for the presence of POAG. The Baltimore Eye Survey found that the prevalence of glaucoma increases dramatically with age, particularly among blacks, exceeding 11% in those aged 80 years or older (Table 4-2). In the Collaborative Initial Glaucoma Treatment Study (CIGTS), visual field defects were 7 times more likely to develop in patients aged 60 years or older than in those younger

Table 4-1 Controlled Clinical Trials With Published Results

Name/Date of Published Results	Study Design	Recruitment (No. of Patients)	Follow-up Duration (Years)	Finding
Scottish Glaucoma Trial/1989	Newly diagnosed POAG: medicine vs trabeculectomy	116	3–5	Trabeculectomy lowered IOP more and was associated with less visual field loss than was medicine.
Moorfields Primary Treatment Trial/1994	Newly diagnosed POAG: medicine vs laser trabeculoplasty vs trabeculectomy	168	5+	Trabeculectomy lowered IOP the most and was associated with less visual field loss.
Glaucoma Laser Trial (GLT)/1990	Newly diagnosed POAG: medicine vs laser trabeculoplasty	271	2.5–5.5	Initial laser trabeculoplasty is at least as effective as initial treatment with topical timolol maleate to reduce IOP and preserve vision.
Glaucoma Laser Trial Follow-up Study/1995	Participants in the GLT	203	6–9	Confirmed GLT findings with extended follow-up.
Fluorouracil Filtering Surgery Study/1989, 1996	Patients at high risk of surgical failure: results of trabeculectomy with or without 5-fluorouracil	213	5+	Greater reduction in IOP and reduced failure rate with adjunctive 5-fluorouracil.
Collaborative Normal-Tension Glaucoma Study (CNTGS)/1998	NTG patients randomized to observation or to 30% reduction of IOP	230	5+	Lowering IOP at least 30% reduced rate of visual field progression from 35% to 12%.

Study	No. of Patients	Years	Conclusions
Advanced Glaucoma Intervention Study (AGIS)/1998	591 (789 eyes)	4–7	After 5 years, white patients had less progression (field and acuity loss) if treated with trabeculectomy first. Black patients had less progression if treated with ALT first. Mean IOP of low teens limits glaucoma progression.
			POAG after medical treatment failure with no previous surgery: laser trabeculoplasty vs trabeculectomy
Collaborative Initial Glaucoma Treatment Study (CIGTS)/2001	607	5	Lowering IOP with medication was as effective as lowering IOP with trabeculectomy in limiting glaucoma progression.
			Newly diagnosed POAG: medication vs trabeculectomy
Ocular Hypertension Treatment Study (OHTS)/2002, 2007	1637	5	Advanced age; increased cup–disc ratio, IOP, and PSD; and reduced CCT were risk factors for glaucoma development; lowering IOP by 22.5% reduced the development of glaucoma from 9.5% to 4.4% over 5 years.
			Ocular hypertensive patients: medication vs observation
Early Manifest Glaucoma Trial (EMGT)/2002	255	6	Lowering IOP by 25% reduced risk of glaucoma progression from 62% to 45% over 5 years.
			Newly diagnosed glaucoma: betaxolol and ALT vs observation
European Glaucoma Prevention Study (EGPS)/2005, 2007	1077	5	Medical therapy lowered IOP by 22%; placebo lowered IOP by 19%. No difference in rates of glaucoma development. OHTS prediction model for development of POAG was validated in the EGPS placebo group.
			OHT patients randomized to medical therapy with dorzolamide or placebo

Modified from Preferred Practice Patterns Committee, Glaucoma Panel. *Primary Open-Angle Glaucoma.* San Francisco: American Academy of Ophthalmology; 2000.

Table 4-2 Prevalence of Definite Primary Open-Angle Glaucoma by Age and Race

Age (Years)	No. Screened	No. of Cases	Observed Rate/100 (95% CI)*	Adjusted Rate/100 (95% CI)
Whites				
40–49	543	1	0.18 (0.02–1.03)	0.92 (0–2.72)
50–59	618	2	0.32 (0.03–1.17)	0.41 (0–0.98)
60–69	915	7	0.77 (0.31–1.57)	0.88 (0.14–1.62)
70–79	631	18	2.85 (1.70–4.50)	2.89 (1.44–4.34)
≥80	206	4	1.94 (0.49–4.95)	2.16 (0.05–4.26)
Total	2913	32	1.10 (0.75–1.55)	1.29 (0.80–1.78)
Blacks				
40–49	632	6	0.95 (0.35–2.07)	1.23 (0.23–2.24)
50–59	699	25	3.58 (2.32–5.26)	4.05 (2.47–5.63)
60–69	614	31	5.05 (3.42–7.17)	5.51 (3.57–7.46)
70–79	349	27	7.74 (4.94–10.54)	9.15 (5.83–12.48)
≥80	101	11	10.89 (4.81–16.97)	11.26 (4.52–18.00)
Total	2395	100	4.18 (3.38–4.98)	4.74 (3.81–5.67)

* CI = confidence interval

Modified from Tielsch JM, Sommer A, Katz J, et al. Racial variations in the prevalence of primary open-angle glaucoma. The Baltimore Eye Survey. *JAMA*. 1991;266:369–374.

than 40 years. Although increased IOP with age has been observed in many populations and may account for part of the relationship between age and glaucoma, studies in Japan have shown a relationship between glaucoma and age even with no increase in IOP in the population. Thus, age appears to be an independent risk factor for the development of glaucoma. The Ocular Hypertension Treatment Study (OHTS) found an increased risk of open-angle glaucoma with age (per decade), of 43% in the univariate analysis and 22% in the multivariate analysis.

Black race is another important risk factor for POAG (see Table 4-2). The prevalence of POAG is 3 to 4 times greater in blacks than in others. Blindness from glaucoma is at least 4 times more common in blacks than in whites. Glaucoma is more likely to be diagnosed at a younger age and likely to be at a more advanced stage at the time of diagnosis in black vs white patients. In the OHTS, black patients were more likely than white patients to develop glaucoma in a univariate analysis (59%), but this relationship was not present after corneal thickness and baseline vertical cup–disc ratio were factored into the multivariate analysis (black patients had thinner corneas and larger baseline vertical cup–disc ratios on average).

Positive family history is also a risk factor for glaucoma. The Baltimore Eye Survey found that the relative risk of having POAG is increased approximately 3.7-fold for individuals who have a sibling with POAG. A Finnish twin cohort study showed a 10.2% inheritance for chronic open-angle glaucoma.

Wilson MR, Martone JF. Epidemiology of chronic open-angle glaucoma. In: Ritch R, Shields MB, Krupin T. *The Glaucomas*. 2nd ed. St Louis: Mosby; 1996:chap 35, pp 753–768.

CLINICAL TRIAL 4-1

Ocular Hypertension Treatment Study Essentials

Purpose: To evaluate the safety and efficacy of topical ocular hypotensive medications in preventing or delaying the onset of visual field loss and/or optic nerve damage in subjects with ocular hypertension.

Participants: 1637 patients with ocular hypertension recruited between 1994 and 1996.

Study Design: Multicenter randomized controlled clinical trial comparing observation with medical therapy for ocular hypertension.

Results 2002: Topical ocular hypotensive medication was effective in delaying or preventing the onset of POAG: a 22.5% decrease in IOP in the treatment group (vs 4.0% in controls) was associated with a reduction of the development of POAG from 9.5% in controls to 4.4% in treated patients at 60 months' follow-up. Topical medications were generally well tolerated.

Increased risk of the onset of POAG was associated with increased age (10 years: 22% increase in relative risk), vertical and horizontal cup–disc ratio (0.1 increase: 32% and 27% increases in relative risk, respectively), pattern standard deviation (0.2 dB increase: 22% increase in relative risk), and IOP at baseline (1 mm Hg increase: 10% increase in relative risk). Central corneal thickness (CCT) was found to be a powerful predictor for the development of POAG (the relative risk of POAG increased 81% for every 40 μm thinner).

OHTS subjects had thicker corneas than the general population. Black subjects had thinner corneas than white subjects had in the study. The effect of CCT may influence the accuracy of applanation tonometry in the diagnosis, screening, and management of patients with glaucoma and ocular hypertension.

Results 2007: The same predictors for the development of POAG were identified independently in both the OHTS observation group and the European Glaucoma Prevention Study (EGPS) placebo group, including baseline age, IOP, CCT, cup–disc ratio, and Humphrey visual field pattern standard deviation. The OHTS prediction model was validated in the EGPS placebo group.

Associated Disorders

Certain conditions, including myopia, diabetes mellitus, cardiovascular disease, and retinal vein occlusion, have been associated with glaucoma. These conditions are not as strongly associated with glaucoma as age, race, and family history. Some of these conditions are discussed in greater detail elsewhere in the BCSC series. See also Section 1, *Update on General Medicine* (diabetes and cardiovascular disease), and Section 12, *Retina and Vitreous* (diabetes and retinal vein occlusion).

CLINICAL TRIAL 4-2

Early Manifest Glaucoma Trial Essentials

Purpose: To compare immediate lowering of IOP with observation in the progression of newly detected open-angle glaucoma.

Participants: Newly diagnosed patients aged 50 to 80 years with early glaucomatous visual field defects were identified mainly from a population-based screening of more than 44,000 residents of Malmö and Helsingborg, Sweden. Exclusion criteria were advanced visual field loss; mean IOP greater than 30 mm Hg or any IOP greater than 35 mm Hg; visual acuity less than 0.5 (20/40). Two hundred fifty-five patients were randomized between 1993 and 1997.

Study Design: Multicenter randomized controlled clinical trial comparing observation with betaxolol and laser trabeculoplasty for open-angle glaucoma.

Results: At 6 years, 62% of untreated patients showed progression, whereas 45% of treated patients progressed. Treatment reduced IOP by 25%. In a univariate analysis, risk factors for progression included no treatment, age, higher IOP, exfoliation, more-severe visual field defect, and bilateral glaucoma. In multivariate analyses, progression risk was halved by treatment (HR = 0.50; 95% CI, 0.35–0.71). Progression risk decreased by approximately 10% with each millimeter of mercury of IOP reduction from baseline to the first follow-up visit. The percentage of patient follow-up visits with disc hemorrhages was also related to progression (HR = 1.02 per percent higher; 95% CI, 1.01–1.03).

Myopia

An association has been reported between POAG and myopia. It is possible that individuals with myopia may be at increased risk for the development of glaucoma. Another possible explanation is that the association between myopia and POAG is influenced by selection bias, because people who have refractive errors are more likely to seek eye care and thus have a higher probability than individuals with emmetropia of having glaucoma detected early. An association between myopia and the development of glaucoma was not observed in OHTS.

The concurrence of POAG and myopia may complicate both diagnosis and management. Disc evaluation is particularly complicated in the presence of myopic fundus changes, such as tilting of the disc and posterior staphylomas, which may make an assessment of cupping difficult. Myopia-related retinal changes can cause visual field abnormalities apart from any glaucomatous process. High refractive error may also make it difficult to perform accurate perimetric measurement and to interpret visual field abnormalities. In addition, the magnification of the disc associated with the myopic refractive error interferes with optic disc evaluation.

Wong TY, Klein BE, Klein R, Knudtson M, Lee KE. Refractive errors, intraocular pressure, and glaucoma in a white population. *Ophthalmology.* 2003;110:211–217.

Diabetes mellitus

Studies have reported a higher prevalence of both elevated mean IOP and POAG among persons with diabetes. Also, glaucoma patients have been reported to have a higher prevalence of abnormal glucose metabolism. Some authorities believe that small-vessel involvement in diabetes may cause the optic nerve to become more susceptible to pressure-related damage. Whether diabetes is an independent risk factor for POAG development remains controversial. Diabetes was not associated with an increased risk of progression to glaucoma in OHTS, though patients with retinopathy were not enrolled in the trial.

Cardiovascular disease

Associations between POAG and blood pressure or perfusion pressure of the eye have been reported. The hypothesis that systemic hypertension, with its possible microcirculatory effects on the optic nerve, may increase susceptibility to glaucoma is biologically plausible. Recent evidence suggests that lower systolic perfusion pressure, lower systolic blood pressure, and cardiovascular disease history are risk factors for glaucoma progression, and these factors may be important in the development of some cases of glaucoma. Evidence

CLINICAL TRIAL 4-3

Collaborative Initial Glaucoma Treatment Study Essentials

Purpose: To determine whether patients with newly diagnosed open-angle glaucoma are better treated by initial treatment with medications or by immediate filtering surgery.

Participants: 607 patients with open-angle glaucoma (primary, pigmentary, or pseudoexfoliative) recruited between 1993 and 1997.

Study Design: Multicenter randomized controlled clinical trial comparing initial medical with initial surgical therapy for open-angle glaucoma.

Results: Initial medical and initial surgical therapy resulted in similar visual field outcomes after up to 5 years of follow-up. Early visual acuity loss was greater in the surgery group, but the differences between groups converged over time.

The quality of life (QOL) impact reported by the 2 treatment groups was very similar. The most persistent QOL finding was the increased impact of local eye symptoms reported by the surgical group compared with the medical group.

The overall rate of progression was lower than in many clinical trials, potentially the result of more aggressive IOP goals and the stage of the disease. Individualized target IOPs were determined according to a formula that accounted for baseline IOP and visual field loss. Over the course of follow-up, IOP in the medical therapy group averaged 17–18 mm Hg (IOP reduction of approximately 38%), whereas that in the surgery group averaged 14–15 mm Hg (IOP reduction of approximately 46%). The rate of cataract removal was greater in the surgically treated group.

is accumulating that suggests vascular circulatory and autoregulatory abnormalities in individuals with glaucoma. Ongoing research into the pathophysiology of glaucoma may expand on these findings in the future. Systemic hypotension may also predispose the optic nerve to damage through reduced perfusion.

> Leske MC, Heijl A, Hyman L, Bengtsson B, Dong L, Yang Z, EMGT Group. Predictors of long-term progression in the Early Manifest Glaucoma Trial. *Ophthalmology.* 2007;114(11): 1965–1972.

Retinal vein occlusion

Patients with central retinal vein occlusion (CRVO) may present with elevated IOP and glaucoma. They may have preexisting POAG or other types of glaucoma. After CRVO, patients may develop angle-closure glaucoma or, at a later stage, neovascular glaucoma. Glaucoma and OHT are risk factors for the development of CRVO. In susceptible individuals, eyes with elevated IOP are at risk of developing CRVO. Thus, elevated IOP in the fellow eye of an eye affected with retinal vein occlusion must be kept as low as reasonably possible.

CLINICAL TRIAL 4-4

Advanced Glaucoma Intervention Study (AGIS) Essentials

Purpose: To compare the clinical outcomes of 2 treatment sequences: argon laser trabeculoplasty–trabeculectomy–trabeculectomy (ATT) and trabeculectomy–argon laser trabeculoplasty–trabeculectomy (TAT).

Participants: 789 eyes of 591 patients with medically uncontrolled open-angle glaucoma recruited from 1988 to 1992.

Study Design: Multicenter randomized controlled clinical trial comparing 2 treatment sequences (ATT and TAT) for patients with open-angle glaucoma uncontrolled by medical therapy.

Results

AGIS 4 and AGIS 13: Black patients had less combined visual acuity and visual field loss if treated with the ATT sequence. White patients had less combined visual acuity and visual field loss at 7 years if treated with the TAT sequence. In the first years of follow-up in the white patients, the TAT group had greater visual acuity loss than the ATT group, but by 7 years the groups' acuities were equivalent.

AGIS 5: Encapsulated blebs were slightly more common in patients with prior argon laser trabeculoplasty (ALT), but this difference was not statistically significant. The 4-week postoperative mean IOP was higher in eyes with encapsulated blebs than without; with resumption of medical therapy, eyes with and without encapsulated blebs had similar IOP after 1 year.

AGIS 6: Visual function scores improved after cataract surgery. Adjustment for cataract did not alter the findings of previous AGIS studies.

AGIS 7: Lower IOP was associated with less visual field loss. Eyes with average IOP of 14 mm Hg or less during the first 18 months, or eyes with

IOP of 18 mm Hg or less at all visits throughout the study had significantly less visual field loss.

AGIS 8: Approximately half of the study patients developed cataract in the first 5 years of follow-up. Trabeculectomy increases the relative risk of cataract formation by 78%.

AGIS 9: Trabeculectomy retards the progression of glaucoma more effectively in white patients than in black patients. ALT was slightly more effective in blacks than in whites.

AGIS 10: Assessment of optic nerve findings showed good intraobserver but poor interobserver agreement.

AGIS 11: ALT failure is associated with younger age and higher IOP. Trabeculectomy failure was associated with younger age, higher IOP, diabetes, and postoperative complications such as particularly elevated IOP and marked inflammation.

AGIS 12: Risk factors for sustained decrease of visual field included better baseline visual fields, male sex, worse baseline visual acuity, and diabetes. Risk factors for sustained decrease of visual acuity included better baseline visual acuity, older age, and less formal education.

AGIS 14: In patients with worsening of the visual field, 1 confirmatory test within 6 months has a 72% probability of indicating a persistent defect. When the number of confirmatory tests is increased from 1 to 2, the percentage of eyes that show a persistent defect increases from 72% to 84%.

Prognosis

Most POAG patients will retain useful vision for their entire lives. The incidence of blindness has been variously reported and has been estimated at 27% and 9%, unilateral vs bilateral, at 20 years after diagnosis (Hattenhauer and colleagues). The prevalence of bilateral blindness has been estimated at 8% in blacks and 4% in whites (Quigley and Vitale). Patients at greatest risk of blindness have visual field loss at the time of diagnosis of glaucoma.

Treatment with medications, lasers, and surgeries to lower IOP has been shown to significantly slow or possibly halt the progression of the disease. Many clinical trials have confirmed the efficacy of IOP reduction and compared various treatments at various points in the clinical course (see Table 4-1 and Clinical Trials 4-1 through 4-4). In the Early Manifest Glaucoma Trial, a 25% reduction in IOP reduced progression from 62% to 45% of patients at 6 years' follow-up. The CIGTS showed relatively equivalent outcomes between initial surgery and initial medications for glaucoma treatment after 5 years, with significant visual field progression in only 10%–13% of participants. In the Advanced Glaucoma Intervention Study (AGIS), the group of patients in whom IOP was always less than 18 mm Hg did not show progressive visual field loss; patients with average IOP of 14 mm Hg or less during the first 18 months fared better than those with average IOP greater than 17.5 mm Hg (AGIS 7).

The AGIS Investigators. Advanced Glaucoma Intervention Study (AGIS): 4. Comparison of treatment outcomes within race: seven-year results. *Ophthalmology.* 1998;105:1146–1164.

The AGIS Investigators. Advanced Glaucoma Intervention Study (AGIS): 7. The relationship between control of intraocular pressure and visual field deterioration. *Am J Ophthalmol.* 2000;130:429–440.

Hattenhauer MG, Johnson DH, Ing HH, et al. The probability of blindness from open-angle glaucoma. *Ophthalmology.* 1998;105:2099–2104.

Oliver JE, Hattenhauer MG, Herman D, et al. Blindness and glaucoma: a comparison of patients progressing to blindness from glaucoma with patients maintaining vision. *Am J Ophthalmol.* 2002;133:764-772.

Preferred Practice Patterns Committee, Glaucoma Panel. *Primary Open-Angle Glaucoma.* San Francisco: American Academy of Ophthalmology; 2005.

Quigley HA, Vitale S. Models of open-angle glaucoma prevalence and incidence in the United States. *Invest Ophthalmol Vis Sci.* 1997;38:83–91.

Wilson MR, Brandt JD. Update on glaucoma clinical trials. *Focal Points: Clinical Modules for Ophthalmologists.* San Francisco: American Academy of Ophthalmology; 2003, module 9.

Open-Angle Glaucoma Without Elevated IOP (Normal-Tension Glaucoma, Low-Tension Glaucoma)

Considerable controversy remains about whether normal-tension glaucoma represents a distinct disease entity or is simply POAG with IOP within the average range. Because IOP is a continuous variable with no firm dividing line between normal and abnormal, many authorities believe the terms *low-tension glaucoma* and *normal-tension glaucoma* should be abandoned. This debate is likely to persist. Whatever the outcome, the concept of normal-tension glaucoma has undeniably had a strong influence on the classification and understanding of glaucoma.

Clinical Features

As previously emphasized, elevated IOP is an important risk factor in the development of glaucoma, but it is not the only risk factor. In normal-tension glaucoma, other risk factors, most of which are currently unknown, may play a more important role. Many authorities have hypothesized that local vascular factors may have a significant part in the development of this disorder. Studies have suggested that patients with normal-tension glaucoma show a higher prevalence of vasospastic disorders such as migraine headache and Raynaud phenomenon, ischemic vascular diseases, autoimmune diseases, and coagulopathies compared with patients who have high-tension glaucoma. However, these findings have not been consistent. Vascular autoregulatory defects have also been described in studies of eyes with normal-tension glaucoma.

The condition is characteristically bilateral and progressive, often despite the lowering of IOP. Studies have indicated that in glaucomatous eyes with normal but asymmetric IOP, the worse damage usually occurs in the eye with the higher IOP. The Collaborative Normal-Tension Glaucoma Study (CNTGS) found that lowering IOP by at least 30% reduced the rate of visual field progression from 35% to 12%, confirming that IOP has a clear role in this disease. However, because some patients did progress despite the reduction in IOP, other factors may be operative as well. In addition, progression of the visual field loss, when it did occur, tended to be slow. It should be noted that the protective effect of IOP reduction was evident only after adjusting for the effect of cataracts, which were more frequent in the treated group.

Another area of considerable debate concerns patterns of optic disc damage and visual field loss in normal-tension glaucoma compared with those of POAG. In eyes matched for total visual field loss, the neuroretinal rim has been reported to be thinner, especially inferiorly and inferotemporally, in persons with normal-tension glaucoma. Varied patterns of peripapillary atrophy may also be characteristic for normal-tension glaucoma. Some authorities have separated normal-tension glaucoma into 2 groups based on disc appearance:

- a *senile sclerotic group* with shallow, pale sloping of the neuroretinal rim (primarily in older patients with vascular disease)
- a *focal ischemic group* with deep, focal notching in the neuroretinal rim

The visual field defects in normal-tension glaucoma tend to be more focal, deeper, and closer to fixation, especially early in the course of the disease, compared with those commonly seen in POAG. A dense paracentral scotoma encroaching on fixation is not an unusual finding as the initial defect. Although many reports have described these differences between groups of patients with normal-tension glaucoma and those with POAG, others have failed to confirm them. In any individual patient, there is no characteristic abnormality of the optic disc or visual field that is diagnostic for normal-tension glaucoma.

Cartwright MJ, Anderson DR. Correlation of asymmetric damage with asymmetric intraocular pressure in normal-tension glaucoma (low-tension glaucoma). *Arch Ophthalmol.* 1988; 106:898–900.

Collaborative Normal-Tension Glaucoma Study Group. Comparison of glaucomatous progression between untreated patients with normal-tension glaucoma and patients with therapeutically reduced intraocular pressures. *Am J Ophthalmol.* 1998;126:487–497.

Differential Diagnosis

Normal-tension glaucoma can be mimicked by many conditions, as summarized in Table 4-3. Several of these conditions can cause arcuate-type visual field defects; some may be progressive. The diagnosis of normal-tension glaucoma is one of exclusion. Great care must be taken to distinguish normal-tension glaucoma from these other etiologies, because appropriate treatment may vary greatly. Diurnal IOP measurement is useful to determine peak IOP, which aids in determining target IOP.

Elevated IOP can be obscured in patients taking systemic medication, particularly systemic beta-blockers, and by artifactually low tonometric readings caused, for example, by reduced scleral rigidity and corneal thickness. Assessment of CCT is recommended in patients suspected of having normal-tension glaucoma, because a thin central cornea may lead to artifactually low IOP readings. In studies to date, the average CCT has ranged between 510 and 520 μm in patients with normal-tension glaucoma vs 530 and 545 μm in unaffected patients. Decreased corneal thickness in patients who have undergone refractive surgery may be associated with underestimation of IOP and difficulty in the

---

Table 4-3 Differential Diagnosis of Normal-Tension Glaucoma

Undetected high-tension glaucoma
  Primary open-angle glaucoma with diurnal IOP variation
  Intermittent IOP elevation
    Angle-closure glaucoma
    Glaucomatocyclitic crisis
  Previously elevated IOP
    Past secondary glaucoma (eg, corticosteroid-induced glaucoma, uveitic glaucoma,
      pigmentary glaucoma, previous trauma)
    Normalized IOP in an eye with previously elevated IOP
  Use of medication that may cause IOP lowering (systemic beta-blocker)
  Tonometric error (reduced corneal thickness, low scleral rigidity)

Nonglaucomatous optic nerve disease
  Congenital anomalies (coloboma, optic nerve pits)
  Compressive lesions of optic nerve and chiasm
  Shock optic neuropathy
  Anterior ischemic optic neuropathy
  Retinal disorders (ie, retinal detachment, retinoschisis, vascular occlusions, chorioretinitis,
    syphilis)
  Optic nerve drusen

---

diagnosis of normal-tension vs high-tension glaucoma. Many patients with myopia may have anomalous discs or myopic visual field changes, further complicating the diagnosis of glaucoma. Other conditions to consider in the differential diagnosis include normalized IOP in an eye with previously elevated IOP, intermittent angle-closure glaucoma, and previous corticosteroid-induced or other secondary glaucoma.

Diagnostic Evaluation

It is difficult to know how often glaucomatous damage occurs with IOP in the normal range. Population-based epidemiologic studies have suggested that as many as 30%–50% of eyes with POAG may have IOP below 21 mm Hg on a single reading. Repeated testing would undoubtedly have detected elevated IOP in many of these eyes. The prevalence of normal-tension glaucoma appears to vary among different populations. Studies have suggested that among Japanese patients, a particularly high proportion of open-angle glaucoma occurs with IOP in the normal range. Among clinic-based patients, a diagnosis of normal-tension glaucoma is influenced by how thoroughly other possible causes of optic neuropathy are considered and eliminated.

Before making a diagnosis of normal-tension glaucoma, the clinician should measure the patient's IOP by applanation tonometry at various times during the day. Gonioscopy should be performed to rule out angle closure, angle recession, or evidence of previous intraocular inflammation. Careful stereoscopic disc evaluation is essential to rule out other congenital or acquired disc anomalies, such as optic nerve coloboma, drusen, and physiologically enlarged cups. The clinician must also consider the patient's medical history, particularly any record of cardiovascular disease and low blood pressure caused by hemorrhage, myocardial infarction, or shock. Visual field loss consistent with glaucoma has been noted after a decrease in blood pressure following a hypotensive crisis. However, damage secondary to such a specific precipitating event tends to be stable and does not progress once the underlying problem has been corrected. Similarly, a prior episode of prolonged, elevated IOP, such as that related to the use of topical steroids in susceptible individuals, may create optic nerve damage that later mimics normal-tension glaucoma but is not progressive. Most cases of normal-tension glaucoma are not caused by a sudden precipitating event.

Sometimes a diagnosis cannot be established on the basis of a single or even multiple ophthalmic examinations, particularly if findings or risk factors are atypical, such as unilateral disease, decreased central vision, dyschromatopsia, young age, afferent defect, neuroretinal rim pallor, or visual field loss not consistent with the optic disc appearance. In such cases, medical and neurologic evaluation should be considered, including tests for anemia, heart disease, syphilis, and temporal arteritis or other causes of systemic vasculitis. Auscultation and palpation of the carotid arteries should be performed, and noninvasive tests of carotid circulation may be helpful. Increasing attention is being focused on assessment of ocular blood flow, but techniques for these measurements are generally still investigational. Evaluation of the optic nerve in the chiasmal region with computed tomography (CT) or magnetic resonance imaging (MRI) may be warranted in some cases to rule out compressive lesions, especially if the visual field loss is at all suggestive of congruous, bitemporal, or other neurologic defects (see also BCSC Section 5, *Neuro-Ophthalmology*).

Greenfield DS, Siatkowski RM, Glaser JS, Schatz NJ, Parrish RK 2nd. The cupped disc. Who needs neuroimaging? *Ophthalmology.* 1998;105:1866–1874.

Prognosis and Therapy

Therapy for normal-tension glaucoma can be difficult. It is generally initiated for normal-tension glaucoma unless the optic neuropathy is determined to be stable. The results of the Collaborative Normal-Tension Glaucoma Study support aggressive reduction in IOP by at least 30% in an attempt to reduce progressive visual field loss. The criteria for initiating therapy in this study were visual field loss threatening fixation, disc hemorrhage, and documented visual field or optic nerve progression. This study demonstrated that disease in some patients (65%) did not progress over the length of the study despite the lack of treatment, whereas in others (12%) it did progress despite aggressive reduction in IOP, revealing the extremely variable clinical course of normal-tension glaucoma. The potential role of neuroprotective agents is experimental and remains under investigation. The goal of therapy should be to use the treatments currently available to achieve an IOP that is as low as possible, without the development of complications.

Systemic medications such as calcium channel blockers (CCBs) are advocated by some authorities because of the possible beneficial effects of increasing capillary perfusion of the optic nerve head. If systemic treatment with calcium channel blockers is undertaken, it should be coordinated with the patient's primary care physician because of possible side effects. Systemic hypotension, a possible complication of this therapy, may adversely affect ocular blood flow. Use of antihypertensive medications such as beta-blockers may be associated with nocturnal hypotension, which may also alter ocular blood flow.

As with POAG, topical medical therapy is the most common initial approach in treating normal-tension glaucoma. As with all glaucomas, it might be useful for the ophthalmologist to change or add medications to one eye at a time so the contralateral eye can be used as a control to assess therapeutic response. Prostaglandin analogs may help achieve the target reduction of IOP. It has been suggested that prostaglandin analogs may be capable of achieving low IOP, even below episcleral venous pressure. Other medications, including topical beta-blockers, carbonic anhydrase inhibitors, and α_2-agonists, may also help achieve the goal of lowering IOP in individual patients. The benefits of these medications' non–IOP-lowering effects, such as neuroprotection or ocular circulation enhancement, have not been demonstrated.

If medications are inadequate in controlling the disease, laser trabeculoplasty can be effective in reducing IOP. Glaucoma filtering surgery may be indicated in an attempt to obtain the lowest IOP. An antifibrotic agent, 5-fluorouracil or mitomycin C, may be used to improve the success rate of filtering surgery and to reduce the postoperative and long-term IOP in these patients with low target IOPs (see Chapter 8).

Bhandari A, Crabb DP, Poinoosawmy D, Fitzke FW, Hitchings RA, Noureddin BN. Effect of surgery on visual field progression in normal-tension glaucoma. *Ophthalmology.* 1997;104(7):1131–1137.

Collaborative Normal-Tension Glaucoma Study Group. Comparison of glaucomatous progression between untreated patients with normal-tension glaucoma and patients with therapeutically reduced intraocular pressures. *Am J Ophthalmol.* 1998;126:487–497.

Collaborative Normal-Tension Glaucoma Study Group. The effectiveness of intraocular pressure reduction in the treatment of normal-tension glaucoma. *Am J Ophthalmol.* 1998;126: 498–505.

Mikelberg FS. Normal tension glaucoma. *Focal Points: Clinical Modules for Ophthalmologists.* San Francisco: American Academy of Ophthalmology; 2000, module 12.

The Glaucoma Suspect

A glaucoma suspect is defined as an adult who has one of the following findings in at least 1 eye:

- an optic nerve or nerve fiber layer defect suggestive of glaucoma (enlarged cup–disc ratio, asymmetric cup–disc ratio, notching or narrowing of the neuroretinal rim, a disc hemorrhage, or suspicious alteration in the nerve fiber layer)
- a visual field abnormality consistent with glaucoma
- an elevated IOP greater than 21 mm Hg

Usually, if 2 or more of these findings are present, the diagnosis of POAG is supported, especially in the presence of other risk factors, such as age older than 50 years, family history of glaucoma, and black race. Diagnosis of a glaucoma suspect is also dependent on a normal open angle on gonioscopy.

A frequent finding warranting this diagnosis is OHT. Estimates of the prevalence of OHT vary considerably; some authorities believe it may be as high as 8 times that of definite POAG. Analysis of studies that have observed individuals with elevated IOP for variable periods indicates that the higher the baseline IOP, the greater the risk of developing glaucoma. However, it is important to note that even among individuals with elevated IOP, the majority never develop glaucoma.

Differentiating between diagnoses of OHT and early POAG is often difficult. The ophthalmologist must look carefully for signs of early damage to the optic nerve, such as focal notching, asymmetry of cupping, splinter disc hemorrhage, nerve fiber layer dropout, or subtle visual field defects. The increasing use of short-wavelength and frequency-doubling automated perimetry may improve our ability to recognize early glaucomatous visual field loss in these patients (see Chapter 3). If these signs of optic nerve damage are present, the diagnosis of early POAG should be considered and treatment initiated. However, in uncertain cases, the ophthalmologist should not hesitate to closely monitor patients without therapy to confirm either initial findings or progressive change in order to better establish the diagnosis prior to initiating therapy.

There is no clear consensus about whether elevated IOP should be treated in the absence of signs of early damage. Some clinicians select and treat those individuals thought to be at greatest risk for developing glaucoma after assessing all risk factors.

The OHTS identified elevated IOP, reduced CCT, and increased cup–disc ratio as important risk factors for the development of glaucoma in patients with ocular hypertension. The OHTS included patients with IOP between 24 and 32 mm Hg and randomized patients to observation or to the reduction of IOP by topical medications (Fig 4-1). In OHTS, 4.4% of patients treated (with topical antiglaucoma medications to reduce IOP 20%) progressed to glaucoma during a 5-year period, based on the development of optic nerve or visual field damage. More than twice as many of the untreated observation group, 9.5%, progressed. Thus, topical medications were definitively shown to reduce the risk of glaucoma in patients with OHT; however, most untreated patients did not get worse over a 5-year period. Each millimeter of elevated baseline IOP increased the risk of glaucomatous change by 10%. For each 0.1 increment in vertical cup–disc ratio, the risk was increased by 32%.

CCT has been recognized to affect the IOP measurement, probably because a thicker cornea resists indentation by applanation, resulting in a higher measured IOP. However, the increase in risk of progression to glaucoma was not fully explained in OHTS by the anticipated artifactual change in measured IOP from differences in CCT. Other potential risk factors such as myopia, diabetes mellitus, family history, migraine, and high or low blood pressure were not confirmed in this study to be significant risk factors in the univariate or multivariate analysis. As mentioned previously, black race was found to increase the risk of developing glaucoma in the univariate but not in the multivariate analysis, apparently as a result of the thinner average corneal thickness and greater baseline vertical cup–disc ratio in this population.

The clinician must weigh all available data in assessing the patient's risk for developing glaucoma and deciding whether to treat elevated IOP. The following risk factors should be considered:

- level of IOP
- CCT (corneal pachymetry)
- cup–disc ratio
- family history of glaucoma
- race
- age
- associated disease states (diabetes mellitus, systemic hypertension, and cardiovascular disease)

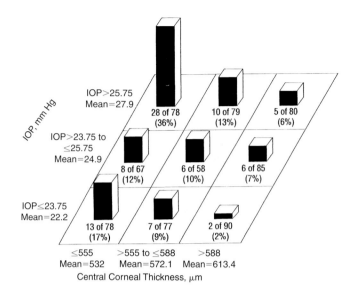

Figure 4-1 The percentage of participants in the observation group who developed POAG (median follow-up, 72 months) grouped by baseline intraocular pressure (IOP) of ≤23.75 mm Hg, >23.75 mm Hg to ≤25.75 mm Hg, and >25.75 mm Hg and by central corneal thickness measurements of ≤555 μm, >555 μm to ≤588 μm, and >588 μm. These percentages are not adjusted for length of follow-up. The means are not identical to those given in the text, which includes all participants in the Ocular Hypertension Treatment Study rather than just the observation group. *(From Wilson RM, Brandt JD, Update on glaucoma clinical trials.* Focal Points: Clinical Modules for Ophthalmologists. *San Francisco: American Academy of Ophthalmology; 2003, module 9. Reprinted with permission from Gordon MO, Beiser JA, Brandt JD, et al. The Ocular Hypertension Treatment Study: baseline factors that predict the onset of primary open-angle glaucoma.* Arch Ophthalmol. *2002;120:718:Fig 1. Copyrighted 2002, American Medical Association.)*

Based on the findings of the examination and the results of the OHTS study, an assessment of the patient's risk of developing glaucoma can be derived. The clinician and the patient can together decide if this risk warrants the inconvenience, cost, and potential side effects of therapy. Care must be taken that the risks and morbidity of therapy do not exceed the risks of the disease. Additional factors that may affect the decision to start ocular antihypertensive therapy include the desires of the patient, patient compliance and availability for follow-up visits, reliability of visual fields, and ability to examine the optic disc.

Gordon MO, Beiser JA, Brandt JD, et al. The Ocular Hypertension Treatment Study: baseline factors that predict the onset of primary open-angle glaucoma. *Arch Ophthalmol.* 2002;120:714–720.

Kass MA, Heuer DK, Higginbotham EJ, et al. The Ocular Hypertension Treatment Study: a randomized trial determines that topical ocular hypotensive medication delays or prevents the onset of primary open-angle glaucoma. *Arch Ophthalmol.* 2002;120:701–713.

Preferred Practice Patterns Committee, Glaucoma Panel. *Primary Open-Angle Glaucoma Suspect.* San Francisco: American Academy of Ophthalmology; 2002.

Wilson MR, Brandt JD. Update on glaucoma clinical trials. *Focal Points: Clinical Modules for Ophthalmologists.* American Academy of Ophthalmology; 2003, module 9.

Secondary Open-Angle Glaucoma

Exfoliation Syndrome

Exfoliation syndrome (pseudoexfoliation) is characterized by the deposition of a distinctive fibrillar material in the anterior segment of the eye. Histologically, this material has been found in and on the lens epithelium and capsule, pupillary margin, ciliary epithelium, iris pigment epithelium, iris stroma, iris blood vessels, and subconjunctival tissue. The material has also been identified in other parts of the body. Although its origin is not known precisely, the material probably arises from multiple sources as part of a generalized basement membrane disorder. Histochemically, the material resembles elastic microfibrils and other extracellular matrix components.

Deposits occur in a targetlike pattern on the anterior lens capsule and are best seen after pupil dilation. A central area and a peripheral zone of deposition are usually separated by an intermediate clear area, where iris movement presumably rubs the material from the lens (Fig 4-2). The material is often visible on the iris at the edge of the pupil. Deposits also occur on the zonular fibers of the lens, ciliary processes, inferior anterior chamber angle, and corneal endothelium (Fig 4-3). In aphakic individuals, these deposits may be seen on the anterior hyaloid as well.

The chamber angle is often characterized by a trabecular meshwork that is heavily pigmented with brown pigment, usually in a variegated fashion. An inferior pigmented deposition, scalloped in nature, is often present anterior to the Schwalbe line. This

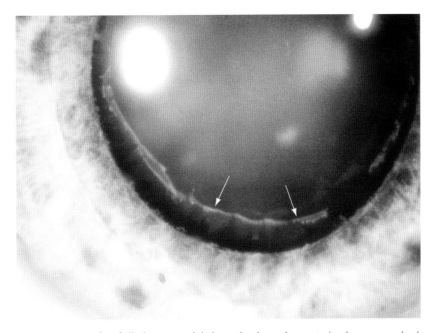

Figure 4-2 Evidence of exfoliative material deposited on the anterior lens capsule *(arrows)*. Exfoliative material may also be deposited on other structures within the anterior segment, including the iris, ciliary processes, peripheral retina, and the conjunctiva.

pigmented line is often referred to as the *Sampaolesi line* (Fig 4-4). The chamber angle is often narrow, presumably as a result of anterior movement of the lens–iris diaphragm related to zonular weakness.

In addition to the typical deposits and pigmentation, other anterior segment abnormalities are noted. Fine pigment deposits often appear on the iris surface, and peripupillary atrophy with transillumination of the pupillary margin is common. A more scattered, diffuse depigmentation may also occur, with transillumination defects over the entire sphincter region. The pupil often dilates poorly. Phacodonesis and iridodonesis are not uncommon; they are related to zonular weakness, which may predispose affected eyes to zonular dehiscence; vitreous loss; and other complications, including lens dislocation, during and after cataract surgery (see also BCSC Section 11, *Lens and Cataract*). Iris angiography has demonstrated abnormalities of the iris vessels with fluorescein leakage.

Exfoliation syndrome may be monocular or binocular with varying degrees of asymmetry. Often the disorder is clinically apparent in only 1 eye, although the uninvolved fellow eye often develops the syndrome at a later time. Exfoliation syndrome is associated with open-angle glaucoma in all populations, but the prevalence varies considerably. In Scandinavian countries, exfoliation syndrome accounts for more than 50% of cases of open-angle glaucoma. The odds of the exfoliation syndrome leading to glaucoma vary widely, and range up to 40% over a 10-year period. This syndrome is strongly age-related: it is rarely seen in persons younger than 50 years and occurs most commonly in individuals older than 70 years.

The open-angle glaucoma associated with exfoliation syndrome is thought to be caused by the fibrillar material obstructing flow through, and causing damage to, the trabecular meshwork. Exfoliation glaucoma differs from POAG in often presenting monocularly and showing greater pigmentation of the trabecular meshwork. Furthermore, the IOP is often higher, with greater diurnal fluctuations than in POAG, and the overall prognosis is worse. Laser trabeculoplasty can be very effective, but the response may not last as long as with POAG. Lens extraction does not alleviate the condition. Trabeculectomy results are similar to those with POAG, but there may be an increase in postoperative inflammation. In fact, increased ocular inflammation can be seen following all ocular surgery in patients with this condition.

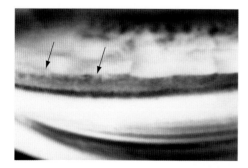

Figure 4-3 Exfoliative debris *(arrows)* collecting on iris processes in inferior anterior chamber angle. *(Courtesy of Steven T. Simmons, MD.)*

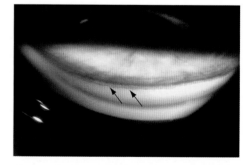

Figure 4-4 The Sampaolesi line *(arrows)* in the inferior anterior chamber angle of a patient who has exfoliation syndrome. *(Courtesy of L. J. Katz, MD.)*

Ritch R. Perspective on exfoliation syndrome. *J Glaucoma.* 2001;10(Suppl 1):S33–S35.

Ritch R. Exfoliation syndrome. In: Ritch R, Shields MB, Krupin T, eds. *The Glaucomas.* 2nd ed. St Louis: Mosby; 1996:chap 47, pp 993–1022.

Schlötzer-Schrehardt U, Naumann GO. Ocular and systemic pseudoexfoliation syndrome. *Am J Ophthalmol.* 2006;141(5):921–937.

Zenkel M, Poschl E, von der Mark K, et al. Differential gene expression in pseudoexfoliation syndrome. *Invest Ophthalmol Vis Sci.* 2005;46:3742–3752.

Pigmentary Glaucoma

The *pigment dispersion syndrome* consists of pigment deposition on the corneal endothelium in a vertical spindle pattern (Krukenberg spindle; Fig 4-5), in the trabecular meshwork, and on the lens periphery, and, typically, midperipheral iris transillumination defects. The spindle pattern on the posterior cornea is caused by the aqueous convection currents and subsequent phagocytosis of pigment by the corneal endothelium. The presence of Krukenberg spindles is not absolutely necessary to make the diagnosis of pigment dispersion syndrome, and it may occur in other diseases such as exfoliation syndrome. Characteristic spokelike loss of the iris pigment epithelium occurs that is manifested as transillumination defects in the iris midperiphery (Fig 4-6). The peripheral iris transillumination defects appear in front of the lens zonular fibers, suggesting that mechanical contact between the zonular fibers and the iris causes the iris pigment release.

Gonioscopy reveals a homogeneous, densely pigmented trabecular meshwork with speckled pigment at or anterior to the Schwalbe line (Fig 4-7), often forming a Sampaolesi line. The midperipheral iris is often concave in appearance, bowing posterior toward the zonular fibers. When the eye is dilated, pigment deposits can be seen on the zonular fibers, the anterior hyaloid, and the lens capsule near the equator of the lens (Zentmayer line; Fig 4-8).

This syndrome does not universally lead to glaucoma. An individual with pigment dispersion syndrome may never develop elevated IOP, and various studies have suggested that the risk of an affected individual developing glaucoma is approximately 25%–50%. Pigmentary glaucoma occurs most commonly in white males who have myopia and who are between the ages of 20 and 50 years. Affected females tend to be older than affected males.

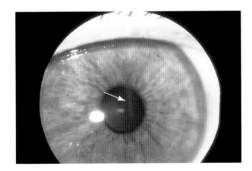

Figure 4-5 Krukenberg spindle *(arrow). (Courtesy of L. J. Katz, MD.)*

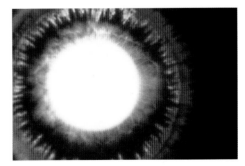

Figure 4-6 Classic spokelike iris transillumination defects seen in pigment dispersion syndrome. *(Courtesy of L. J. Katz, MD.)*

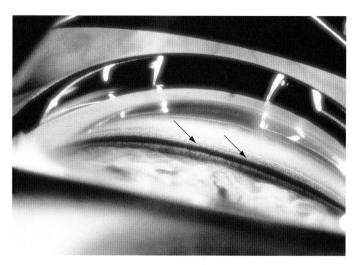

Figure 4-7 Characteristic heavy, uniform pigmentation of the trabecular meshwork *(arrows)* seen in the pigment dispersion syndrome and pigmentary glaucoma. *(Courtesy of M. Roy Wilson, MD.)*

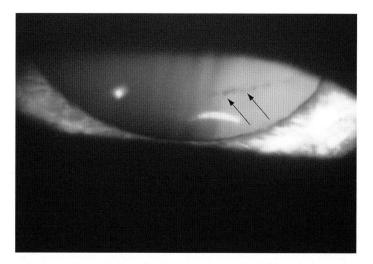

Figure 4-8 In pigment dispersion syndrome, pigment deposits can be seen on the anterior hyaloid (Zentmayer line), the posterior lens capsule *(arrows),* and the lens zonules, on gonioscopy in the dilated eye. *(Courtesy of Steven T. Simmons, MD.)*

Pigmentary glaucoma is characterized by wide fluctuations in IOP, which can exceed 50 mm Hg in untreated eyes. High IOP often occurs when pigment is released into the aqueous humor, such as following exercise or pupillary dilation. Symptoms may include halos, intermittent visual blurring, and ocular pain.

Posterior bowing of the iris with "reverse pupillary block" configuration is noted in many eyes that have pigmentary glaucoma. This iris configuration may result in greater contact of the zonular fibers with the posterior iris surface, with a subsequent increase of pigment release. Laser iridectomy has been proposed as a means of minimizing posterior bowing of the iris (Fig 4-9). However, its effectiveness in treating pigmentary glaucoma has not been established.

With age, the signs and symptoms of pigment dispersion may decrease in some individuals, possibly as a result of normal growth of the lens and an increase in physiologic pupillary block, moving the iris forward, away from contact with the zonular fibers. Loss of accommodation may also be a factor. As pigment dispersion is reduced, the deposited pigment may fade from the trabecular meshwork, anterior iris surface, and corneal endothelium. Transillumination defects may also gradually disappear.

Medical treatment is often successful in reducing IOP. Patients respond reasonably well to laser trabeculoplasty, although the effect may be short-lived. The heavy trabecular pigmentation allows increased absorption of laser energy, in turn allowing lower energy levels for trabeculoplasty. Spikes in IOP may be seen more frequently with higher energy settings in pigment dispersion syndrome following laser trabeculoplasty. Filtering surgery is usually successful; however, extra care is warranted, because young patients with myopia may be at increased risk of hypotony maculopathy.

Liebmann JM. Pigmentary glaucoma: new insights. *Focal Points: Clinical Modules for Ophthalmologists.* San Francisco: American Academy of Ophthalmology; 1998, module 2.

Reistad CE, Shields MB, Campbell DG, Ritch R, Wang JC, Wand M; American Glaucoma Society Pigmentary Glaucoma Iridotomy Study Group. The influence of peripheral iridotomy on the intraocular pressure course in patients with pigmentary glaucoma. *J Glaucoma.* 2005;14:255–259.

Yang JW, Sakiyalak D, Krupin T. Pigmentary glaucoma. *J Glaucoma.* 2001;10(5 Suppl 1): S30–S32.

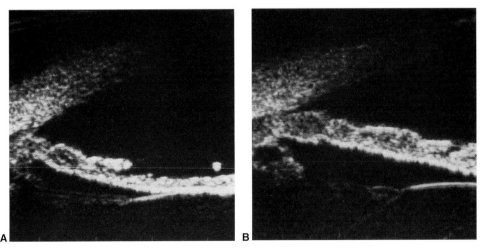

Figure 4-9   A, Ultrasound biomicroscopy image of concave iris configuration in pigmentary glaucoma, pre–laser treatment. **B,** Same eye, post–laser treatment. *(Courtesy of Charles J. Pavlin, MD.)*

Lens-Induced Glaucoma

The lens may cause both open-angle and angle-closure glaucomas, and these are summarized in Table 4-4. The open-angle, lens-induced glaucomas are divided into 3 clinical entities:

- phacolytic glaucoma
- lens particle glaucoma
- phacoantigenic glaucoma

See also BCSC Section 9, *Intraocular Inflammation and Uveitis,* and Section 11, *Lens and Cataract.*

Phacolytic glaucoma

Phacolytic glaucoma is an inflammatory glaucoma caused by the leakage of lens protein through the capsule of a mature or hypermature cataract (Fig 4-10). As the lens ages, its protein composition becomes altered, with an increased concentration of high-molecular-weight lens protein. In a mature or hypermature cataract, these proteins are released through microscopic openings in the lens capsule. The proteins precipitate a secondary glaucoma as these lens proteins, phagocytizing macrophages, and other inflammatory debris obstruct the trabecular meshwork.

The clinical picture usually involves an elderly patient with a history of poor vision who has sudden onset of pain, conjunctival hyperemia, and worsening vision. Examination reveals a markedly elevated IOP, microcystic corneal edema, prominent cell and flare reaction without keratic precipitates (KP), and an open anterior chamber angle (Fig 4-11). The lack of KP helps distinguish phacolytic glaucoma from phacoantigenic glaucoma. Cellular debris may be seen layering in the anterior chamber angle, and a pseudohypopyon may be present. Large white particles (clumps of lens protein) may also be seen in the anterior chamber. A mature or hypermature (morgagnian) cataract is present, often

Table 4-4 Lens-Induced Glaucomas

Open-angle	Angle-closure (see Chapter 5)
Phacolytic glaucoma	Phacomorphic glaucoma
Lens particle glaucoma	Ectopia lentis
Phacoantigenic glaucoma	

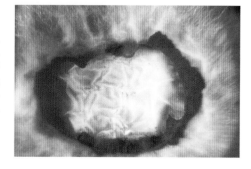

Figure 4-10 Characteristic appearance of hypermature cataract with wrinkling of the anterior lens capsule, which results from loss of cortical volume. Extensive posterior synechiae are present, confirming the presence of previous inflammation. *(Courtesy of Steven T. Simmons, MD.)*

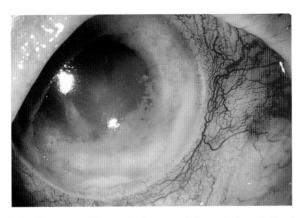

Figure 4-11 Phacolytic glaucoma. The typical presentation of phacolytic glaucoma is conjunctival hyperemia, microcystic corneal edema, mature cataract, and prominent anterior chamber reaction, as demonstrated in this photograph. Note lens protein deposits on endothelium and layering in the angle, creating a pseudohypopyon. *(Courtesy of George A. Cioffi, MD.)*

with wrinkling of the anterior lens capsule representing loss of volume and the release of lens material (see Fig 4-10). Although medications to control the IOP should be used immediately, definitive therapy requires cataract extraction.

Lens particle glaucoma

Lens particle glaucoma occurs when lens cortex particles obstruct the trabecular meshwork following cataract extraction, capsulotomy, or ocular trauma. The extent of the glaucoma depends on the quantity of lens material released, the degree of inflammation, the ability of the trabecular meshwork to clear the lens material, and the functional status of the ciliary body, which is often altered following surgery or trauma.

Lens particle glaucoma usually occurs within weeks of the initial surgery or trauma, but it may occur months or years later (Fig 4-12). Clinical findings include free cortical material in the anterior chamber, elevated IOP, moderate anterior chamber reaction, microcystic corneal edema, and, with time, the development of posterior synechiae and peripheral anterior synechiae.

If possible, medical therapy should be initiated to control the IOP while the residual lens material resorbs. Appropriate therapy includes medications to decrease aqueous formation, mydriatics to inhibit posterior synechiae formation, and topical corticosteroids to

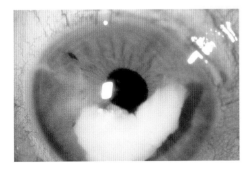

Figure 4-12 Lens particle glaucoma. Despite the large amount of lens cortex remaining in the anterior chamber following cataract surgery, this eye is relatively quiet; the IOP remained normal. *(Courtesy of the Wills Eye Hospital slide collection, 1986.)*

reduce inflammation. If the glaucoma cannot be controlled, surgical removal of the lens material is necessary.

Phacoantigenic glaucoma

Phacoantigenic glaucoma (previously known as *phacoanaphylaxis*) is a rare entity in which patients become sensitized to their own lens protein following surgery or penetrating trauma, resulting in a granulomatous inflammation. The clinical picture is quite variable, but most patients present with a moderate anterior chamber reaction with KP on both the corneal endothelium and the anterior lens surface. In addition, a low-grade vitritis, synechial formation, and residual lens material in the anterior chamber may be found. Glaucomatous optic neuropathy, although it may occur, is not common in eyes with phacoantigenic glaucoma. Phacoantigenic glaucoma is treated medically with corticosteroids and aqueous suppressants, which are used to reduce inflammation and IOP. If medical treatment is unsuccessful, residual lens material should be removed.

Intraocular Tumors

A variety of tumors can cause unilateral chronic glaucoma. Many of the tumors described in this section are discussed in greater detail in BCSC Section 4, *Ophthalmic Pathology and Intraocular Tumors*. The glaucoma can result from several different mechanisms, depending on the size, type, and location of the tumor:

- direct tumor invasion of the anterior chamber angle
- angle closure by rotation of the ciliary body or by anterior displacement of the lens–iris diaphragm (see Chapter 5)
- intraocular hemorrhage
- neovascularization of the angle
- deposition of tumor cells, inflammatory cells, and cellular debris within the trabecular meshwork

Choroidal melanomas and other choroidal and retinal tumors tend to cause secondary angle-closure glaucoma as the result of a forward shift in the lens–iris diaphragm and closure of the anterior chamber angle. Inflammation caused by necrotic tumors may cause posterior synechiae, which can exacerbate this angle closure through a pupillary block mechanism. Choroidal melanomas, medulloepitheliomas, and retinoblastomas can also cause anterior segment neovascularization, which can result in angle closure.

The most common cause of glaucoma in primary or metastatic tumors of the ciliary body is direct invasion of the anterior chamber angle. This glaucoma can be exacerbated by anterior segment hemorrhage and inflammation, which further obstruct outflow. Necrotic tumor and tumor-filled macrophages may cause obstruction of the trabecular meshwork and result in a secondary open-angle glaucoma. Tumors causing glaucoma in adults include uveal melanoma, metastatic carcinoma, lymphomas, and leukemia. Glaucoma in children is associated with retinoblastoma, juvenile xanthogranuloma, and medulloepithelioma.

Grostern RJ, Brown SVL. Glaucoma associated with intraocular tumors. In: Higginbotham E, Lee D, eds. *Management of Difficult Glaucomas*. Boston: Butterworth Heinemann; 2004:343–351.

Shields CL, Materin MA, Shields JA, Gershenbaum E, Singh AD, Smith A. Factors associated with elevated intraocular pressure in eyes with iris melanoma. *Br J Ophthalmol*. 2001;85:666–669.

Ocular Inflammation and Secondary Open-Angle Glaucoma

Inflammatory glaucoma is a secondary glaucoma that often combines components of open-angle and angle-closure disease. In uveitis, elevated IOP occurs when the trabecular dysfunction exceeds the ciliary body hyposecretion seen with acute inflammation. Often the ocular inflammation is nonspecific. When the inflammation is accompanied by increased IOP, the physician's dilemma is whether the cause of the increased IOP is the active inflammation and insufficient anti-inflammatory therapy, chronic structural damage related to the underlying inflammation, or corticosteroid therapy.

Open-angle inflammatory glaucoma may be caused by a variety of mechanisms:

- edema of the trabecular meshwork
- trabecular meshwork endothelial cell dysfunction
- blockage of the trabecular meshwork by fibrin and inflammatory cells
- prostaglandin-mediated breakdown of the blood–aqueous barrier
- blockage of Schlemm's canal by inflammatory cells
- steroid-induced reduction in aqueous outflow through the trabecular meshwork

Most cases of anterior uveitis are idiopathic, but uveitides commonly associated with open-angle inflammatory glaucoma include herpes zoster iridocyclitis, herpes simplex keratouveitis, toxoplasmosis, rheumatoid arthritis, and pars planitis. See also BCSC Section 9, *Intraocular Inflammation and Uveitis*.

The presence of KP suggests iritis as the cause of IOP elevation. Gonioscopic evaluation may reveal subtle trabecular meshwork precipitates. Sometimes, peripheral anterior synechiae (PAS) or posterior synechiae with iris bombé may develop, resulting in angle closure. The treatment of inflammatory glaucoma is complicated by the fact that corticosteroid therapy may increase IOP, either by reducing inflammation and improving aqueous production or by decreasing outflow. Miotic agents should be avoided in patients with iritis, because they may aggravate the inflammation and cause posterior synechiae. Prostaglandin analogs may exacerbate inflammation in poorly controlled uveitis and herpetic keratitis. In uveitic glaucomas, inadequately controlled inflammation with elevated IOP is often mistaken for steroid-induced glaucoma. In the face of active inflammation, elevated IOP should be presumed to be inflammation-related rather than steroid-induced.

Glaucomatocyclitic crisis

Glaucomatocyclitic crisis (Posner-Schlossman syndrome), an uncommon form of open-angle inflammatory glaucoma, is characterized by recurrent bouts of markedly increased IOP and low-grade anterior chamber inflammation. First described by Posner and Schlossman in 1948, the condition most frequently affects middle-aged patients and usually presents with unilateral blurred vision and mild eye pain. The iritis is mild, with few KP that are small, discrete, and round in nature and that usually resolve spontaneously within a few weeks. KP may be seen on the trabecular meshwork on gonioscopy, suggesting a "trabeculitis." The IOP is usually markedly elevated, in the 40–50 mm Hg range, and corneal edema may be present. In between bouts, the IOP usually returns to normal, but, with increasing numbers of attacks, a chronic secondary glaucoma may develop, resulting in visual loss. The etiology of the disease remains unknown. There is no evidence that chronic suppressive therapy with topical nonsteroidal anti-inflammatory agents or mild steroids is effective in preventing attacks. Recurrent attacks of acute angle-closure glaucoma have been mistaken for this condition.

Fuchs heterochromic iridocyclitis

Fuchs heterochromic iridocyclitis, a relatively rare, chronic form of iridocyclitis, is characterized by iris heterochromia with loss of iris pigment in the affected eye; low-grade anterior chamber reaction with small, stellate KP; posterior subcapsular cataracts; and secondary open-angle glaucoma. The condition is insidious and unilateral, affecting the hypochromic eye, and presents equally in middle-aged men and women. The secondary open-angle glaucoma occurs in approximately 15% of the cases. Gonioscopy reveals multiple fine vessels that cross the trabecular meshwork (Fig 4-13). These vessels, unlike those in iris neovascularization, do not appear to be associated with a fibrous membrane and usually do not lead to PAS and secondary angle closure, although in rare cases the neovascularization may be progressive. These vessels are fragile and may cause an anterior chamber hemorrhage, either spontaneously or with trauma, including cataract or glaucoma surgery.

The glaucoma does not correspond to the degree of inflammation and may be difficult to control. Corticosteroids are generally not effective in treating this condition. Medical therapy starts with aqueous suppressants, which are often effective in controlling IOP.

Elevated Episcleral Venous Pressure

Episcleral venous pressure is an important factor in the regulation of IOP. Normal episcleral venous pressure is 8–10 mm Hg, but it can be raised by a variety of clinical entities that either obstruct venous outflow or involve arteriovenous malformations. A partial list of entities that increase episcleral venous pressure is presented in Table 4-5.

Patients may note a chronic red eye without discomfort or allergic symptoms. Occasionally, a distant history of significant head trauma may suggest the cause of a carotid-cavernous sinus or dural fistula. However, most cases are idiopathic, often without angiographic abnormalities, and may be familial. Clinically, patients with increased epi-

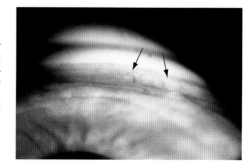

Figure 4-13 Fuchs heterochromic iridocyclitis. Fine vessels *(arrows)* are seen crossing the trabecular meshwork. This neovascularization is not accompanied by a fibrovascular membrane and does not result in peripheral anterior synechiae formation and secondary angle closure. *(Courtesy of Steven T. Simmons, MD.)*

Table 4-5 Causes of Increased Episcleral Pressure

> **Arteriovenous malformations**
> Arteriovenous fistula
> > Dural
> > Carotid-cavernous sinus
> Orbital varix
> Sturge-Weber syndrome
> **Venous obstruction**
> Retrobulbar tumor
> Thyroid-associated orbitopathy
> **Superior vena cava syndrome**
> **Idiopathic (familial)**

scleral venous pressure present with tortuous, dilated episcleral veins (Fig 4-14). These vascular changes may be unilateral or bilateral depending on the location of the vascular anomaly. The anterior segment appears normal in most of these patients, except for elevated IOP and often the gonioscopic finding of blood in Schlemm's canal. Rarely, signs of ocular ischemia or venous stasis may be present. Sudden, severe carotid-cavernous fistulas may be accompanied by proptosis and other orbital or neurologic signs. These cases may require neuroradiologic intervention.

Medications that reduce aqueous humor formation are more effective than drugs that increase trabecular aqueous outflow. Prostaglandin analogs may be effective in some patients. Laser trabeculoplasty is not effective unless there are secondary changes in the outflow channels. Glaucoma filtering surgery may be complicated by a ciliochoroidal effusion or a suprachoroidal hemorrhage.

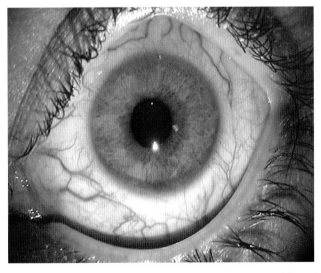

Figure 4-14 Prominent episcleral vessels are seen in a patient with idiopathic elevated episcleral venous pressure. *(Courtesy of Keith Barton, MD.)*

Accidental and Surgical Trauma

Nonpenetrating, or blunt, trauma to the eye causes a variety of anterior segment injuries:

- hyphema
- angle recession (cleavage)
- iridodialysis
- iris sphincter tear
- cyclodialysis
- lens subluxation

A combination of posttraumatic inflammation, presence of blood and red blood cells (RBCs), and direct injury to the trabecular meshwork often results in elevated IOP initially after trauma. This elevation tends to be short in duration but may be protracted, with the risk of corneal blood staining (Fig 4-15) and glaucomatous optic nerve damage.

Open-angle glaucoma is one of the long-term sequelae of *siderosis* or *chalcosis* from a retained intraocular metallic foreign body in penetrating or perforating injuries. Chemical injuries, particularly alkali, may cause acute secondary glaucoma as a result of inflammation, shrinkage of scleral collagen, release of chemical mediators such as prostaglandins, direct damage to the chamber angle, or compromise of the anterior uveal circulation. Trabecular damage or inflammation may cause glaucoma to develop months or years after a chemical injury.

Hyphema

Glaucoma may result from hyphema through several mechanisms (Fig 4-16). Increased IOP is more common following recurrent hemorrhage or rebleeding following a traumatic hyphema. The reported frequency of rebleeding following hyphema varies considerably in the literature, probably because of differences in study populations, with an average incidence of 5%–10%. Rebleeding usually occurs within 3–7 days of the initial hyphema and

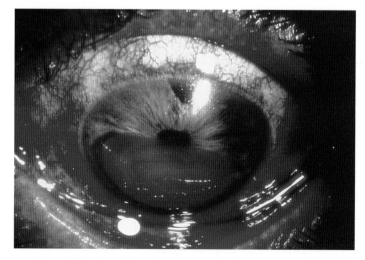

Figure 4-15 Corneal blood staining following trauma. *(Courtesy of Steven T. Simmons, MD.)*

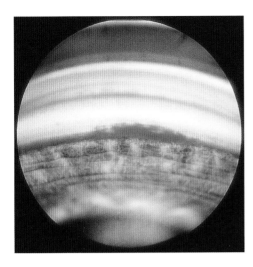

Figure 4-16 A small hyphema seen gonio-scopically in the inferior chamber angle with layering of blood on the trabecular meshwork. *(Courtesy of Steven T. Simmons, MD.)*

may be related to normal clot retraction and lysis. In general, the larger the hyphema, the higher the incidence of increased IOP, although small hemorrhages may also be associated with marked elevation of IOP, especially in the already compromised angle. Increased IOP is a result of obstruction of the trabecular meshwork with RBCs, inflammatory cells, debris, and fibrin, and of direct injury to the trabecular meshwork from the blunt trauma.

Individuals with sickle cell hemoglobinopathies have an increased incidence of elevated IOP following hyphema and are more susceptible to complications from hyphema, including optic neuropathy. Normal RBCs generally pass through the trabecular meshwork without difficulty. However, in the sickle cell hemoglobinopathies (including sickle trait), the RBCs tend to sickle in the anterior chamber, because of the acidity of the stagnant aqueous humor. These more rigid cells have great difficulty passing out of the eye through the trabecular meshwork. Even small amounts of blood in the anterior chamber may therefore result in marked elevations of IOP. In addition, the optic nerves of patients with sickle cell disease are much more sensitive to elevated IOP and are prone to ischemic injuries, such as anterior ischemic optic neuropathy and central retinal artery occlusion, as a result of compromised microvascular perfusion.

In general, the patient with an uncomplicated hyphema should be managed conservatively, with an eye shield, limited activity, and head elevation. Topical and systemic corticosteroids may reduce associated inflammation, although their effect on rebleeding is debatable. If significant ciliary spasm or photophobia occurs, cycloplegic agents may be helpful, but they have no proven benefit for prevention of rebleeding. Systemic administration of aminocaproic acid has been shown to reduce rebleeding in some studies. However, this has not been confirmed in all studies, and systemic adverse effects, such as hypotension, syncope, abdominal pain, and nausea, can be significant and limit the use of aminocaproic acid. Also, discontinuation of aminocaproic acid may be associated with clot lysis and with additional IOP elevation. Patching and bed rest are advocated by some authors, although these precautions are of unproven value.

If the IOP is elevated, aqueous suppressants and hyperosmotic agents are recommended. It has been suggested that patients with sickle cell hemoglobinopathies avoid carbonic anhydrase inhibitors, because these agents may increase the sickling tendency in the anterior chamber by increasing aqueous acidity; however, this relationship has not been firmly established. Physicians should be aware of the potential of systemic carbonic anhydrase inhibitors and hyperosmotic agents to induce sickle crises in susceptible individuals who are significantly dehydrated. Both drugs may enhance sickling, as each may exacerbate dehydration. Adrenergic agonists with significant α_1-agonist effects (apraclonidine, dipivefrin, epinephrine) should also be avoided in sickle cell disease because of concerns regarding anterior segment vasoconstriction. Parasympathomimetic agents should be avoided in all patients with hyphemas.

Clinicians should have a lower threshold for surgical intervention in sickle cell patients, given the increased risk of complications from elevated IOP. If the hyphema or corneal staining significantly obstructs vision, amblyopia could result. The possibility of amblyopia may justify early surgical intervention in very young children. If surgery for increased IOP becomes necessary, an anterior chamber irrigation or washout procedure is commonly performed first. If a total hyphema is present, pupillary block may occur, and an iridectomy is helpful at the time of the washout. If the IOP remains uncontrolled, a trabeculectomy may be required. Some surgeons prefer to perform a trabeculectomy as the initial surgical procedure with the anterior chamber washout in order to obtain immediate control of IOP and relief of any pupillary block.

Campagna JA. Traumatic hyphema: current strategies. *Focal Points: Clinical Modules for Ophthalmologists.* San Francisco: American Academy of Ophthalmology; 2007, module 10.

Hemolytic and ghost cell glaucoma

Hemolytic and/or ghost cell glaucoma may develop after a vitreous hemorrhage. In *hemolytic glaucoma,* hemoglobin-laden macrophages block the trabecular outflow channels. Red-tinged cells are seen floating in the anterior chamber, and a reddish brown discoloration of the trabecular meshwork is often present.

Ghost cell glaucoma is a secondary open-angle glaucoma caused by degenerated RBCs (ghost cells) blocking the trabecular meshwork. Ghost cells are RBCs that have lost their intracellular hemoglobin and appear as small, khaki-colored cells. They are less pliable than normal RBCs (Fig 4-17). As a result of their loss of pliability, ghost cells remain longer in the anterior chamber, causing obstruction of the trabecular meshwork and secondary glaucoma. The cells develop within 1–3 months of a vitreous hemorrhage. They gain access to the anterior chamber through a disrupted hyaloid face, which can occur from previous surgery (pars plana vitrectomy, cataract extraction, or capsulotomy), trauma, or spontaneous disruption.

Clinically, patients present with increased IOP and a history of vitreous hemorrhage resulting from trauma, surgery, or preexisting retinal disease. The IOP may be markedly elevated, causing corneal edema. The anterior chamber is filled with small, circulating, tan-colored cells (see Fig 4-17). The cellular reaction appears out of proportion to the aqueous flare, and the conjunctiva tends not to be inflamed unless the IOP is markedly elevated. On gonioscopy, the angle appears normal except for the layering of ghost cells over the trabecular meshwork inferiorly. The vitreous has the appearance of an old hemorrhage, with characteristic khaki coloration and clumps of extracellular pigmentation from degenerated hemoglobin.

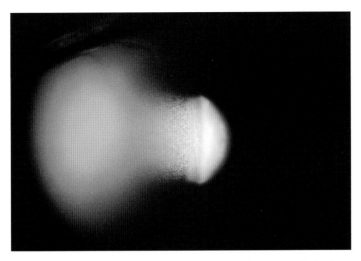

Figure 4-17 Ghost cell glaucoma: the classic appearance of ghost cells in the anterior chamber. These khaki-colored cells are small and can become layered, as is seen in a hyphema and hypopyon. *(Courtesy of Ron Gross, MD.)*

Both hemolytic and ghost cell glaucoma generally resolve once the hemorrhage has cleared. Medical therapy with aqueous suppressants is the preferred initial approach. If medical therapy fails to control marked elevations of IOP, some patients may require irrigation of the anterior chamber, pars plana vitrectomy, and/or a trabeculectomy to control the condition. When a collection of RBCs or ghost cells is present in the vitreous, a pars plana vitrectomy is usually required for effective treatment of elevated IOP.

Traumatic, or angle-recession, glaucoma

An angle recession, or cleavage, is due to a tear in the ciliary body, usually between the longitudinal and circular muscle fibers. Angle recessions are often associated with injury to the trabecular meshwork as well. Angle-recession glaucoma is a chronic, unilateral secondary open-angle glaucoma that may occur soon after ocular trauma or may develop months to years later. It resembles POAG in presentation and clinical course but can usually be distinguished by its classic gonioscopic findings (Figs 4-18, 4-19):

- brown-colored, broad angle recess
- absent or torn iris processes
- white, glistening scleral spur
- depression in the overlying trabecular meshwork
- PAS at the border of the recession

The degree of angle involvement and underlying patient predisposition are important factors in determining whether a secondary glaucoma will develop. A significant proportion (up to 50%) of fellow eyes may develop increased IOP, suggesting that perhaps many eyes with angle-recession glaucoma may have been predisposed to open-angle glaucoma.

Angle-recession glaucoma should be considered in a patient presenting with unilateral elevation in IOP. The patient's history may reveal the contributing incident; however,

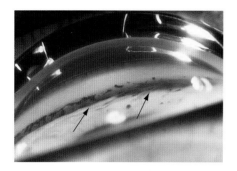

Figure 4-18 An angle recession occurs when the ciliary body is torn, usually between the longitudinal and circular fibers of the ciliary body. There is a deepened angle recess as a result of a tear in the ciliary body *(arrows)*. *(Courtesy of Joseph Krug, MD.)*

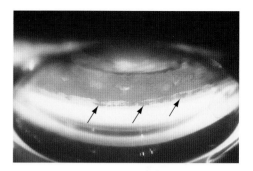

Figure 4-19 Typical angle appearance of an angle recession. Torn iris processes *(arrows)*; a whitened, increasingly visible scleral spur; and a localized depression in the trabecular meshwork are seen. *(Courtesy of Steven T. Simmons, MD.)*

often this has been forgotten. Careful examination may show findings consistent with previous trauma, such as corneal scars, tears in the pupil margin, changes in the angle as above, focal anterior subcapsular cataracts, and a loose or subluxated lens. The clinician may compare gonioscopic findings in the affected eye with findings in the fellow eye to help identify areas of recession.

A greater extent of angle recession is associated with a greater risk of glaucoma. Even with substantial angle recession, this risk is not high, but all eyes with angle recession must be followed because it is not possible to predict which eyes will develop glaucoma. Although the risk of developing glaucoma decreases appreciably after several years, the risk is still present even 25 years or more following injury, and these eyes should continue to be examined annually.

The treatment of angle-recession glaucoma is often initiated with aqueous suppressants, prostaglandin analogs, and α_2-adrenergic agonists. Miotics may be useful, but paradoxical responses with increased IOP may occur. Laser trabeculoplasty has a limited role and a reduced chance of success. Trabeculectomy may be required to control the IOP in patients not responding to medical therapy.

Surgical trauma

Operative procedures such as cataract extraction, filtering surgery, or corneal transplantation may be followed by an increase in IOP. Similarly, laser surgery—including trabeculoplasty, iridectomy, and posterior capsulotomy—may be complicated by posttreatment IOP elevation. Although the IOP may rise as high as 50 mm Hg or more, these elevations are usually transient, lasting from a few hours to a few days. The exact mechanism is not always known, but pigment release, presence of inflammatory cells and debris, mechanical deformation of the trabecular meshwork, and angle closure may all be implicated.

In addition, agents used as adjuncts to intraocular surgery may cause secondary IOP elevations. For example, the injection of viscoelastic substances such as sodium hyaluronate into the anterior chamber may result in a transient and possibly severe postoperative increase in IOP. Dispersive viscoelastics (sodium hyaluronate), especially in higher-molecular-weight forms, may be more likely to cause IOP increases than retentive visco-elastic agents (chondroitin sulfate).

Such postoperative pressure elevation can cause considerable damage to the optic nerve of a susceptible individual, even in a short time. Eyes with preexisting glaucoma are at particular risk of further damage. Elevated IOP may increase the risk of retinal and optic nerve ischemia. It is thus important to measure IOP soon after surgery or laser treatment. If a substantial rise in IOP does occur, therapy may be required. Usually, use of β-adrenergic antagonists, α_2-adrenergic agonists, or carbonic anhydrase inhibitors is adequate. However, hyperosmotic agents, and even paracentesis, are sometimes necessary. Persistent elevation of IOP may necessitate filtering surgery.

The implantation of an intraocular lens (IOL) can lead to a variety of secondary glaucomas:

- uveitis-glaucoma-hyphema (UGH) syndrome
- secondary pigmentary glaucoma (Fig 4-20)
- pseudophakic pupillary block (see Chapter 5)

Uveitis-glaucoma-hyphema (UGH) syndrome is a form of secondary inflammatory glaucoma caused by chronic irritation that is usually the result of a malpositioned or rotating anterior chamber IOL. Characterized by chronic inflammation, secondary iris neovascularization, and recurrent hyphemas, this condition often results in an intractable form of secondary glaucoma following the chafing of the iris by the IOL or erosion of the lens haptics through the iris or ciliary body. This condition may also occur following implantation of a posterior chamber or suture-fixated IOL. Gonioscopy and ultrasound biomicroscopy (UBM) may be helpful in revealing the IOL's exact relation to the iris and ciliary body. Persistent or recurrent cases often require lens repositioning or lens exchange, which can be technically challenging, because many of these eyes may have synechiae and/or an open posterior capsule. This syndrome may be mimicked in patients with neovascularization of the internal lip of a corneoscleral wound. These patients may have recurrent spontaneous hyphemas, which can lead to elevated IOP. Argon laser ablation of the vessels may successfully resolve these cases.

Jarstad JS, Hardwig PW. Intraocular hemorrhage from wound neovascularization years after anterior segment surgery (Swan syndrome). *Can J Ophthalmol.* 1987;22:271–275.

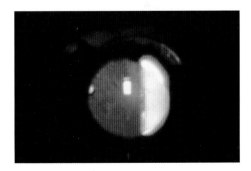

Figure 4-20 Secondary pigmentary glaucoma. Superior iris transillumination is seen in this photograph caused by the underlying optic and haptic of the posterior chamber IOL. The release of iris pigmentation can lead to trabecular meshwork dysfunction and secondary glaucoma. *(Courtesy of Wills Eye Hospital slide collection, 1986.)*

Glaucoma and penetrating keratoplasty

Secondary glaucoma is a common complication of penetrating keratoplasty, and it occurs with increased frequency in the aphakic/pseudophakic patient and with repeat grafts. Wound distortion of the trabecular meshwork and a progressive angle closure are the most common causes of long-standing glaucoma, and attempts to minimize these secondary glaucomas with different-sized donor grafts, peripheral iridectomies, and surgical repair of the iris sphincter have been only partially successful. Alternative procedures, such as lamellar stromal or endothelial grafts, may be associated with a lower percentage of patients having elevated IOP. BCSC Section 8, *External Disease and Cornea,* discusses penetrating keratoplasty in detail.

Schwartz Syndrome (Schwartz-Matsuo Syndrome)

Rhegmatogenous retinal detachments typically lower IOP, presumably as a result of increased outflow by active pumping of fluid through the exposed retinal pigment epithelium. Schwartz first described elevated IOP in association with a rhegmatogenous retinal detachment, and Matsuo later demonstrated photoreceptor outer segments in the aqueous humor in a group of similar patients. The postulated mechanism of IOP elevation is that a chronic rhegmatogenous retinal detachment leads to the liberation of photoreceptor outer segments, which, migrating through the retinal tear, reach the anterior chamber and impede aqueous outflow through the trabecular meshwork. The photoreceptor segments may be mistaken for an anterior chamber inflammatory reaction or pigment. The IOP tends to normalize after successful retinal reattachment.

Drugs and Glaucoma

Corticosteroid-induced glaucoma is an open-angle glaucoma caused by prolonged use of topical, periocular, intravitreal, inhaled, or systemic corticosteroids. It mimics POAG in its presentation and clinical course. Approximately one-third of all patients demonstrate some responsiveness to corticosteroids, but only a small percentage will have a clinically significant elevation in IOP. The type and potency of the agent, the means and frequency of its administration, and the susceptibility of the patient all affect the duration of time before the IOP rises and the extent of this rise. A high percentage of patients with POAG demonstrate this response to topical corticosteroids. Systemic administration of corticosteroids may also raise IOP in some individuals, though less frequently than topical administration. The elevated IOP is a result of an increased resistance to aqueous outflow in the trabecular meshwork. See also BCSC Section 9, *Intraocular Inflammation and Uveitis,* Chapter 6, for a discussion of corticosteroids.

Corticosteroid-induced glaucoma may develop at any time during long-term corticosteroid administration. IOP thus needs to be monitored regularly in patients receiving corticosteroid treatment. Some corticosteroid preparations such as fluorometholone (FML), rimexolone (Vexol), medrysone (HMS), or loteprednol (Lotemax) are less likely to raise IOP than are prednisolone or dexamethasone. However, even weaker corticosteroids or lower concentrations of stronger drugs can raise IOP in susceptible individuals.

A corticosteroid-induced rise in pressure may cause glaucomatous optic nerve damage in some patients. This condition can mimic POAG in patients of any age.

The cause of the elevation in IOP is not always related to the use of a corticosteroid and may be instead related to underlying ocular disease such as anterior uveitis. After use of the corticosteroid is discontinued, the IOP usually decreases with a time course similar to or slightly longer than that of the onset of elevation. However, unmasked POAG or secondary open-angle inflammatory glaucoma may remain.

Patients with excessive levels of endogenous corticosteroids (eg, Cushing syndrome) can also develop increased IOP. When the corticosteroid-producing tumor or hyperplastic tissue is excised, IOP generally returns to normal.

After treatment with periocular injection of corticosteroid, patients may develop increased IOP. Medical therapy may be used to lower the IOP. Although many patients respond to medical therapy, some may require excision of the depot of corticosteroid or filtering surgery.

Intravitreal corticosteroid injection may be associated with transient elevation of IOP in more than 50% of patients. Up to 25% of these patients may require topical medications to control IOP, and 1%–2% may require filtration surgery. In contrast, intravitreal implants that release corticosteroid are frequently associated with elevated IOP, often requiring patients to undergo filtration surgery as therapy. In patients with corticosteroid-induced elevation of IOP unresponsive to medical therapy, surgical treatment has a high success rate.

Cycloplegic drugs can increase IOP in individuals with open angles. Routine dilation for ophthalmoscopy may increase IOP; those at greater risk include patients with POAG, exfoliation syndrome, or pigment dispersion syndrome, and those on miotic therapy.

Epstein DL, Allingham RR, Schuman JS, eds. *Chandler and Grant's Glaucoma*. 4th ed. Baltimore: Williams & Wilkins; 1997.

Shields MB. *Shields' Textbook of Glaucoma*. 5th ed. Philadelphia: Lippincott Williams & Wilkins; 2005.

CHAPTER 5

Angle-Closure Glaucoma

Introduction

Of the nearly 67 million patients with glaucoma worldwide, it has been estimated that one-half are affected by angle-closure glaucoma. Primary angle-closure glaucoma (PACG) is a common form of glaucoma and a leading cause of bilateral blindness. PACG is the predominant form of glaucoma in East Asia and is responsible for 91% of the bilateral blindness in China, affecting more than 1.5 million Chinese.

The modern history of PACG dates back more than 150 years. In 1856, von Graefe performed an iridectomy on a staphylomatous eye and demonstrated the first cure for acute "inflammatory glaucoma." However, the pathophysiology of primary angle closure and how the iridectomy brought about this cure remained in question for another century. In 1873, Leber wrote that aqueous was secreted from the ciliary processes, traveled through the pupil, and entered into the anterior chamber. He felt that the forward movement of the iris could lead to elevated IOP and angle-closure glaucoma. In the later part of the 19th century, Weber and later Priestly Smith hypothesized that angle closure occurred as a result of swelling of the ciliary processes, which pushed the iris forward over the trabecular meshwork. In 1920, Edward Curran proposed the mechanism of pupillary block and the importance of an iridectomy in breaking this impeded aqueous flow. His initial observations and theories on PACG were finally accepted in 1951, following papers and presentations by Joseph Haas, Harold Scheie, and Paul Chandler, confirming the principle of "relative pupillary block." Advances in gonioscopy prior to 1940, by Barkan, Trantas, Koeppe, Salzmann, and Troncoso, further helped define and distinguish the angle-closure glaucomas. The development of the Goldmann lens in 1938 allowed more universal use of gonioscopy, further advancing our knowledge and understanding of the anterior chamber angle.

Accurate assessment of the anatomy of the anterior chamber angle is perhaps the most fundamental factor in classifying the various forms of glaucoma. Further, knowledge of the angle anatomy is essential for proper treatment. Thus, the clinician must be skilled at gonioscopy to determine whether aqueous has complete, unimpeded access to the trabecular meshwork and to identify cases in which the peripheral iris impedes free flow of aqueous to the meshwork. In primary open-angle glaucoma, while the resistance to aqueous outflow is known to be increased, structures proximal to the trabecular meshwork do not add to the resistance to aqueous outflow and the pathologic resistance to outflow resides in the meshwork itself. Conversely, in the angle-closure glaucomas, the primary pathology is anatomic, proximal to the trabecular meshwork. Specifically, in such cases, the peripheral iris impedes the access of aqueous to the trabecular meshwork.

The angle-closure glaucomas include a large and diverse group of diseases. While the various forms of angle closure are unified by the presence of peripheral anterior synechiae and/or iridotrabecular apposition, the mechanism of iris apposition or synechiae formation is varied. Moreover, the clinical presentation of angle closure varies from the dramatic presentation of acute angle-closure glaucoma to the insidious and initially asymptomatic presentation of chronic angle-closure glaucoma. The patient in acute angle closure often presents to the emergency room in acute distress, often with vague symptomatology including headache, nausea, vomiting, and general malaise. Such non-ocular complaints may mask the fact that the inciting pathology is ocular in origin. In either presentation, acute or chronic, the physician must identify the anatomic changes that have occurred and the underlying pathophysiology that has precipitated these changes in order to initiate the appropriate therapy. Early diagnosis and treatment of most forms of angle-closure glaucoma can be invaluable, if not curative. Accordingly, understanding and identification of the pathophysiology is essential if proper treatment is to be initiated. Also, screening patients at greatest risk for angle closure can be beneficial in reducing the number of patients who develop these diseases and in reducing the risk of blindness.

Traditionally, the angle-closure glaucomas are separated into 2 main categories: primary and secondary angle closure. Each category is further divided by the symptomatology, etiology, and duration of each of the diseases.

In *primary* angle closure, there is no underlying pathology; there is only an anatomic predisposition. In *secondary* angle closure, an underlying pathologic cause, such as an intumescent lens, iris neovascularization, chronic inflammation, corneal endothelial migration, or epithelial downgrowth, initiates the angle closure.

Foster PJ, Johnson GJ. Glaucoma in China: how big is the problem? *Br J Ophthalmol.* 2001;85:1277–1282.

Kim YY, Jung HR. Clarifying the nomenclature for primary angle-closure glaucoma. *Surv Ophthalmol.* 1997;42:125–136.

Lowe RF. A history of primary angle closure glaucoma. *Surv Ophthalmol.* 1995;40:163–170.

Pathogenesis and Pathophysiology of Angle Closure

Angle closure is defined by the apposition of the peripheral iris to the trabecular meshwork and the resulting reduced drainage of aqueous humor through the anterior chamber angle. In considering the underlying pathogenesis of angle closure, it is important to assess the relative and absolute size and position of each of the anterior segment structures and the pressure gradients between the posterior and anterior chambers. In the setting of a narrow angle, any region of apposition of the iris to the trabecular meshwork is abnormal and requires further assessment.

Conceptually, the mechanism of angle closure falls into 2 categories (Table 5-1):

- mechanisms that push the iris forward from behind
- mechanisms that pull the iris forward into contact with the trabecular meshwork

Table 5-1 **Underlying Mechanisms of Angle Closure**

Iris pushed forward from behind, into the angle:
- relative pupillary block
- absolute pupillary block
- aqueous misdirection (malignant glaucoma)
- ciliary body swelling, inflammation, or cysts
- anteriorly located ciliary processes (plateau iris configuration/syndrome)
- choroidal swelling, serous or hemorrhagic choroidal detachments or effusions
- posterior segment tumors or space-occupying lesions (silicone oil, gas bubble)
- contracting retrolental tissue (retinopathy of prematurity)
- anteriorly displaced lens
- encircling retinal bands/buckles

Iris pulled forward into contact with the angle:
- contraction of inflammatory membrane or fibrovascular tissue
- migration of corneal endothelium (iridocorneal endothelial [ICE] syndrome)
- fibrous ingrowth
- epithelial downgrowth
- iris incarceration in traumatic wound or surgical incision

Pupillary Block

Pupillary block is the most frequent cause of angle closure and is the underlying cause of most cases of primary angle closure. The flow of aqueous from the posterior chamber through the pupil is impeded, and this obstruction creates a pressure gradient between the posterior and anterior chambers, causing the peripheral iris to bow forward against the trabecular meshwork (Fig 5-1). Pupillary block is maximal when the pupil is in the mid-dilated position. Though rare, absolute pupillary block occurs when there is no movement of aqueous through the pupil as a result of 360° of posterior synechiae (secluded pupil). These posterior synechiae can form between the iris and the crystalline lens, an intraocular lens, capsular remnants, and/or the vitreous face. Relative pupillary block occurs when there is restricted movement of aqueous through the pupil because of iris contact with the

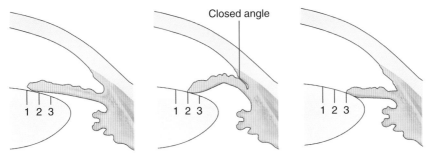

Figure 5-1   *1,* The pupil is constricted and the angle is open. *2,* The pupil is in the mid-dilated position. Pupillary block is maximal in this position and as a result the iris is bowed anteriorly and the angle narrows. *3,* The pupil is more completely dilated and the relative pupillary block is diminished, with a return to a flatter iris configuration. If full-blown angle closure occurs, the iris may stay in the mid-dilated position until the angle closure attack is broken. *(Redrawn with permission from Quigley HA, Friedman DS, Congdon NG. Possible mechanisms of primary angle-closure and malignant glaucoma. J Glaucoma. 2003;12:171. © 2003 Lippincott Williams & Wilkins, Inc. Illustration by Cyndie C. H. Wooley.)*

lens, intraocular lens, capsular remnants, anterior hyaloid, or vitreous space–occupying substance (air, silicone oil). Relative and absolute pupillary block are broken by an unobstructed peripheral iridectomy.

Angle Closure Without Pupillary Block

Angle closure may occur without pupillary block. Iridotrabecular apposition or synechiae can result from the iris and/or lens being pushed, rotated, or pulled forward for a variety of reasons, as outlined in Table 5-1. Each of these underlying mechanisms can usually be identified by a comprehensive examination, including gonioscopy. Many patients may present with multiple underlying causes for their angle closure.

Lens-Induced Angle-Closure Glaucoma

Intumescent or dislocated lenses (complete zonular dehiscence) may increase pupillary block and cause angle closure. Angle closure from an unusually large or intumescent lens is often referred to as *phacomorphic glaucoma*. With lens subluxation (partial zonular dehiscence), as in Marfan syndrome, exfoliation syndrome, or homocystinuria, pupillary block from the lens or vitreous may occur. Lens block describes an underlying mechanism of primary angle closure, in which the lens's increased anterior-posterior excursion is due to weakened or lax zonules ("mobile lens syndrome"). This may result in a tendency of the lens to rotate forward, especially in the prone position, aggravating the relative pupillary block and the angle closure.

Iris-Induced Angle Closure

Iris-induced angle closure occurs when the peripheral iris is the cause of the iridotrabecular apposition. This can occur with an anterior iris insertion into the scleral spur; a thick peripheral iris, which on dilatation "rolls" into the trabecular meshwork; and/or anteriorly displaced ciliary processes, which may secondarily rotate the peripheral iris forward (plateau iris) into the meshwork. Another example of iris-induced angle closure is seen in aniridia, where the rudimentary iris leaflets rotate into the angle, resulting in secondary angle closure.

Primary Angle Closure

Primary angle closure is a complex disease entity that is a leading cause of glaucoma worldwide. Relative pupillary block is considered to be the underlying cause of more than 90% of cases of primary angle closure, although plateau iris and lens block (anterior lens movement) have been implicated as causes or partial causes of chronic primary angle closure, especially in East Asia.

Risk Factors for Developing Primary Angle Closure

Race

The prevalence of PACG in patients older than age 40 varies greatly depending on race: 0.1%–0.6% in whites, 0.1%–0.2% in blacks, 2.1%–5.0% in the Inuit, 0.4%–1.4% in East Asians, 0.3%

in the Japanese, and 2.3% in a mixed ethnic group in South Africa. Some of these differences can be explained by the difference in the biometric parameters (anterior chamber depth, axial length) of the different white and Inuit populations, whereas the increased incidence in the Chinese and East Asian populations cannot be explained by biometric parameters alone. In addition, some races present more commonly with acute forms (whites), whereas Africans and Asians present more frequently with asymptomatic chronic disease. It has become increasingly clear that the burden of angle-closure glaucoma is greater in Asian countries.

Bonomi L, Marchini G, Marraffa M, et al. Epidemiology of angle-closure glaucoma: prevalence, clinical types, and association with peripheral anterior chamber depth in the Egna-Neumarket Glaucoma Study. *Ophthalmology*. 2000;107:998–1003.

Congdon N, Wang F, Tielsch JM. Issues in the epidemiology and population-based screening of primary angle-closure glaucoma. *Surv Ophthalmol*. 1992;36:411–423.

Dandona L, Dandona R, Mandal P, et al. Angle-closure glaucoma in an urban population in southern India: the Andhra Pradesh Eye Disease Study. *Ophthalmology*. 2000;107:1710–1716.

Erie JC, Hodge DO, Gray DT. The incidence of primary angle-closure glaucoma in Olmstead County, Minnesota. *Arch Ophthalmol*. 1997;115:177–181.

Foster PJ, Oen FT, Machin D, et al. The prevalence of glaucoma in Chinese residents of Singapore: a cross-sectional population survey of the Tanjong Pagar district. *Arch Ophthalmol*. 2000;118:1105–1111.

Quigley HA, Broman AT. The number of people with glaucoma worldwide in 2010 and 2020. *Br J Ophthalmol*. 2006;90:262–267.

Rotchford AP, Johnson GJ. Glaucoma in Zulus: a population-based cross-sectional survey in a rural district in South Africa. *Arch Ophthalmol*. 2002;120:471–478.

Ocular biometrics

Patients who develop primary angle closure have small, "crowded" anterior segments and short axial lengths. The most important factors predisposing to angle closure are a shallow anterior chamber, a thick lens, increased anterior curvature of the lens, a short axial length, and a small corneal diameter and radius of curvature. An anterior chamber depth (ACD) of less than 2.5 mm predisposes patients to primary angle closure, whereas most patients with primary angle closure have an ACD of less than 2.1 mm. With improvements in biometry techniques, a clear association between ACD and peripheral anterior synechiae (PAS) has been demonstrated. While primary PAS seem to be uncommon with an ACD of greater than 2.4 mm, there is a strong correlation of increasing PAS formation with an ACD shallower than 2.4 mm. However, despite these generalizations, angle closure still occurs with deep anterior chambers in some cases.

Aung T, Nolan WP, Machin D, et al. Anterior chamber depth and the risk of primary angle closure in 2 East Asian populations. *Arch Ophthalmol*. 2005;123:527–532.

Congdon NG, Youlin Q, Quigley H, et al. Biometry and primary angle-closure glaucoma among Chinese, white, and black populations. *Ophthalmology*. 1997;104:1489–1495.

Devereux JG, Foster PJ, Baasanhu J, et al. Anterior chamber depth measurement as a screening tool for primary angle-closure glaucoma in an East Asian population. *Arch Ophthalmol*. 2000;118:257–263.

Marchini G, Pagliarusco A, Toscano A, Tosi R, Brunelli C, Bonomi L. Ultrasound biomicroscopic and conventional ultrasonographic study of ocular dimensions in primary angle-closure glaucoma. *Ophthalmology*. 1998;105:2091–2098.

Age

The prevalence of angle-closure glaucoma increases with each decade after 40 years of age. This increased incidence with age has been explained by the increasing thickness of the lens, its forward movement with age, and the resultant increase in iridolenticular contact. Primary angle-closure glaucoma is rare in individuals younger than 40 years, and the etiology of angle closure in young individuals is most often related to structural or developmental anomalies rather than relative pupillary block.

> Ritch R, Chang BM, Liebmann JM. Angle closure in younger patients. *Ophthalmology.* 2003;110:1880–1889.

Gender

Primary angle closure has been reported 2 to 4 times more commonly in women than in men, irrespective of race. In studies assessing ocular biometry, women tend to have smaller anterior segments and axial lengths than do men. This difference does not appear to be large enough to explain this sexual predilection.

Family history

The incidence of primary angle closure is increased in first-degree relatives of affected individuals. In whites, the prevalence of primary angle closure in first-degree relatives has been reported to be between 1% and 12%, whereas in a Chinese population survey, the risk was 6 times greater in patients with any family history. In the Inuit, the relative risk in patients with a family history is increased 3.5 times compared with the general Inuit population.

Refraction

Primary angle closure occurs more commonly in patients with hyperopia, irrespective of race. Increasing rates of myopia, especially in Asia, have influenced the prevalence of this disease. Angle closure occurring in patients with significant myopia should alert the clinician to search for secondary mechanisms such as microspherophakia or phacomorphic closure related to nuclear sclerotic cataract.

Acute Primary Angle Closure

Acute primary angle closure (PAC) occurs when IOP rises rapidly as a result of relatively sudden blockage of the trabecular meshwork by the iris. It is typically manifested by ocular pain, headache, blurred vision, rainbow-colored halos around lights, nausea, and vomiting. The rise in IOP to relatively high levels causes corneal epithelial edema, which is responsible for the visual symptoms. Signs of acute angle closure include

- high IOP
- iris bombé
- mid-dilated, sluggish, and irregularly shaped pupil
- corneal epithelial edema
- congested episcleral and conjunctival blood vessels
- shallow anterior chamber
- a mild amount of aqueous flare and cells

Definitive diagnosis depends on the gonioscopic verification of angle closure. Gonioscopy should be possible in almost all cases of acute angle closure, although medical treatment of elevated IOP and clearing of corneal edema with topical glycerin may be necessary to enable visualization of the chamber angle. Dynamic gonioscopy may help the physician determine whether the iris–trabecular meshwork blockage is reversible (appositional closure) or irreversible (synechial closure), and it may also be therapeutic in breaking the attack of acute angle closure. Gonioscopy of the fellow eye in a patient with PAC usually reveals a narrow, occludable angle. When performing gonioscopy, the clinician should observe the effect that the examination light has on the angle recess. For example, the pupillary constriction stimulated by the slit-lamp beam itself may open the angle and the narrow recess may go unrecognized (Fig 5-2).

During an acute attack, the IOP may be high enough to cause glaucomatous optic nerve damage, ischemic nerve damage, and/or retinal vascular occlusion. PAS can form rapidly, and IOP-induced ischemia may produce sector atrophy of the iris. Such atrophy releases pigment and causes pigmentary dusting of the iris surface and corneal endothelium. Iris ischemia, specifically of the iris sphincter muscle, may cause the pupil to become permanently fixed and dilated. *Glaukomflecken,* characteristic small anterior subcapsular lens opacities, may also develop as a result of ischemia. These findings are helpful in the detection of previous episodes of acute angle-closure glaucoma.

The definitive treatment for acute angle closure is an iridectomy, laser or surgical; this procedure is discussed in detail in Chapter 8, Surgical Therapy for Glaucoma. Mild attacks may be broken by cholinergic agents (pilocarpine 1%–2%), which induce miosis that pulls the peripheral iris away from the trabecular meshwork. Stronger miotics should be avoided, as they may increase the vascular congestion of the iris or rotate the lens–iris

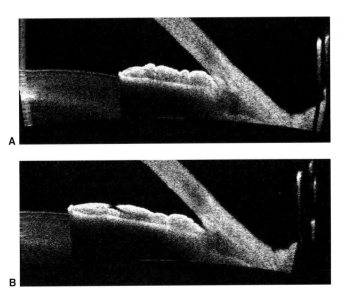

Figure 5-2 Ultrasound biomicroscopy of a narrow angle. **A,** Angle closure is evident when the angle is imaged with lights off. **B,** The same angle is much more open when imaged with lights on. *(Courtesy of Yaniv Barkana, MD.)*

diaphragm more anteriorly, increasing the pupillary block. Moreover, when the IOP is markedly elevated (eg, above 40–50 mm Hg), the pupillary sphincter may be ischemic and unresponsive to miotic agents alone. In this case, the patient should be treated with other agents such as β-adrenergic antagonists; α_2-adrenergic agonists; prostaglandin analogs; and oral, topical, or intravenous carbonic anhydrase inhibitors. When necessary, a hyperosmotic agent may be administered orally or intravenously. Such treatment is used to reduce IOP to the point where the miotic agent will constrict the pupil and open the angle. Globe compression and dynamic gonioscopy have also been described to treat acute angle-closure glaucoma. Nonselective adrenergic agonists or medications with significant α_1-adrenergic activity (apraclonidine) should be avoided to prevent further pupillary dilation and iris ischemia.

In most cases of primary angle-closure glaucoma, the fellow eye shares the anatomic predisposition for increased pupillary block and is at high risk for developing acute angle closure. This is especially true if the inciting mechanism included a systemic sympathomimetic agent such as a nasal decongestant or an anticholinergic. In addition, the pain and emotional upset resulting from the involvement of the first eye may increase sympathetic flow to the fellow eye and produce pupillary dilation. It is recommended that a peripheral iridectomy be performed in the other eye if a similar angle configuration is present. If the contralateral eye has a significantly different angle configuration, secondary angle-closure glaucomas must be strongly considered in the differential diagnosis. In general, PAC is a bilateral disease, and its occurrence in a patient whose fellow eye has a deep chamber angle raises the possibility of a secondary cause, such as a posterior segment mass, zonular insufficiency, or the ICE syndrome.

An untreated fellow eye in a patient who has had an acute angle-closure attack has a 40%–80% chance of developing an acute attack of angle closure over the next 5–10 years. Long-term pilocarpine administration is not effective in preventing acute attacks in many cases. Thus, prophylactic iridectomy should be performed in the contralateral eye unless the angle clearly appears to be non-occludable.

Laser iridectomy is the treatment of choice for primary angle closure secondary to pupillary block. Surgical iridectomy is indicated when laser iridectomy cannot be accomplished. Once an iridectomy has been performed, the pupillary block is relieved and the pressure gradient between the posterior and anterior chambers is normalized, which in most cases allows the iris to fall away from the trabecular meshwork. As a result the anterior chamber deepens and the angle opens. If a laser iridectomy cannot be performed, the acute attack may be broken in one of two ways: the peripheral iris may be flattened with a laser iridoplasty or the pupillary block may be relieved with a laser pupilloplasty. In such cases, a peripheral iridectomy should be accomplished once the attack is broken and the cornea is of adequate clarity. Following resolution of the acute attack, it is important to reevaluate the angle by gonioscopy to assess the degree of residual synechial angle closure and to confirm the reopening of at least part of the angle.

Improved IOP does not necessarily mean that the angle has opened, because the IOP may remain low for weeks following acute angle closure as a result of ciliary body ischemia and reduced aqueous production. Thus, IOP may be a poor indicator of angle function or anatomy. Repeat or serial gonioscopy is therefore essential for follow-up of the patient to be certain that the angle has adequately opened.

Seah SK, Foster PJ, Chew PT, et al. Incidence of acute primary angle-closure glaucoma in Singapore: an island-wide survey. *Arch Ophthalmol.* 1997;115:1436–1440.

Subacute or Intermittent Angle Closure

Subacute (intermittent or prodromal) angle closure is a condition characterized by episodes of blurred vision, halos, and mild pain caused by elevated IOP. These symptoms resolve spontaneously, especially during sleep-induced miosis, and IOP is usually normal between the episodes, which occur periodically over days, weeks, or months. These episodes are often confused with headaches or migraines. The correct diagnosis can be made only with a high index of suspicion and gonioscopy. The typical history and the gonioscopic appearance of a narrow chamber angle with or without PAS help establish the diagnosis. Laser iridectomy is the treatment of choice in subacute angle closure. This condition can progress to chronic angle closure or to an acute attack that does not resolve spontaneously. With improvements in phacoemulsification, especially in terms of anterior chamber stabilization and fluidic control, primary lensectomy is increasingly recognized as an effective treatment for this disorder. Goniosynechialysis may be performed in conjunction with lensectomy to help open the angle and improve trabecular outflow.

Chronic Angle Closure

Chronic angle closure may develop after acute angle closure in which synechial closure persists. It may also develop when the chamber angle closes gradually and IOP rises slowly as angle function progressively becomes compromised. The latter form of chronic angle closure, in which there is gradual asymptomatic angle closure, is the most common. This disease tends to be diagnosed in its later stages and is a major cause of blindness in Asia. In discussions of the mechanism of chronic primary angle closure, the term *creeping angle closure* is often used. Creeping angle closure defines the slow formation of PAS, which advance circumferentially, moving the iris insertion gradually forward onto the trabecular meshwork. The cause of the phenomenon is uncertain, but evidence suggests that multiple mechanisms are involved, including pupillary block, abnormalities in iris thickness and position, and plateau iris configuration.

In chronic angle-closure glaucoma, permanent PAS are present, as determined by dynamic gonioscopy. The clinical course resembles that of open-angle glaucoma in its lack of symptoms, modest elevation of IOP, progressive glaucomatous optic nerve damage, and characteristic visual field loss. The diagnosis of chronic angle-closure glaucoma is frequently overlooked, and it is commonly confused with chronic open-angle glaucoma. Gonioscopic examination of all glaucoma patients is important to enable the ophthalmologist to make the correct diagnosis.

Even if miotics and other agents lower the IOP, an iridectomy is necessary to relieve the pupillary block component and reduce the potential for further permanent synechial angle closure. Without an iridectomy, the closure of the angle usually progresses and makes the glaucoma more difficult to control. Even with a patent peripheral iridectomy, progressive angle closure can occur, and repeated periodic gonioscopy is imperative. An iridectomy with or without long-term use of ocular hypotensive medication will control the disease for most chronic angle-closure glaucoma patients. Others may require subsequent filtering surgery or goniosynechialysis.

No clinical test can reliably determine whether an iridectomy alone will control the disease for an individual patient. However, because laser iridectomy is a relatively low-risk procedure compared with other surgical procedures, it should be performed prior to a more invasive or risky operative procedure. Individuals with extensive PAS and elevated IOP following acute angle closure may be helped by argon laser gonioplasty or goniosynechialysis.

Alsagoff Z, Aung T, Ang LP, Chew PT. Long-term clinical course of primary angle-closure glaucoma in an Asian population. *Ophthalmology.* 2000;107:2300–2304.

Ritch R, Lowe RF. Angle closure glaucoma: clinical types. In: Ritch R, Shields MB, Krupin T, eds. *The Glaucomas.* 2nd ed. St Louis: Mosby; 1996:chap 38, pp 821–840.

Ritch R, Lowe RF. Angle closure glaucoma: mechanisms and epidemiology. In: Ritch R, Shields MB, Krupin T, eds. *The Glaucomas.* 2nd ed. St Louis: Mosby; 1996:chap 37, pp 801–819.

The Occludable, or Narrow, Anterior Chamber Angle

The nomenclature pertaining to the narrow anterior chamber angle may be somewhat misleading. For example, a narrow angle is not synonymous with a diagnosis of glaucoma, but rather an anatomic description. Only a small percentage of patients with shallow anterior chambers develop angle-closure glaucoma. Many clinicians have attempted to predict which asymptomatic patients with normal IOP will develop angle closure by performing a variety of provocative tests. These tests are designed to precipitate a limited form of angle closure, which can then be detected by gonioscopy and IOP measurement. The methods commonly used include pharmacologic pupillary dilation and prone-darkroom testing. An IOP increase of 8 mm Hg or more is considered positive. An asymmetric pressure rise between the 2 eyes with a corresponding degree of angle closure is also considered a positive sign. Provocative testing has not been validated in a prospective study, thus it is rarely used.

The decision to treat an asymptomatic patient with narrow angles rests on the clinical judgment of the ophthalmologist and the accurate assessment of the anterior chamber angle. Any patient with narrow angles, regardless of the results of provocative testing, should be advised of the symptoms of angle closure, of the need for immediate ophthalmic attention if symptoms occur, and of the value of long-term periodic follow-up. An iridectomy is not necessary in all patients with a suspicious or borderline narrow angle. If patients with a narrow angle have documented appositional or near appositional closure, PAS, increased segmental trabecular meshwork pigmentation, a history of previous angle closure, a positive provocative test result, or a significant risk of angle closure (anterior chamber depth of less than 2.0 mm, strong family history), then the angle should be considered occludable and an iridectomy is strongly considered.

Various factors that cause pupillary dilation may induce angle closure. These factors include a variety of drugs, as well as pain, emotional upset, or fright. In predisposed eyes with shallow anterior chambers, either mydriatic or miotic agents can precipitate acute angle closure. Mydriatic agents include not only dilating drops but also systemic medications that cause dilation. The effect of miotics is to pull the peripheral iris away from the chamber angle. However, miotics may also cause the zonular fibers of the lens to relax, allowing the lens–iris diaphragm to move forward. Furthermore, their use results in an increase in the amount of iris–lens contact, thus potentially increasing pupillary block. For these reasons, miotics, especially the cholinesterase inhibitors, may induce or aggravate angle closure. Gonioscopy should be repeated soon after miotic drugs are administered to patients with narrow angles.

A number of systemic medications that possess adrenergic (sympathomimetic) or anticholinergic (parasympatholytic) activity, including allergy and cold medications, antidepressants, and some urological drugs, carry warnings against use by patients with glaucoma. These drugs have the potential for precipitating angle closure in susceptible individuals. Although systemic administration generally does not raise intraocular drug levels to the same degree as does topical administration, even slight mydriasis in a patient with a critically narrow chamber angle can induce angle closure. The ophthalmologist should strongly consider performing an iridectomy in select patients with potentially occludable angles and warn such patients of the increased risk if they take the medication.

Dapiprazole and thymoxamine are alpha-receptor blockers that reverse pharmacologic dilation more rapidly than does placebo. While the use of dapiprazole following pupillary dilation does not eliminate the possibility of precipitating angle closure, it does reduce the overall time that the pupil is dilated, as well as the critical period when the pupil is mid-dilated.

Foster PJ, Devereux JG, Alsbirk PH, et al. Detection of gonioscopically occludable angles and primary angle-closure glaucoma by estimation of limbal chamber depth in Asians: modified grading scheme. *Br J Ophthalmol.* 2000;84:186–192.

Plateau Iris

Plateau iris represents an atypical configuration of the anterior chamber angle that may result in acute or chronic angle-closure glaucoma. Angle closure in plateau iris is most often caused by anteriorly positioned ciliary processes that critically narrow the anterior chamber recess by pushing the peripheral iris forward. A component of pupillary block is often present. The angle may be further compromised following dilation of the pupil as the peripheral iris bunches up and obstructs the trabecular meshwork. Plateau iris may be suspected if the central anterior chamber appears to be of normal depth and the iris plane appears to be rather flat for an eye with angle closure. This suspicion can be confirmed with gonioscopy or ultrasound biomicroscopy. The ophthalmologist should also consider plateau iris if angle closure occurs in younger patients with myopia. The diagnosis of plateau iris can only be made by gonioscopy or another angle imaging technique. The condition will be missed if the examiner relies solely on the slit-lamp exam or the Van Herick method of angle examination.

The management of plateau iris relies on proper diagnosis, followed by a laser iridectomy to remove any component of pupillary block. Eyes with plateau iris remain predisposed to angle closure despite a patent iridectomy as a result of the peripheral iris anatomy.

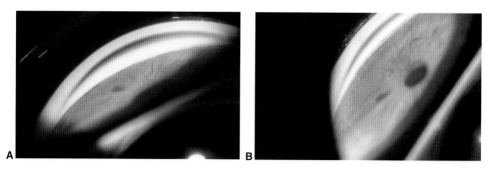

Figure 5-3 **A,** Plateau iris syndrome with a flat iris plane and closed angle. **B,** Plateau iris syndrome with an open angle following laser peripheral iridoplasty. *(Courtesy of M. Roy Wilson, MD.)*

PAS have been reported to begin at the Schwalbe line and then to extend in a posterior direction over the trabecular meshwork, scleral spur, and angle recess. The reverse is seen in pupillary block–induced angle closure in which PAS form in the posterior to anterior direction. These patients may be treated with long-term miotic therapy. However, argon laser peripheral iridoplasty may be more useful in individuals with this condition to flatten and thin the peripheral iris (Fig 5-3). Repeat gonioscopy is necessary as the threat of chronic angle closure may remain despite measures to deepen the angle recess.

Pavlin CJ, Foster FS. Plateau iris syndrome: changes in angle opening associated with dark, light, and pilocarpine administration. *Am J Ophthalmol.* 1999;128:288–291.

Secondary Angle Closure With Pupillary Block

Lens-Induced Angle Closure

Phacomorphic glaucoma

The mechanism of phacomorphic glaucoma is typically multifactorial. However, by definition a significant component of the pathological angle narrowing is related to the acquired mass effect of the cataractous lens itself. As with primary angle closure, relative pupillary block often plays an important role in this condition. Among the distinguishing features between primary angle closure and phacomorphic angle closure is the rapidity of onset of the anatomic predisposition. The anatomic predisposition tends to occur slowly in patients with primary angle closure, typically occurring in patients with hyperopia who undergo progressive shallowing of the anterior chamber as a result of increasing relative pupillary block and anteroposterior lens diameter. In contrast, the process in phacomorphic glaucoma is often much more rapid and on occasion may be precipitated by marked lens swelling (intumescence) as a result of cataract formation and the development of pupillary block in an eye that is otherwise not anatomically predisposed to closure (Figs 5-4, 5-5). Distinguishing between primary angle closure and phacomorphic angle closure is not always straightforward and may not be necessary since the treatment for both conditions is similar, but disparities between the 2 eyes in anterior chamber depth, gonioscopy, and degree of cataract should suggest a phacomorphic process (Fig 5-6). (See

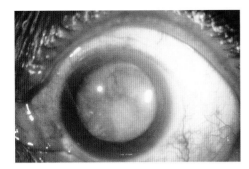

Figure 5-4 Phacomorphic glaucoma. Lens intumescence precipitates pupillary block and secondary angle closure in an eye not anatomically predisposed to angle closure. *(Courtesy of Steven T. Simmons, MD.)*

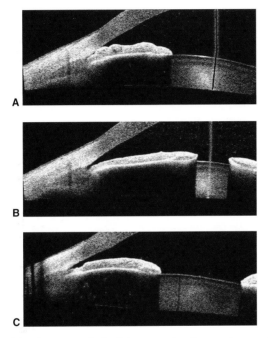

Figure 5-5 Phacomorphic glaucoma. **A,** In this example, the angle remains narrow despite a patent iridectomy. **B,** The angle is transiently made deeper by instillation of pilocarpine. **C,** In this case, a more long-term solution is accomplished by thinning the peripheral iris with argon laser iridoplasty. Lensectomy is also a viable treatment strategy. *(Courtesy of Yaniv Barkana, MD.)*

also BCSC Section 11, *Lens and Cataract.*) A laser iridectomy followed by cataract extraction in a quiet eye is the preferred treatment. In many cases the iridectomy may be unnecessary if cataract surgery is planned in the near future.

Ectopia lentis

Ectopia lentis is defined as displacement of the lens from its normal anatomic position (Fig 5-7). With forward displacement, pupillary block may occur resulting in iris bombé, shallowing of the anterior chamber angle, and secondary angle closure. This may present clinically as an acute event with pain, conjunctival hyperemia, and loss of vision, or as a chronic angle-closure glaucoma with PAS formation secondary to repeated attacks. Two

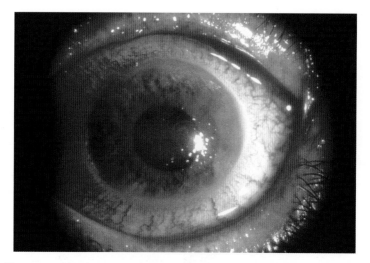

Figure 5-6 Phacomorphic glaucoma often presents clinically as acute angle-closure glaucoma. Disparities in the anterior chamber depths and degree of cataract between the 2 eyes can help the clinician distinguish between a phacomorphic process and primary angle-closure glaucoma. *(Courtesy of Steven T. Simmons, MD.)*

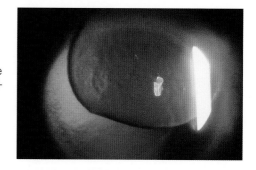

Figure 5-7 Ectopia lentis: dislocation of the lens into the anterior chamber through a dilated pupil. *(Courtesy of Ron Gross, MD.)*

laser iridectomies 180° apart is the treatment of choice to relieve the pupillary block and temporize until more definitive lensectomy, if indicated from a visual function standpoint. Lens extraction is usually indicated to restore visual acuity and reduce recurrent lens block and the possible development of chronic angle closure. A list of conditions causing this entity is given in Table 5-2.

Microspherophakia, a congenital disorder in which the lens has a spherical or globular shape, may cause pupillary block and angle-closure glaucoma (Fig 5-8). Treatment with cycloplegia may tighten the zonule, flatten the lens, and pull it posteriorly, breaking the pupillary block. Miotics may make the condition worse by increasing the pupillary block and by rotating the ciliary body forward, loosening the zonule and allowing the lens to become more globular. Microspherophakia is often familial and may occur as an isolated condition or as part of either Weill-Marchesani or Marfan syndrome. Finally, the most common form of acquired zonular insufficiency and crystalline lens subluxation occurs in the exfoliation syndrome (Fig 5-9).

Table 5-2 Common Causes of Ectopia Lentis

Exfoliation
Trauma
Marfan syndrome
Homocystinuria
Microspherophakia
Weill-Marchesani syndrome

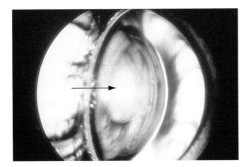

Figure 5-8 Ectopia lentis. In a case of microspherophakia, the lens *(arrow)* is trapped anteriorly by the pupil, resulting in iris bombé and a dramatic shallowing of the anterior chamber. *(Courtesy of G. L. Spaeth, MD.)*

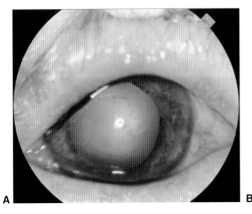

A

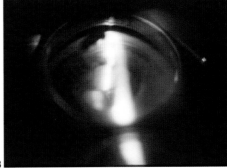

B

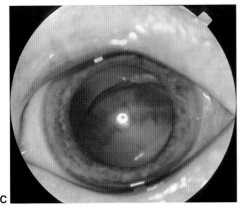

C

Figure 5-9 The exfoliation syndrome is a common cause of subluxation of the crystalline lens. **A,** Right eye of patient with complete dislocation of the lens. **B,** Gonioscopic view of the same eye reveals that the dislocated lens is in the inferior vitreous cavity. **C,** Left eye of same patient showing subluxation of the lens. *(Courtesy of Thomas W. Samuelson, MD.)*

Aphakic or pseudophakic angle-closure glaucoma

Pupillary block may occur in *aphakic* and *pseudophakic* eyes. An intact vitreous face can block the pupil and/or an iridectomy in aphakic or pseudophakic eyes or in a phakic eye with a dislocated lens. Generally, the anterior chamber shallows and the iris demonstrates considerable bombé configuration. Treatment with mydriatic and cycloplegic agents may restore the aqueous flow through the pupil but may also make the performing of a laser iridectomy difficult initially. Topical β-adrenergic antagonists, α_2-adrenergic agonists, carbonic anhydrase inhibitors, and hyperosmotic agents can be effective in reducing IOP prior to the placement of an iridectomy. One or more laser iridectomies may be required.

A variant of this problem occurs with *anterior chamber intraocular lenses.* Pupillary block develops with apposition of the iris, vitreous face, and/or lens optic. The lens haptic or vitreous may obstruct the iridectomy or the pupil, and the peripheral iris bows forward around the anterior chamber IOL to occlude the chamber angle. The central chamber remains deep in this instance, because the lens haptic and optic prevent the central portions of the iris and vitreous face from moving forward. Laser iridectomies, often multiple, are required to relieve the block.

Pupillary block may also occur following posterior capsulotomy when vitreous obstructs the pupil. A condition referred to as *capsular block* may also be seen whereby retained viscoelastic or fluid in the capsular bag pushes a posterior chamber IOL anteriorly, which may narrow the angle.

Secondary Angle Closure Without Pupillary Block

A number of disorders can lead to secondary angle closure without pupillary block, and several are discussed in this section. This form of secondary angle closure may occur through 1 of 2 mechanisms:

- contraction of an inflammatory, hemorrhagic, or vascular membrane, band, or exudate in the angle, leading to PAS
- forward displacement of the lens–iris diaphragm, often accompanied by swelling and anterior rotation of the ciliary body

Neovascular Glaucoma

This common, severe type of secondary angle-closure glaucoma is caused by a variety of disorders characterized by retinal or ocular ischemia or ocular inflammation (Table 5-3). The most common causes are diabetes mellitus, central retinal vein occlusion, and ocular ischemic syndrome. The disease is characterized by fine arborizing blood vessels on the surface of the iris, pupil margin, and trabecular meshwork, which are accompanied by a fibrous membrane. The contraction of the fibrovascular membrane results in the formation of PAS, leading to the development of secondary angle-closure glaucoma. In some cases, a fibrous membrane may be evident without active angle neovascularization. Moreover, angle vessels may be present without vessels on the iris surface.

Table 5-3 Disorders Predisposing to Neovascularization of the Iris and Angle

Systemic vascular disease	Other ocular disease
Carotid occlusive disease*	Chronic uveitis
Carotid artery ligation	Chronic retinal detachment
Carotid cavernous fistula	Endophthalmitis
Giant cell arteritis	Stickler syndrome
Takayasu (pulseless) disease	Retinoschisis
Ocular vascular disease	**Intraocular tumors**
Diabetic retinopathy*	Uveal melanoma
Central retinal vein occlusion*	Metastatic carcinoma
Central retinal artery occlusion	Retinoblastoma
Branch retinal vein occlusion	Reticulum cell sarcoma
Sickle cell retinopathy	**Ocular therapy**
Coats disease	Radiation therapy
Eales disease	
Retinopathy of prematurity	**Trauma**
Persistent fetal vasculature	
Syphilitic vasculitis	
Anterior segment ischemia	

* Most common causes

Neovascularization of the anterior segment usually presents in a classic pattern that starts with fine vascular tufts at the pupil (Fig 5-10). As these vessels grow, they extend radially over the iris. The neovascularization crosses the ciliary body and scleral spur as fine single vessels that then branch as they reach and involve the trabecular meshwork (Fig 5-11). Often the trabecular meshwork takes on a reddish coloration. With contraction of the fibrovascular membrane, PAS develop and coalesce, gradually closing the angle (Fig 5-12). Because the fibrovascular membrane typically does not grow over healthy corneal endothelium, the PAS end at the Schwalbe line, distinguishing this

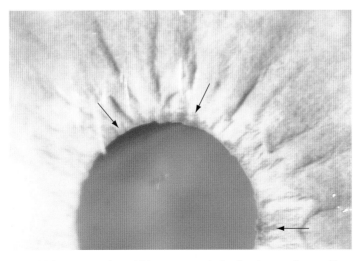

Figure 5-10 The initial presentation of iris neovascularization is usually small vascular tufts at the pupillary margin. *(Courtesy of Steven T. Simmons, MD.)*

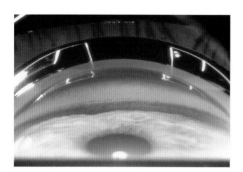

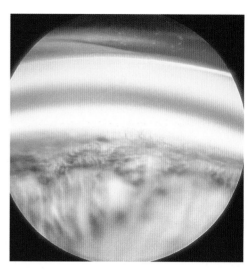

Figure 5-11 Initially, the iris neovascularization crosses the angle recess and scleral spur as single vessels that then branch over the trabecular meshwork. *(Courtesy of Tom Richardson, MD.)*

Figure 5-12 Iris neovascularization. With progressive angle involvement, PAS develop with contraction of the fibrovascular membrane, resulting in secondary neovascular glaucoma. *(Courtesy of Steven T. Simmons, MD.)*

condition from other secondary angle-closure glaucomas that result from an abnormal corneal endothelium, such as ICE syndrome, which is discussed in the following section (Figs 5-13, 5-14).

Clinically, patients often present with an acute or subacute glaucoma associated with reduced vision, pain, conjunctival injection, microcystic corneal edema, and high IOP. While performing gonioscopy in patients suspected of having neovascularization, the clinician may find it helpful to use a bright slit-lamp beam of light and high magnification in order to best visualize these fine vessels.

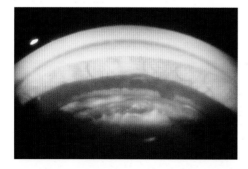

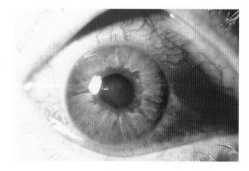

Figure 5-13 With end-stage neovascular glaucoma, total angle closure occurs, obscuring the iris neovascularization. The PAS end at the Schwalbe line because the fibrovascular membrane does not grow over healthy corneal endothelium. *(Courtesy of Steven T. Simmons, MD.)*

Figure 5-14 With growth, iris neovascularization extends from the pupillary margin radially toward the anterior chamber angle. *(Courtesy of Steven T. Simmons, MD.)*

Rarely, anterior segment neovascularization may occur without demonstrable retinal ischemia, as in Fuchs heterochromic iridocyclitis and other types of uveitis, exfoliation syndrome, or isolated iris melanomas. When an ocular cause cannot be found, carotid artery occlusive disease should be considered. In establishing a correct diagnosis, it is important to distinguish dilated iris vessels associated with inflammation from newly formed abnormal blood vessels.

Because the prognosis for neovascular glaucoma is poor, prevention and early diagnosis are desirable. Gonioscopy is vitally important to the early diagnosis because angle neovascularization can occur without iris neovascularization. In central retinal vein occlusion (CRVO), approximately 10% of patients develop angle neovascularization alone. The most common cause of iris neovascularization is ischemic retinopathy, and retinal ablation should be performed whenever possible. The treatment of choice when the ocular media are clear is panretinal photocoagulation. When cloudy media prevent laser therapy, panretinal cryotherapy should be considered, as an alternative to vitrectomy to clear the media with endophotocoagulation or subsequent panretinal photocoagulation. Frequently, marked involution of the neovascularization occurs. The resulting decrease in neovascularization after retinal ablation may reduce or normalize the IOP, depending on the degree of synechial closure that has occurred. Even in the presence of total synechial angle closure, panretinal photocoagulation may improve the success rate of subsequent glaucoma surgery by eliminating the angiogenic stimulus and may decrease the risk of hemorrhage at the time of surgery. More recently, antiproliferative agents have been successfully employed to promote regression of the neovascular tissue prior to filtering surgery (Figs 5-15, 5-16).

Medical management of neovascular glaucoma yields variable success but often is a temporizing measure until more definitive surgical or laser treatment is undertaken. Topical β-adrenergic antagonists, α_2-adrenergic agonists, carbonic anhydrase inhibitors, cycloplegics, and corticosteroids may be useful in reducing IOP and decreasing inflammation either as a chronic remedy or prior to filtration surgery. Filtering surgery has a better chance of success once the neovascularization has regressed after panretinal photocoagulation. The use of the antimetabolites 5-fluorouracil and mitomycin C has been shown to

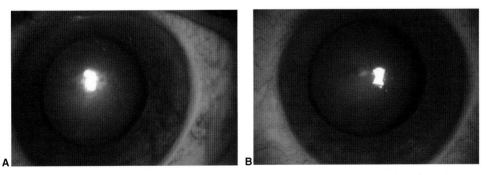

Figure 5-15 **A,** Slit-lamp photograph of florid iris neovascularization taken 15 minutes before injection of bevacizumab. **B,** Regression of iris neovascularization 4 days after treatment with bevacizumab. *(Courtesy of Nicholas P. Bell, MD.)*

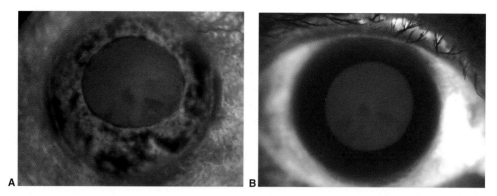

Figure 5-16 **A,** Fluorescein angiogram of pronounced iris neovascularization before injection of bevacizumab. **B,** Regression of iris neovascularization 1 month after injection of bevacizumab. *(Courtesy of Eugene Eng, MD.)*

increase the success rate and decrease the final IOP following trabeculectomy in patients with neovascular glaucoma. A variety of aqueous shunts have also been successfully implanted to control the IOP in neovascular glaucoma and, in many cases, an aqueous shunt is the surgical procedure of choice. If these therapies fail, either endoscopic or transscleral cyclophotocoagulation, or less often, cyclocryotherapy, may help reduce the IOP.

Heuer DK, Lloyd MA. Management of glaucomas with poor surgical prognoses. *Focal Points: Clinical Modules for Ophthalmologists.* San Francisco: American Academy of Ophthalmology; 1995, module 1.

Iliev ME, Domig D, Wolf-Schnurrbursch U, Wolf S, Sarra GM. Intravitreal bevacizumab (Avastin) in the treatment of neovascular glaucoma. *Am J Ophthalmol.* 2006;142:1054–1056.

Jonas JB, Spandau UH, Schlichtenbrede F. Intravitreal bevacizumab for filtering surgery. *Ophthalmic Res.* 2007;39:121–122.

McGrath DJ, Ferguson JG, Sanborn GE. Neovascular glaucoma. *Focal Points: Clinical Modules for Ophthalmologists.* San Francisco: American Academy of Ophthalmology; 1997, module 7.

Sivak-Callcott JA, O'Day DM, Gass JD, Tsai JC. Evidence-based recommendations for the diagnosis and treatment of neovascular glaucoma. *Ophthalmology.* 2001;108:1767–1776.

Iridocorneal Endothelial Syndrome

Iridocorneal endothelial (ICE) syndrome is a group of disorders characterized by abnormal corneal endothelium that causes variable degrees of iris atrophy, secondary angle-closure glaucoma, and corneal edema. BCSC Section 8, *External Disease and Cornea,* discusses the corneal aspects of ICE syndrome. Three clinical variants have been described:

- Chandler syndrome
- essential/progressive iris atrophy
- iris nevus/Cogan-Reese syndrome

The condition is clinically unilateral, presents between 20 and 50 years of age, and occurs more often in women. No consistent association has been found with another ocular or systemic disease, and familial cases are very rare. Patients present with decreased vision, pain secondary to corneal edema or secondary angle-closure glaucoma, or an abnormal iris appearance. In each of the 3 clinical variants, the corneal endothelium appears abnormal and takes on a beaten bronze appearance, similar to corneal guttae seen in Fuchs corneal endothelial dystrophy. Microcystic corneal edema may be present without elevated IOP, especially in Chandler syndrome. The unaffected eye may have subclinical irregularities of the corneal endothelium without other manifestations of the disease.

High PAS are characteristic of ICE syndrome (Fig 5-17), and these often extend anterior to the Schwalbe line. The PAS are caused by the contraction of the single or multiple layers of endothelial cells and surrounding collagenous-fibrillar tissue that extend from the peripheral cornea over the trabecular meshwork and iris. These PAS result in synechial closure of the anterior chamber angle and lead to an angle-closure glaucoma. Similar to neovascular glaucoma, the degree of angle closure does not always correlate to the elevation in IOP, because some angles may be functionally closed by the endothelial membrane without overt synechial formation.

Various degrees of iris atrophy and corneal changes distinguish the specific clinical entities. The "progressive iris atrophy" variant of ICE syndrome is characterized by severe progressive iris atrophy resulting in heterochromia, corectopia, ectropion uveae, iris stromal and pigment epithelial atrophy, and hole formation (Fig 5-18). In Chandler syndrome, minimal iris atrophy and corectopia occur, and the corneal and angle findings predominate (Fig 5-19).

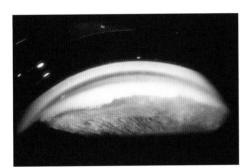

Figure 5-17 The classic high PAS seen in ICE syndrome. These PAS extend anterior to the Schwalbe line in this patient with progressive iris atrophy. With angle closure, the secondary glaucoma occurs. *(Courtesy of Steven T. Simmons, MD.)*

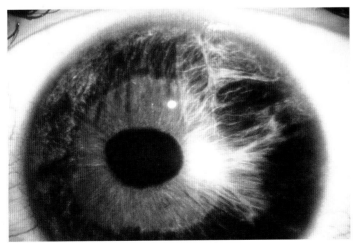

Figure 5-18 ICE syndrome. Corectopia and hole formation are typical findings in progressive iris atrophy. *(Courtesy of Steven T. Simmons, MD.)*

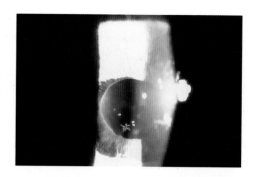

Figure 5-19 Ectropion uveae in a patient with Chandler syndrome. *(Courtesy of Steven T. Simmons, MD.)*

Chandler syndrome is the most common of the clinical variants and makes up approximately 50% of the cases of ICE syndrome. The iris atrophy tends to be less severe in Cogan-Reese syndrome. This condition is distinguished by tan pedunculated nodules or diffuse pigmented lesions on the anterior iris surface.

Glaucoma occurs in approximately 50% of patients with ICE syndrome, and the glaucoma tends to be more severe in progressive iris atrophy and Cogan-Reese syndrome. In the 3 clinical variations, corneal endothelial abnormalities are seen with a fine, hammered metal appearance to the posterior cornea. In this condition, the corneal endothelium migrates posterior to the Schwalbe line onto the trabecular meshwork. Electron microscopy has shown this endothelial layer to vary in thickness, with areas of single and multiple endothelial layers, and to contain surrounding collagenous and fibrillar tissue. Unlike normal corneal endothelium, filopodial processes and cytoplasmic actin filaments are present, supporting the migratory nature of these cells. PAS are formed when this migratory endothelium and its surrounding collagenous, fibrillar tissue contract. A viral cause has been postulated for the mechanism of ICE syndrome after lymphocytes were seen on the corneal endothelium of affected patients.

The diagnosis of ICE syndrome must always be considered in young to middle-aged patients who present with unilateral, secondary angle-closure glaucoma. It is particularly important to maintain a high index of suspicion as this condition may mimic primary open-angle glaucoma when the iris and corneal features are subtle. Specular microscopy can confirm the diagnosis by demonstrating an asymmetric loss of endothelial cells and atypical endothelial cell morphology in the involved eye. Therapy is directed toward the corneal edema and secondary glaucoma. Hypertonic saline solutions and medications to reduce the IOP, when elevated, can be effective in controlling the corneal edema. The angle-closure glaucoma can be treated medically with aqueous suppressants. Miotics are ineffective, and the role of prostaglandin analogs remains uncertain. When medical therapy fails, filtering surgery (trabeculectomy or an aqueous shunt) can be effective. Late failures have been reported with trabeculectomy secondary to endothelialization of the fistula. These can be reopened in some cases with the Nd:YAG laser. Laser trabeculoplasty has no useful role in treating glaucoma related to ICE syndrome.

Tumors

Tumors in the posterior segment of the eye or anterior uveal cysts may cause a unilateral secondary angle-closure glaucoma. Primary choroidal melanomas, ocular metastases, and retinoblastoma are the most common tumors to cause secondary angle closure. The mechanism of the angle-closure glaucoma is determined by the size, location, and pathology of the tumor. Choroidal and retinal tumors tend to shift the lens–iris diaphragm forward as the tumors enlarge, causing secondary angle closure. Breakdown of the blood–aqueous barrier and inflammation from tissue necrosis can result in posterior and peripheral anterior synechiae formation, further exacerbating other underlying mechanisms of angle closure. Iris neovascularization can occur frequently with retinoblastomas, medulloepitheliomas, and choroidal melanomas, resulting in secondary angle closure and neovascular glaucoma.

Inflammation

Secondary angle-closure glaucoma can result from ocular inflammation. Fibrin and increased aqueous proteins from the breakdown of the blood–aqueous barrier may predispose to the formation of posterior synechiae (Fig 5-20) and PAS. If left untreated, these posterior synechiae can result in a secluded pupil, iris bombé, and secondary angle closure (Fig 5-21).

Inflammation may prompt PAS to form through peripheral iris edema, organization of inflammatory debris in the angle, and the bridging of the angle by large keratic precipitates (sarcoidosis). Unlike primary angle closure, in which the PAS occur preferentially in the superior angle, with inflammatory etiologies they occur most frequently in the inferior angle (Fig 5-22). These PAS tend to be nonuniform in shape and height, which further differentiates inflammatory disease from primary angle closure (Fig 5-23). Ischemia secondary to inflammation may rarely cause rubeosis iridis and neovascular glaucoma.

Ocular inflammation can lead to the shallowing and closure of the anterior chamber angle by uveal effusion, resulting in anterior rotation of the ciliary body. Significant posterior uveitis causing massive exudative retinal detachment or choroidal effusions may lead to angle-closure glaucoma through forward displacement of the lens–iris diaphragm. Treatment is primarily directed at the underlying cause of the uveitis. Aqueous suppressants and corticosteroids are the primary agents for reducing elevated IOP and preventing synechial angle closure.

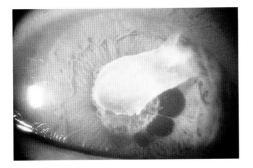

Figure 5-20 Inflammatory glaucoma. A fibrinous anterior chamber reaction and posterior synechiae formation are shown in a patient with ankylosing spondylitis. *(Courtesy of Steven T. Simmons, MD.)*

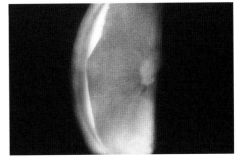

Figure 5-21 Inflammatory glaucoma. A secluded pupil is shown in a patient with longstanding uveitis with classic iris bombé and secondary angle closure. *(Courtesy of Steven T. Simmons, MD.)*

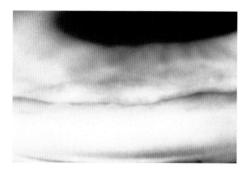

Figure 5-22 Inflammatory glaucoma. Keratic precipitates can be seen bridging the inferior anterior chamber angle in this patient with long-standing uveitis, resulting in the formation of PAS. *(Courtesy of Joseph Krug, MD.)*

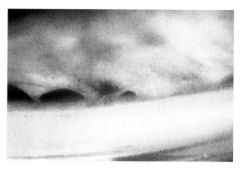

Figure 5-23 Inflammatory glaucoma. PAS in uveitis occur preferentially in the inferior anterior chamber angle and are nonuniform in height and shape, as demonstrated in this photograph. *(Courtesy of Joseph Krug, MD.)*

Interstitial keratitis may be associated with open-angle or angle-closure glaucoma. The angle closure may be caused by chronic inflammation and PAS formation or by multiple cysts of the iris pigment epithelium.

> Samples JR. Management of glaucoma secondary to uveitis. *Focal Points: Clinical Modules for Ophthalmologists.* San Francisco: American Academy of Ophthalmology; 1995, module 5.

Aqueous Misdirection

Aqueous misdirection is also known as *malignant glaucoma, ciliary block glaucoma,* and *posterior aqueous diversion syndrome.* This rare but potentially devastating form of glaucoma usually presents following ocular surgery in patients with a history of angle closure or PAS. It may also occur spontaneously in eyes with an open angle following cataract surgery or various laser procedures. The disease presents with uniform flattening of both the central and peripheral anterior chamber, which is typically markedly asymmetrical to the fellow eye (Fig 5-24). This is in contrast to acute primary angle-closure glaucoma, which presents with iris bombé and shallow peripheral anterior chamber (Fig 5-25). Classically, the condition is thought to result from anterior rotation of the ciliary body and posterior misdirection of the aqueous, in association with a relative block to aqueous movement at the level of the lens equator, vitreous face, and ciliary processes. More recently, some have proposed that primary angle closure and malignant glaucoma may result from the simultaneous presence of several factors including a small eye, a propensity for choroidal expansion, and reduced vitreous fluid conductivity. Undoubtedly, the improved ability to image the angle, choroid, and lens–iris diaphragm with high-resolution ultrasound will improve our understanding of the physiological mechanism of these complex disorders.

Clinically, the anterior chamber is shallow or flat with anterior displacement of the lens, pseudophakos, or vitreous face. Ciliary processes are seen to be rotated anteriorly and may be seen through an iridectomy to come in contact with the lens equator. Optically clear "aqueous" zones may be seen in the vitreous, highlighting the underlying pathology. In the early postoperative setting, aqueous misdirection is often difficult to distinguish from choroidal effusion, pupillary block, or suprachoroidal hemorrhage. Often the level

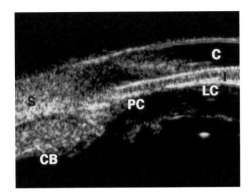 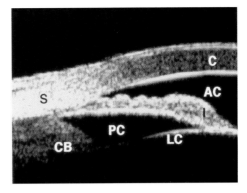

Figure 5-24 Aqueous misdirection seen by UBM. Expansion of the vitreous pushes the lens and ciliary body forward, causing a uniform shallowing of the anterior chamber. The central portion of the anterior lens capsule *(LC)* is nearly in contact with the cornea *(C)*. PC = posterior chamber; *CB* = ciliary body; *I* = iris; *S* = sclera. *(From Lundy DC. Ciliary block glaucoma.* Focal Points: Clinical Modules for Ophthalmologists. *San Francisco: American Academy of Ophthalmology; 1999, module 3. Courtesy of Jeffrey M. Liebmann, MD.)*

Figure 5-25 Acute angle closure seen by UBM. Pupillary block leads to forward bowing of the peripheral iris. The peripheral chamber is shallow, whereas the central chamber depth is relatively deep. *C* = cornea; *AC* = anterior chamber; *PC* = posterior chamber; *LC* = lens capsule; *CB* = ciliary body; *I* = iris; *S* = sclera. *(From Lundy DC. Ciliary block glaucoma.* Focal Points: Clinical Modules for Ophthalmologists. *San Francisco: American Academy of Ophthalmology; 1999, module 3. Courtesy of Jeffrey M. Liebmann, MD.)*

of IOP, time frame following surgery, patency of an iridectomy, or presence of a choroidal effusion or suprachoroidal hemorrhage help the clinician make the appropriate diagnosis and initiate treatment. In some cases, unfortunately, the clinical picture is difficult to interpret and surgical intervention may be required to make the diagnosis.

Medical management includes the triad of intensive cycloplegic therapy; aggressive aqueous suppression with β-adrenergic antagonists, α_2-adrenergic agonists, and carbonic anhydrase inhibitors; and shrinking of the vitreous with hyperosmotic agents. Miotics should not be used and can make aqueous misdirection worse. In aphakic and pseudophakic eyes, the anterior vitreous can be disrupted with the Nd:YAG laser. Argon laser photocoagulation of the ciliary processes has reportedly been helpful in treating this condition; this procedure may alter the adjacent vitreous face. Approximately 50% of patients can be controlled medically, whereas the other half will require surgical intervention. The definitive surgical treatment is a vitrectomy with anterior hyaloid disruption combined with an anterior chamber deepening procedure. BCSC Section 12, *Retina and Vitreous,* discusses vitrectomy in greater detail.

Lundy DC. Ciliary block glaucoma. *Focal Points: Clinical Modules for Ophthalmologists.* San Francisco: American Academy of Ophthalmology; 1999, module 3.

Quigley HA, Friedman DS, Congdon NG. Possible mechanisms of primary angle-closure and malignant glaucoma. *J Glaucoma.* 2003;12:167–180.

Nonrhegmatogenous Retinal Detachment and Uveal Effusions

A nonrhegmatogenous retinal detachment occurs as a result of subretinal fluid in which no retinal break is present. A suprachoroidal effusion or hemorrhage refers to blood or fluid in the potential space between the choroid and the sclera. Retinoblastoma, Coats disease, metastatic carcinoma, choroidal melanoma, suprachoroidal hemorrhage, choroidal effusion/detachment, infections (HIV), and subretinal neovascularization in age-related macular degeneration with extensive effusion or hemorrhage can cause nonrhegmatogenous retinal detachments or suprachoroidal mass effect that may result in secondary angle closure related to forward displacement of the lens–iris diaphragm. See BCSC Section 12, *Retina and Vitreous,* for further discussion.

In a *rhegmatogenous retinal detachment,* the subretinal fluid can escape through the retinal tear and equalize the hydraulic pressure on both sides of the retina. In a non-rhegmatogenous retinal detachment, by contrast, the subretinal fluid accumulates and becomes a space-occupying lesion in the vitreous, which may progressively push the retina forward against the lens like a hydraulic press. The fluid or hemorrhage may accumulate rapidly, and as it pushes the bullous retinal detachment forward to a retrolenticular position, in severe cases it can flatten the anterior chamber completely. The retina may be dramatically visible behind the lens on slit-lamp examination.

Epithelial and Fibrous Downgrowth

Epithelial and fibrous proliferation are rare surgical complications that can cause devastating secondary glaucomas. Epithelial and fibrous downgrowth occurs when epithelium and/or connective tissue invades the anterior chamber through a defect in a wound site. Fortunately, improved surgical and wound closure techniques have greatly reduced the incidence of these entities (Fig 5-26). Fibrous ingrowth is more prevalent than epithelial downgrowth, progresses more slowly, and is often self-limited. Risk factors for the development of these entities include prolonged inflammation, wound dehiscence, delayed wound closure, or a Descemet's membrane tear.

Epithelial proliferation can be present in 3 forms: "pearl" tumors of the iris, epithelial cysts, and epithelial ingrowth. The latter 2 often cause secondary glaucoma. Epithelial cysts appear as translucent, nonvascular anterior chamber cysts that originate from the surgical or traumatic wound. Epithelial ingrowth presents as a grayish, sheetlike growth on the trabecular meshwork, iris, ciliary body, and posterior surface of the cornea. It is often associated with wound incarceration, wound gape, ocular inflammation, and corneal edema (Figs 5-27, 5-28). The epithelial downgrowth consists of nonkeratinized, stratified, squamous epithelium with an avascular subepithelial connective tissue layer. Underlying tissues undergo disorganization and destruction with epithelial contact.

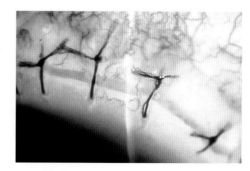

Figure 5-26 Epithelial and fibrous proliferation. This corneoscleral wound gape occurred following cataract extraction with silk closure of the incision. Improved surgical and wound closure techniques have greatly reduced the incidence of epithelial and fibrous proliferation. *(Courtesy of Wills Eye Hospital slide collection, 1986.)*

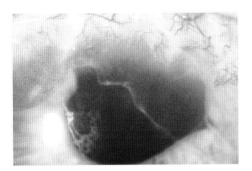

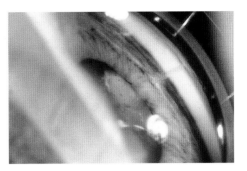

Figure 5-27 Epithelial ingrowth appears as a grayish, sheetlike growth on the endothelial surface of the cornea, usually originating from a surgical incision or traumatic wound. The epithelial ingrowth shown here originated from a cataract incision. *(Courtesy of Steven T. Simmons, MD.)*

Figure 5-28 Epithelial ingrowth. The precipitating causes of epithelial ingrowth include vitreous incarceration in corneal and scleral wounds, as seen in this photograph, as well as wound gape, ocular inflammation, and hypotony secondary to choroidal effusions. *(Courtesy of Steven T. Simmons, MD.)*

The argon laser produces characteristic white burns on the epithelial membrane on the iris surface, which helps to confirm the diagnosis of epithelial downgrowth and to determine the extent of involvement. If the diagnosis remains in question, a cytologic examination of an aqueous aspirate can be performed. Radical surgery is sometimes necessary to remove the intraocular epithelial membrane and the affected tissues and to repair the fistula, but the prognosis remains poor; thus the decision to intervene is made based on the extent of disease, the visual potential, the status of the fellow eye, and social-medical circumstances relevant to the affected individual.

Fibrovascular tissue may also proliferate into an eye from a penetrating wound. Unlike epithelial proliferation, fibrous ingrowth progresses slowly and is often self-limited. A common cause of corneal graft failure, fibrous ingrowth appears as a thick, gray-white, vascular, retrocorneal membrane with an irregular border. The ingrowth often involves the angle, resulting in PAS and the destruction of the trabecular meshwork (Fig 5-29). The resultant secondary angle-closure glaucoma is often difficult to control. Medication is the preferred treatment of the secondary glaucomas that present without a pupillary block mechanism, although surgical intervention may be required. See Chapter 7, Medical Management of Glaucoma, and Chapter 8, Surgical Therapy for Glaucoma, for detailed discussion.

Trauma

Angle-closure glaucoma without pupillary block may develop following ocular trauma from the formation of PAS associated with angle recession or from contusion, hyphema, and inflammation. See Chapter 4 for discussion of trauma.

Retinal Surgery and Retinal Vascular Disease

Angle-closure glaucoma may occur following treatment of retinal disorders, and it is important to measure IOP after retinal detachment surgery. Scleral buckling operations, especially encircling bands, can produce shallowing of the anterior chamber angle and frank

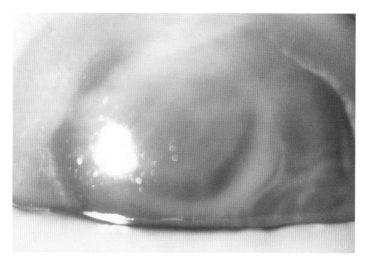

Figure 5-29 Fibrous ingrowth appears as a thick, grayish, vascular retrocorneal membrane that results in high PAS and destruction of the trabecular meshwork. *(Courtesy of Steven T. Simmons, MD.)*

angle-closure glaucoma, often accompanied by choroidal effusion and anterior rotation of the ciliary body, causing a flattening of the peripheral iris with a relatively deep central anterior chamber. Usually, the anterior chamber deepens with the opening of the anterior chamber angle over days to weeks with therapy of cycloplegics, anti-inflammatory agents, β-adrenergic antagonists, carbonic anhydrase inhibitors, and hyperosmotic agents. If medical management is unsuccessful, argon laser iridoplasty, drainage of suprachoroidal fluid, or adjustment of the scleral buckle may be required. Iridectomy is usually of little benefit in this condition. The scleral buckle can impede venous drainage by compressing a vortex vein, increasing episcleral venous pressure and IOP. Such cases may respond only to moving the scleral buckle or releasing tension on the band.

Following a pars plana vitrectomy, angle-closure glaucoma may result from the injection of air, long-acting gases such as sulfur hexafluoride and perfluorocarbons (perfluoropropane and perfluoroethane), or silicone oil. These substances are less dense than water and rise to the top of the eye, and an iridectomy may be beneficial. The iridectomy should be located inferiorly to prevent obstruction of the iridectomy site by the oil or gas. Eyes that have undergone complicated vitreoretinal surgery and have developed elevated IOP require individualized treatment plans. Treatment options include the following:

- removal of silicone oil
- release of the encircling element
- removal of expansile gases
- filtering surgery, including aqueous shunts
- cilioablation

Following panretinal photocoagulation, IOP may become elevated by an angle-closure mechanism. The ciliary body is thickened and rotated anteriorly, and often an anterior annular choroidal detachment occurs. Generally, this secondary glaucoma is self-limited, and therapy is directed at temporary medical management with cycloplegic agents, topical corticosteroids, and aqueous suppressants.

Central retinal vein occlusion (CRVO) sometimes causes early shallowing of the chamber angle, presumably because of swelling of the choroid and ciliary body. In rare cases, the angle becomes sufficiently compromised to cause angle-closure glaucoma. The chamber deepens and the glaucoma resolves over 1 to several weeks. Medical therapy treating the elevated IOP is usually preferred in combination with topical corticosteroids and cycloplegia. However, if the contralateral eye of a patient with CRVO has a potentially occludable anterior chamber angle, the ophthalmologist must consider an underlying pupillary block mechanism and the possible need for bilateral iridectomy.

Nanophthalmos

A nanophthalmic eye is normal in shape but unusually small, with a shortened antero-posterior diameter (<20 mm), a small corneal diameter, and a relatively large lens for the eye volume. Thickened sclera may impede drainage from the vortex veins. These eyes are markedly hyperopic and highly susceptible to angle-closure glaucoma, which occurs at an earlier age than in primary angle closure. Intraocular surgery is frequently complicated by choroidal effusion and nonrhegmatogenous retinal detachment. Choroidal effusion may occur spontaneously, and it can induce angle-closure glaucoma. Laser iridectomy, argon laser peripheral iridoplasty, and medical therapy are the safest ways to manage glaucoma in these patients. Surgery should be avoided if possible because of the high rate of surgical complications. When intraocular surgery is employed, prophylactic posterior sclerotomies may reduce the severity of intraoperative choroidal effusion.

Persistent Fetal Vasculature

Contracting retrolental tissue seen in persistent fetal vasculature (PFV; formerly known as *persistent hyperplastic primary vitreous*) and in retinopathy of prematurity can cause progressive shallowing of the anterior chamber angle with subsequent angle-closure glaucoma. These conditions are discussed in more detail in BCSC Section 6, *Pediatric Ophthalmology and Strabismus,* and Section 12, *Retina and Vitreous.* In PFV, the onset of this complication usually occurs at 3–6 months of age during the cicatricial phase of the disease. However, the angle-closure glaucoma may occur later in childhood.

PFV is usually unilateral and often associated with microphthalmos and elongated ciliary processes. The contracture of the hyperplastic primary vitreous and swelling of a cataractous lens may result in subsequent angle-closure glaucoma.

Flat Anterior Chamber

A flat anterior chamber from any cause can result in the formation of PAS. Debate continues concerning how long a postoperative flat chamber should be treated conservatively before surgical intervention is undertaken. Hypotony in an eye with a postoperative flat chamber following cataract surgery indicates a wound leak until proven otherwise. A Seidel test should be performed to locate the leak. Simple pressure patching or bandage contact lens application will often cause the leak to seal and the chamber to re-form. If the chamber does not re-form, it should be repaired surgically to prevent permanent synechial closure of the angle or other complications of hypotony.

Some ophthalmologists repair the wound leak and re-form a flat chamber following cataract surgery within 24 hours. Others prefer observation in conjunction with corticosteroid therapy for several days to prevent synechiae formation. While iridocorneal contact is well tolerated, if the hyaloid face or an IOL is in contact with the cornea, the chambers should be re-formed without delay to minimize corneal endothelial damage. Early intervention should also be considered in the presence of corneal edema, excessive inflammation, or posterior synechiae formation.

Drug-Induced Secondary Angle-Closure Glaucoma

Topiramate (Topamax), a sulfamate-substituted monosaccharide, is an oral medication prescribed as an antiepileptic and antidepressant. In some patients using this medication, a syndrome characterized by acute myopic shift (>6 D) and acute bilateral angle-closure glaucoma can occur. Patients presenting with this syndrome experience bilateral, sudden loss of vision with acute myopia, bilateral ocular pain, and headache, usually within 1 month of initiating topiramate. Ocular findings of this syndrome include high myopia, a uniformly shallow anterior chamber with anterior iris and lens displacement, microcystic corneal edema, elevated IOP (40–70 mm Hg), a closed anterior chamber angle, and a ciliochoroidal effusion/detachment (Fig 5-30). The underlying mechanism of this syndrome is the ciliochoroidal effusion, which causes the relaxation of zonules and the profound anterior displacement of the lens–iris complex, causing the secondary angle-closure glaucoma and high myopia. The bilateral nature of this form of angle closure should alert the clinician to the possibility of an idiosyncratic response to topiramate. Treatment of this syndrome involves early recognition of the causal systemic medication and immediate discontinuation of the topiramate. In addition to discontinuation of the medica-

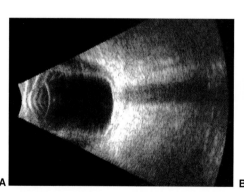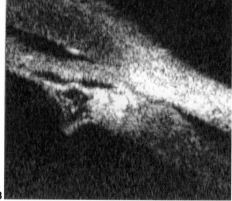

Figure 5-30 **A,** B-scan ultrasound of patient with topiramate-induced angle-closure glaucoma. The choroidal effusion is clearly evident. **B,** Ultrasound view of extremely shallow anterior chamber and closed angle. The posterior choroidal effusion is clearly visible. *(Courtesy of Jonathan Eisengart, MD.)*

tion, medical treatment for the elevated IOP is initiated, generally in the form of aqueous suppressants. Systemic agents such as acetazolamide may also be administered orally or intravenously. Aggressive cycloplegia may help deepen the anterior chamber and relieve the attack. The secondary angle-closure glaucoma usually resolves within 24–48 hours with medical treatment, and the myopia resolves within 1 to 2 weeks of discontinuing the topiramate. Because pupillary block is not an underlying mechanism of this syndrome, a peripheral iridectomy is not indicated. Other sulfonamides, such as acetazolamide, have been reported to cause a similar clinical syndrome.

Epstein DL, Allingham RR, Schuman JS, eds. *Chandler and Grant's Glaucoma*. 4th ed. Baltimore: Williams & Wilkins; 1997.

Ritch R, Shields MB, Krupin T, eds. *The Glaucomas*. 2nd ed. St Louis: Mosby; 1996.

Shields MB. *Textbook of Glaucoma*. 4th ed. Philadelphia: Williams & Wilkins; 2000.

Stamper RL, Lieberman MF, Drake MV, eds. *Becker-Shaffer's Diagnosis and Therapy of the Glaucomas*. 7th ed. St Louis: Mosby; 1999.

CHAPTER 6

Childhood Glaucoma

BCSC Section 6, *Pediatric Ophthalmology and Strabismus,* also discusses the issues covered here.

Definitions and Classification

Primary congenital, or *infantile, glaucoma* is evident either at birth or within the first few years of life. This condition is caused by abnormalities in anterior chamber angle development that obstruct aqueous outflow in the absence of systemic anomalies or other ocular malformation. *Secondary infantile glaucoma* is associated with inflammatory, neoplastic, hamartomatous, metabolic, or other congenital abnormalities. *Primary juvenile glaucoma* is recognized later in childhood (generally after 3 years of age) or in early adulthood.

The term *developmental glaucomas* embraces both primary congenital glaucoma and secondary glaucoma associated with other developmental anomalies, either ocular or systemic. Glaucoma associated with other ocular disorders or with systemic anomalies may be inherited or acquired. The term *buphthalmos* (ox eye) is still used in some diagnostic classification systems to refer to the enlargement of the globe. The developmental glaucomas appear when the onset of elevated IOP occurs before the age of 3 in primary congenital glaucoma or in the pediatric glaucomas associated with other ocular and/or systemic abnormalities.

Epidemiology and Genetics

Glaucoma in the pediatric age group is heterogeneous. Primary congenital glaucoma, which accounts for approximately 50%–70% of the congenital glaucomas, occurs much less frequently than primary adult glaucoma and is believed to be rare (1 in 10,000 births). Of pediatric glaucoma cases, 60% are diagnosed by the age of 6 months and 80% within the first year of life. Approximately 65% of patients are male, and involvement is bilateral in 70% of all cases.

Although some pedigrees suggest an autosomal dominant inheritance, increasingly, more patients show a recessive pattern with incomplete or variable penetrance and possibly multifactorial inheritance. Three major loci of recessively inherited primary congenital glaucoma (*GLC3A, GLC3B,* and *GLC3C*) have been identified on chromosome 2 (2p21), chromosome 1 (1p36), and chromosome 14 (14q24.3), respectively. The genes for primary congenital glaucoma are more prevalent in some ethnic populations than in others. The first gene to be directly implicated in the pathogenesis of primary congenital glaucoma (ie, the cytochrome P4501B1 gene, or *CYP1B1*) was mapped to the 2p21 region. The initial sequence analysis of *CYP1B1* in families previously linked to the GLC3A locus found 3 DNA sequence alterations in several affected individuals. These mutations perfectly segregated with the primary congenital glaucoma phenotype, indicating that *CYP1B1* is the congenital glaucoma gene at the GLC3A locus. Subsequently, reports were made of the *CYP1B1* mutation in families with primary congenital glaucoma in Saudi Arabia, Turkey, Canada, Slovakia, and the United Kingdom. *CYP1B1* is a member of the cytochrome P450 family of drug-metabolizing enzymes.

For parents of pediatric glaucoma patients and for adults whose glaucoma had its onset in childhood, it is advisable to consider genetic counseling.

Pathophysiology

Figure 6-1 shows the normal development, at 11 weeks, of the structures discussed here. Because histopathologic findings in primary congenital glaucoma vary, several theories of pathogenesis have been proposed; these fall into 2 main groups. Some investigators have proposed that a cellular or membranous abnormality in the trabecular meshwork is the primary pathologic mechanism. This abnormality is described as either an anomalous

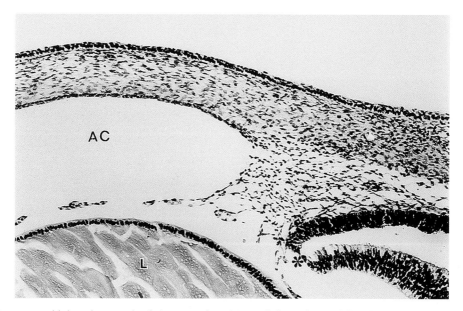

Figure 6-1 Light micrograph of the eye of an 11-week fetus in meridional section. The angular region is poorly defined at this stage and is occupied by loosely arranged, spindle-shaped cells. Schlemm's canal is unrecognizable, and ciliary muscles and ciliary processes are not yet formed; the latter are derived from neural ectodermal fold *(asterisk)*. Corneal endothelium appears continuous with cellular covering of primitive iris. *AC* = anterior chamber. *L* = lens. (Original magnification ×230.) *(Reproduced with permission from Tripathi RC, Tripathi BJ. Functional anatomy of the anterior chamber angle. In: Tasman W, Jaeger EA, eds.* Duane's Foundations of Clinical Ophthalmology. *Philadelphia: Lippincott; 1991.)*

impermeable trabecular meshwork or a Barkan membrane covering the trabecular mesh-work. Other investigators have emphasized a more widespread anterior segment anomaly, including abnormal insertion of the ciliary muscle. These observations are not mutually exclusive.

Although the exact mechanism of primary congenital glaucoma remains unproven, there is little doubt that the disease represents a developmental anomaly of the angle struc-tures. Many of the features of primary congenital glaucoma suggest a developmental arrest in the late embryonic period. See also BCSC Section 2, *Fundamentals and Principles of Ophthalmology,* Part II, Embryology.

Clinical Features and Examination

Characteristic findings of primary congenital glaucoma include the classic triad of pre-senting symptoms in the newborn: *epiphora, photophobia,* and *blepharospasm.* Diagnosis of congenital glaucoma depends on careful clinical evaluation, including measurement of IOP, corneal diameter, and axial length (the latter by ultrasonography and retinos-copy); gonioscopy; and ophthalmoscopy. Optic nerve photography is helpful for future follow-up.

External eye examination may reveal buphthalmos with corneal enlargement greater than 12 mm in diameter during the first year of life. (The normal horizontal corneal diam-eter is 9.5–10.5 mm in full-term newborns and smaller in premature newborns.) Corneal edema may range from mild haze to dense opacification of the corneal stroma because of elevated IOP. Tears in Descemet's membrane, called *Haab striae,* may occur acutely as a result of corneal stretching; these are typically oriented horizontally or concentric to the limbus.

Reduced visual acuity may occur as a result of optic atrophy, corneal clouding, astig-matism, amblyopia, cataract, lens dislocation, or retinal detachment. Amblyopia may be caused by the corneal opacity itself or by refractive error as the eye lengthens under pres-sure and becomes more myopic. The enlargement of the eye causes myopia, whereas tears in Descemet's membrane can cause a large degree of astigmatism. Appropriate measures to prevent or treat amblyopia should be initiated as early as possible.

Often, the clinician can successfully measure the IOP of an infant younger than 6 months without general anesthesia or sedation by performing the measurement while the infant is feeding or immediately thereafter. A complete evaluation of infants requires an examination under anesthesia; however, examination under anesthesia has several im-portant implications. Most general anesthetic agents and sedatives lower IOP. The only exception to this rule is ketamine, which may raise IOP. In addition, infants may become dehydrated in preparation for general anesthesia, also reducing the IOP. The normal IOP in an infant under anesthesia may range from 10 to 15 mm Hg, depending on the tonom-eter. It is therefore essential to measure the IOP as soon as possible after anesthesia has been administered.

Gonioscopy under anesthesia is recommended. The ophthalmologist may find it useful in categorizing the disease and in determining whether a previous goniotomy has been effective or whether it has been covered by peripheral anterior synechiae. In primary childhood glaucoma, the anterior chamber is characteristically deep with a normal appearance to the iris. Findings include a high and flat iris insertion, absence of angle recess, peripheral iris hypoplasia, tenting of the peripheral iris pigment epithelium, and thickened uveal trabecular meshwork. The angle is typically open, with a high insertion of the iris root forming a somewhat scalloped line as a result of abnormal tissue with a shagreened, glistening appearance. This tissue holds the peripheral iris anteriorly. The angle is usually avascular, but loops of vessels from the major arterial circle may be seen above the iris root.

Many of the findings just listed are nonspecific, and the anterior chamber angle of an infant or child without glaucoma differs from that of an adult. Thus, the gonioscopic findings in congenital glaucoma may be difficult to appreciate. If corneal edema prevents an adequate view of the angle, the clinician may improve visibility by removing the epithelium with a scalpel blade or a cotton-tipped applicator soaked in 70% alcohol. Alternatively, the topical application of a hyperosmotic solution is sometimes effective.

Visualization of the optic disc is part of a routine examination and should include both direct and indirect ophthalmoscopy as well as photographs of the disc, when feasible. The optic nerve head of an infant without glaucoma is pink, with a small physiologic cup. Glaucomatous cupping in childhood resembles the cupping seen in adult glaucoma patients, with preferential loss of neural tissue in the superior and inferior poles. But in childhood, unlike adulthood, the scleral canal enlarges in response to elevated IOP, causing enlargement of the cup. Cupping may be reversible if IOP is lowered, and progressive cupping indicates poor control of IOP.

Photographic documentation of the optic disc is useful in following pediatric glaucoma patients. Ultrasonography documents the progression of glaucoma by recording increasing axial length. Following reduction of IOP, the increase in axial length may be minimally reversible, but corneal enlargement may not decrease.

Differential Diagnosis

Many other conditions with similar features are included in the differential diagnosis of primary congenital glaucoma (Table 6-1). Excessive tearing may be caused by an obstruction of the lacrimal drainage system. Ocular abnormalities associated with enlarged corneas include X-linked congenital megalocornea without glaucoma. Tears in Descemet's membrane resulting from birth trauma, often associated with forceps-assisted deliveries, are usually vertical or oblique. Corneal opacification and clouding have many possible causes:

- birth trauma
- dysgeneses (Peters anomaly and sclerocornea)
- dystrophies (congenital hereditary endothelial dystrophy and posterior polymorphous dystrophy)
- choristomas (dermoid and dermislike choristoma)
- intrauterine inflammation (congenital syphilis and rubella)
- inborn errors of metabolism (eg, mucopolysaccharidoses and cystinosis)
- keratomalacia

Table 6-1 Diagnostic Considerations for Symptoms and Signs of Primary Congenital Glaucoma

Excessive tearing
Nasolacrimal duct obstruction
Corneal epithelial defect or abrasion
Conjunctivitis

Corneal enlargement or apparent enlargement
X-linked megalocornea
Exophthalmos
Shallow orbits (eg, craniofacial dysostoses)

Corneal clouding
Birth trauma
Inflammatory corneal disease
Congenital hereditary endothelial dystrophies (CHED), posterior polymorphous dystrophy
Corneal malformations (dermoid tumors, sclerocornea, Peters anomaly)
Keratomalacia
Metabolic disorders with associated corneal abnormalities (mucopolysaccharidoses, sphingolipidoses, cystinoses)
Skin disorders affecting the cornea (congenital ichthyosis and congenital dyskeratosis)
Choristomas (dermis and dermislike choristoma)
Intrauterine inflammation (congenital syphilis and rubella)
Keratitis (eg, herpes)

Optic nerve abnormalities
Optic nerve pit
Optic nerve coloboma
Optic nerve hypoplasia
Optic nerve malformation
Physiologic cupping

- skin disorders that affect the cornea (congenital ichthyosis and congenital dyskeratosis)
- keratitis (eg, herpes)

Long-term Prognosis and Follow-up

Medications have limited long-term value for primary congenital glaucoma in most cases, and surgery is often regarded as the preferred therapy. Medications have a useful role in lowering IOP prior to surgery in order to reduce corneal edema and improve visualization during surgery. The initial procedures of choice are goniotomy or trabeculotomy if the cornea is clear, and trabeculotomy ab externo if the cornea is hazy. The success rates are similar for both procedures in patients with clear corneas.

Trabeculectomy and shunt procedures should be reserved for those cases in which goniotomy or trabeculotomy has failed. Cyclophotocoagulation is necessary in some intractable cases but should be avoided whenever possible because of its potential adverse effects on the lens and the retina.

To control IOP and help clear a cloudy cornea, β-adrenergic antagonists or carbonic anhydrase inhibitors (CAIs) may be used as temporizing therapy prior to surgery. These drugs must be used with caution and at doses appropriate for the child's weight in order to prevent systemic side effects. The parents should be instructed in particular to occlude the nasolacrimal drainage system for at least 3 minutes immediately after administering topical β-adrenergic antagonists and to be alert for apnea and hypotension. Cough may be the first sign that the β-adrenergic antagonists are causing or exacerbating reactive airway disease. Young children given oral CAIs require assessment for possible acidosis, hypokalemia, and feeding problems. Topical CAIs appear to be relatively safe for use in young children. α_2-Adrenergic agonists should be avoided in children because of the risk of central nervous system adverse effects such as apnea. There is debate about how old a child should be before taking α_2-adrenergic agonists, but in no instance should α_2-adrenergic agonists be used in patients younger than 3 years, and they should be used with caution in children younger than 10 years.

Long-term prognosis has greatly improved with the development of effective surgical techniques, particularly for patients who are asymptomatic at birth and present with onset of symptoms before 24 months of age. When symptoms are present at birth or when the disease is diagnosed after 24 months of age, the outlook for surgical control of IOP is more guarded. Even patients whose IOP is usually controlled by surgery may experience late complications such as amblyopia, corneal scarring, strabismus, anisometropia, cataract, lens subluxation, susceptibility to trauma (as occurs in an eye with a thinned sclera), and recurrent glaucoma in the affected or unaffected eye many years later.

Developmental Glaucomas With Associated Ocular or Systemic Anomalies

Associated Ocular Anomalies

Glaucoma may be associated with other ocular abnormalities, including the following conditions:

- microphthalmos
- corneal anomalies (microcornea, megalocornea, cornea plana, sclerocornea, corneal staphyloma)
- anterior segment dysgenesis (Axenfeld-Rieger syndrome, Peters anomaly, iridoschisis)
- aniridia
- lens anomalies (congenital cataracts, lens dislocation, microspherophakia)
- persistent fetal vasculature (persistent hyperplastic primary vitreous)
- congenital ectropion-uvea syndrome

Following are discussions of the more common of these conditions.

Axenfeld-Rieger syndrome

Axenfeld-Rieger (A-R) syndrome is a group of bilateral congenital anomalies that may include abnormal development of the anterior chamber angle, the iris, and the trabecular meshwork. Autosomal dominant inheritance occurs in most cases, but A-R syndrome can also occur sporadically. Approximately 50% of cases are associated with glaucoma. Axenfeld-Rieger syndrome is the result of abnormal development of tissues derived from the neural crest.

Although this syndrome was initially separated into Axenfeld anomaly (posterior embryotoxon with multiple adherent peripheral iris strands), Rieger anomaly (Axenfeld anomaly plus iris hypoplasia and corectopia), and Rieger syndrome (Rieger anomaly plus developmental defects of the teeth or facial bones, including maxillary hypoplasia; redundant periumbilical skin; pituitary abnormalities; or hypospadias), these disorders are now considered variations of the same clinical entity and are combined under the name *Axenfeld-Rieger syndrome.*

The typical corneal abnormality is a posterior embryotoxon (a prominent and anteriorly displaced Schwalbe line), with the remainder of the cornea being normal. Iridocorneal adhesions to the Schwalbe line range from threadlike to broad bands of iris tissue. The iris itself may range from normal to markedly atrophic with corectopia, hole formation, and ectropion uveae. Axenfeld-Rieger syndrome can be distinguished from other conditions that involve abnormalities of the iris, cornea, and anterior chamber, as outlined in Table 6-2.

Peters anomaly

Peters anomaly is a condition of central corneal opacity with adhesions between the central iris and posterior cornea. It is bilateral 80% of the time. The lens may be clear or cataractous. The condition is usually sporadic, although autosomal dominant and autosomal recessive forms have been reported. Approximately 50% of cases are associated with glaucoma.

In Peters anomaly, there is an annular corneal opacity (leukoma) in the central visual axis, with iris strands extending from the collarette to the corneal opacity. This annular corneal opacity corresponds to a central defect in the corneal endothelium and underlying Descemet's membrane. Patients with Peters anomaly may have defects in the posterior stroma, Descemet's membrane, and endothelium without extension of iris strands

Table 6-2 Differential Diagnosis of Axenfeld-Rieger Syndrome

Condition	Differentiating Features
Iridocorneal endothelial syndrome	Unilateral Middle age Corneal endothelial abnormalities
Isolated posterior embryotoxon	Lack of glaucoma, iris changes
Aniridia	Iris hypoplasia Associated corneal and macular changes
Iridoschisis	Lack of angle abnormalities, glaucoma
Peters anomaly	Corneal changes
Ectopia lentis et pupillae	Lack of glaucoma
Oculodentodigital dysplasia	Lack of angle changes, glaucoma

Used with permission from Morrison JC, Pollack IP. *Glaucoma: Science and Practice.* New York: Thieme Medical Publishers; 2003:188.

to the edge of the corneal leukoma. The lens may be in normal position, with or without a cataract, or the lens may be adherent to the posterior layers of the cornea. Patients with corneolenticular adhesions have a higher likelihood of ocular abnormalities such as microcornea and angle anomalies, and of systemic abnormalities, including those of the heart, genitourinary system, musculoskeletal system, ear, palate, and spine.

Aniridia

Aniridia is a bilateral condition characterized by variable iris hypoplasia that often appears as complete absence of the iris. In aniridia, the iris appearance may vary greatly, from a rudimentary stump to a complete, or nearly complete, but thin iris. In addition, patients with aniridia may have limbal stem cell abnormalities that eventually result in a pannus that begins in the peripheral cornea and slowly extends centrally. There may be a role for limbal stem cell transplants in these patients. Cataracts may be present at birth or develop later in life. Many patients with aniridia also have foveal hypoplasia that leads to pendular nystagmus and reduced vision.

Most cases of aniridia are familial and are transmitted in an autosomal dominant form; however, about one-third of cases are isolated sporadic mutations. Approximately 20% of sporadic cases are associated with a chromosomal deletion and an increased risk of Wilms tumor, although relatively few cases of Wilms tumor are seen in the familial form. The aniridia gene locus for both the familial and the sporadic forms is a mutation of the *PAX6* gene on band 13 of the short arm of chromosome 11. Approximately 50%–75% of patients with aniridia develop glaucoma. Though occasionally associated with congenital glaucoma, glaucoma in aniridia usually develops after the rudimentary iris stump rotates anteriorly to progressively cover the trabecular meshwork. This is a gradual process, and glaucoma may not occur until the second decade of life or later.

Although roughly 85% of patients with aniridia have an autosomal dominant form not associated with systemic abnormalities, 2 other types have been described: WAGR syndrome is an autosomal dominant form seen in 13% of aniridia patients and includes *W*ilms tumor, *a*niridia, *g*enitourinary anomalies, and mental *r*etardation; an autosomal recessive form of aniridia, also called *Gillespie syndrome,* is associated with cerebellar ataxia and mental retardation and occurs in 2% of those with aniridia.

Associated Systemic Anomalies and Syndromes

Developmental glaucoma may be associated with other anomalies and multisystem syndromes. Some anomalies are syndromes with known chromosomal abnormalities, systemic disorders of unknown etiology, and ocular congenital disorders. Glaucomas associated with systemic congenital anomalies are summarized in Table 6-3.

A number of systemic disorders are also associated with pediatric glaucoma, including the following:

- Sturge-Weber syndrome
- neurofibromatosis
- Marfan syndrome
- Weill-Marchesani syndrome

Table 6-3 Systemic Congenital Anomalies Associated With Childhood Glaucomas

GLAUCOMA ASSOCIATED WITH SYSTEMIC CONGENITAL SYNDROMES, WITH REPORTED CHROMOSOMAL ABNORMALITIES

Trisomy 21 (Down syndrome, trisomy G syndrome)
Mental deficiency, short stature, cardiac anomalies, hypotonia, atypical facies

Trisomy 13 (Patau syndrome)
Mental retardation, deafness, heart disease, motor seizures

Trisomy 18 (Edwards syndrome, trisomy E syndrome)
Low-set ears, high-arched hard palate, ventricular septal defects, rocker-bottom feet, short sternum, hypertonia

Turner (XO/XX) syndrome
Short stature, postadolescent females with sexual infantilism, webbed neck, mental retardation, congenital deafness, multiple systemic anomalies

GLAUCOMA ASSOCIATED WITH SYSTEMIC CONGENITAL DISORDERS

Lowe (oculocerebrorenal) syndrome
X-linked recessive disease, mental retardation, renal rickets, aminoaciduria, hypotonia, acidemia, cataracts

Stickler syndrome (hereditary progressive arthro-ophthalmopathy)
Autosomal dominant connective tissue dysplasia; ocular, otic, and generalized skeletal abnormalities with high myopia; open-angle glaucoma; cataracts; vitreoretinal degeneration; retinal detachment

Zellweger (cerebrohepatorenal) syndrome
Congenital autosomal recessive syndrome, abnormal facies, cerebral dysgenesis, hepatic interstitial fibrosis, polycystic kidneys, central nervous system abnormalities
Ocular findings: nystagmus, corneal clouding, cataracts, retinal vascular and pigmentary abnormalities, optic nerve head lesions

Hallermann-Streiff syndrome (dyscephalic mandibulo-oculofacial syndrome, François dyscephalic syndrome)
Micrognathia, dwarfism, microphthalmos, cataract, aniridia, optic atrophy

Rubinstein-Taybi (broad-thumb) syndrome
Mental and motor retardation, typical congenital skeletal deformities of large thumbs and first toes
Ocular findings: bushy brows, hypertelorism, epicanthus, anti-mongoloid slant of eyelids, hyperopia, strabismus

Oculodentodigital dysplasia (Meyer-Schwickerath and Weyers syndrome)
Autosomal dominant inheritance, hypoplastic dental enamel, microdontia, bilateral syndactyly, thin nose, microcornea, microphthalmos

Prader-Willi syndrome
Chromosome 15 deletion, muscular hypotonia, hypogonadism, obesity, mental retardation
Ocular findings: ocular albinism, congenital ectropion uveae, iris stromal hypoplasia, angle abnormalities

Cockayne syndrome
Autosomal recessive disorder, dwarfism, mental retardation, progressive wasting, "birdlike" facies
Ocular findings: retinal degeneration, cataracts, corneal exposure, blepharitis, nystagmus, hypoplastic irides, irregular pupils

Fetal alcohol syndrome
Teratogenic effects of alcohol during gestation, facial abnormalities, mental retardation, anterior segment involvement resembling Axenfeld-Rieger syndrome and Peters anomaly, optic nerve hypoplasia

With Sturge-Weber syndrome and neurofibromatosis in particular, upper eyelid involvement is associated with an increased risk of glaucoma. A number of these conditions have ocular findings similar to those of primary congenital glaucoma; in others, the glaucoma is secondary.

Sturge-Weber syndrome

Sturge-Weber syndrome (also known as *encephalotrigeminal angiomatosis*) is usually a unilateral condition with ipsilateral facial cutaneous hemangioma (nevus flammeus or port-wine stain), ipsilateral cavernous hemangioma of the choroid, and ipsilateral leptomeningeal angioma. There is no race or sex predilection, and no inheritance pattern has been established. Glaucoma occurs in 30%–70% of children with this syndrome. When seen in infants with this syndrome, glaucoma is thought to be due to congenital anterior chamber anomalies (similar to congenital glaucoma). Glaucoma developing after the first decade of life is believed to be the result of elevated episcleral venous pressure causing elevated IOP. Involvement of the central nervous system may be associated with seizures, focal neurologic defects, or mental retardation. Surgery should be undertaken with extreme caution in this group of patients, because their risk of choroidal hemorrhage is substantially increased.

Neurofibromatosis

Neurofibromatosis (NF) is the most common phakomatosis. Two forms are recognized. Neurofibromatosis 1 (NF1), also known as *von Recklinghausen disease* or *peripheral neurofibromatosis,* is the most common type, with a prevalence of 1 in 3000–5000 persons. NF1 is localized to band 11 of the long arm of chromosome 17 and is inherited in an autosomal dominant fashion about half the time, with the other cases being sporadic. Ectropion uveae is a common ocular finding whose presence in a neonate should prompt a workup for NF. Other ocular findings include Lisch nodules, optic nerve gliomas, eyelid neurofibromas, and glaucoma. Systemic findings include cutaneous café-au-lait spots, cutaneous neurofibromas, and axillary or inguinal freckling.

Neurofibromatosis 2 (NF2), or *central neurofibromatosis,* is localized to chromosome 22. The principal ocular finding with NF2 is the development of posterior subcapsular cataracts in adolescence or young adulthood. NF2 is not associated with glaucoma. NF2 is defined by the presence of bilateral acoustic neuromas and is frequently accompanied by multiple other nervous system tumors, including meningiomas, schwannomas, and ependymomas, typically involving cranial nerves and spinal cord or nerve roots.

Other Secondary Glaucomas

The causes of secondary glaucoma in infants and children are the same as those in adults: trauma, inflammation, retinopathy of prematurity (angle-closure glaucoma), lens-associated disorders, corticosteroid use, pigmentary glaucoma, and intraocular tumors. Retinoblastoma, juvenile xanthogranuloma, and medulloepithelioma are some of the intraocular tumors known to lead to secondary glaucoma in infants and children. Rubella and congenital cataract are also important associated conditions. It is now recognized that children often develop glaucoma within 3 years of surgery for congenital cataract. They may also develop glaucoma many years after the surgery and require continued follow-up for this reason. Emphasis on removal of all residual cortex during cataract surgery may reduce the occurrence of pediatric aphakic glaucoma following surgery.

Akarsu AN, Turacli ME, Aktan SG, et al. A second locus (GLC3B) for primary congenital glaucoma (Buphthalmos) maps to the 1p36 region. *Hum Mol Genet.* 1996;5(8):1199–1203.

Beck AD. Diagnosis and management of pediatric glaucoma. *Ophthalmol Clin North Am.* 2001;14:501–512.

Higginbotham EJ, Lee DA, eds. *Management of Difficult Glaucoma: A Clinician's Guide.* Boston: Blackwell Scientific Publications; 1994.

Isenberg SJ, ed. *The Eye in Infancy.* 2nd ed. St Louis: Mosby; 1994.

Mandal AK, Netland PA. *The Pediatric Glaucomas.* Philadelphia: Butterworth-Heinemann; 2006.

Plásilová M, Feráková E, Kádasi L, et al. Linkage of autosomal recessive primary congenital glaucoma to the GLC3A locus in Roms (Gypsies) from Slovakia. *Hum Hered.* 1998;48(1):30–33.

Sarfarazi M, Stoilov I, Schenkman JB. Genetics and biochemistry of primary congenital glaucoma. *Ophthalmol Clin North Am.* 2003;16;543–554.

Shields MB. *Textbook of Glaucoma.* 4th ed. Philadelphia: Williams & Wilkins; 2000.

Stamper RL, Lieberman MF, Drake MV, eds. *Becker-Shaffer's Diagnosis and Therapy of the Glaucomas.* 7th ed. St Louis: Mosby; 1999.

Stoilov I, Akarsu AN, Sarfarazi M. Identification of three different truncating mutations in cytochrome P4501B1 *(CYP1B1)* as the principal cause of primary congenital glaucoma (Buphthalmos) in families linked to the GLC3A locus on chromosome 2p21. *Hum Mol Genet.* 1997;6(4):641–647.

Tasman W, Jaeger EA, eds. *Duane's Clinical Ophthalmology.* Philadelphia: Lippincott; 2002.

Walton DS, Katavounidou G. Newborn primary congenital glaucoma: 2005 update. *J Pediatr Ophthalmol Strabismus.* 2005;42(6):333–341.

CHAPTER 7

Medical Management of Glaucoma

Two decisions arise in choosing an appropriate glaucoma therapy: when to treat and how to treat. The risks of therapy must always be weighed against the anticipated benefits.

A patient with early open-angle glaucoma may be difficult to distinguish from a glaucoma suspect. Because the latter has a lower risk of ultimate significant vision loss, the decision of when to treat the glaucoma suspect who has not demonstrated actual nerve damage remains an individual determination for each patient. The Ocular Hypertension Treatment Study (OHTS) has provided invaluable information to assist in this discussion. The first goal of OHTS was to determine the efficacy and safety of lowering IOP (from a baseline of 24–32 mm Hg) in decreasing the risk of development of primary open-angle glaucoma (POAG). A 22.5% decrease in IOP with medications decreased the risk of developing POAG from 9.5% in the observation group to 4.4% in the treatment group at 5 years. There were few safety concerns. The second goal was to identify baseline characteristics that increased the risk of POAG in patients with ocular hypertension. Higher IOP, older age, larger cup–disc diameter, greater pattern standard deviation, and reduced central corneal thickness (CCT) were shown by multivariate analysis to be significant risk factors. Race and family history, as well as other factors, were not found to be independent risk factors by multivariate analysis. The recommendation was made that treatment should be considered in those with a moderate or high risk of developing POAG. The Scoring Tool for Assessing Risk (STAR) was unveiled in 2005 and can be useful in assessing the risk of glaucoma development in an individual patient with untreated ocular hypertension. More recently, a calculator that estimates an ocular hypertensive individual's 5-year risk of developing POAG was found to have high precision. Based on the pooled OHTS-EGPS (European Glaucoma Prevention Study) predictive model, this tool (STAR II) may be helpful in deciding when to initiate preventive treatment.

The goal of currently available glaucoma therapy is to preserve visual function by lowering IOP below a level that is likely to produce further damage to the nerve. The treatment regimen that achieves this goal with the lowest risk, fewest adverse effects, and least disruption of the patient's life, taking into account the cost implications of treatment, should be the one employed. The so-called target pressure should actually be a range, with an upper IOP limit that is unlikely to lead to further damage of the nerve in a given patient. The range should be individualized, based on the IOP at which damage is thought to have occurred, severity of the damage, life expectancy, and associated risk factors.

The more advanced the glaucomatous process on initial presentation, the lower the target range generally needs to be to prevent further progression. This more aggressive target is meant to minimize the risk of progressive glaucoma damage and vision loss. Once the optic nerve is damaged, it is more likely to incur more damage, and if severe visual loss is present, there is greater impact on the patient from any additional damage that may occur. An initial reduction in the IOP of 20% from baseline is suggested. However, reduction of IOP to the target pressure range does not guarantee that progression will not occur. *Therefore, the target pressure range needs to be constantly reassessed and changed as dictated by IOP fluctuations, optic nerve changes, and/or visual field progression.* Several studies have shown that a consistently lower IOP results in a reduced risk of progressive glaucoma damage.

The anticipated benefits of any therapeutic regimen should justify the risks, and regimens associated with substantial adverse effects should be reserved for patients with a high probability of progressive visual loss. For example, it is reasonable to expose a patient to the adverse effects of oral carbonic anhydrase inhibitors (CAIs) when significant damage to the visual field and optic nerve has occurred and the elevated IOP is not controlled by medications with fewer potential adverse effects. When progressive visual field loss or cupping has not been established, however, the physician should exercise caution in subjecting a patient to the risk of the significant adverse effects of these agents.

The interrelationship between medical and surgical therapy is also complex. The treatment of pupillary block angle-closure glaucoma and primary congenital glaucoma is primarily surgical, either laser or incisional, with medical therapy taking a secondary role. Initial treatment of POAG has commonly been medical, with surgery undertaken only if medical treatment fails or is not well tolerated. The Glaucoma Laser Trial (GLT) found that as initial glaucoma therapy, argon laser trabeculoplasty was at least as effective as medications. The Collaborative Initial Glaucoma Treatment Study (CIGTS) reported that medical therapy was essentially equally as effective as surgical therapy in preventing POAG progression. In fact, the rate of progression at 5 years was substantially less than anticipated. This has been attributed to the definition of progression used in the study and to the aggressive IOP lowering obtained in both groups. Surgical therapy is discussed in detail in Chapter 8, Surgical Therapy for Glaucoma.

The Advanced Glaucoma Intervention Study (AGIS): 4. Comparison of treatment outcomes within race: seven-year results. *Ophthalmology.* 1998;105:1146–1164.

The Advanced Glaucoma Intervention Study (AGIS): 7. The relationship between control of intraocular pressure and visual field deterioration. The AGIS Investigators. *Am J Ophthalmol.* 2000;130:429–440.

Kass MA, Heuer DK, Higginbotham EJ, et al. The Ocular Hypertension Treatment Study: a randomized trial determines that topical ocular hypotensive medication delays or prevents the onset of primary open-angle glaucoma. *Arch Ophthalmol.* 2002;120:701–713.

Leske MC, Heijl A, Hussein M, et al. Factors for glaucoma progression and the effect of treatment: the Early Manifest Glaucoma Trial. *Arch Ophthalmol.* 2003;121:48–56.

Lichter PR, Musch DC, Gillespie BW, et al. Interim clinical outcomes in the Collaborative Initial Glaucoma Treatment Study comparing initial treatment randomized to medications or surgery. *Ophthalmology.* 2001;108:1943–1953.

Medeiros FA, Weinreb RN, Sample PA, et al. Validation of a predictive model to estimate the risk of conversion from ocular hypertension to glaucoma. *Arch Ophthalmol.*
2005;123(10):1351–1360.

Ocular Hypertension Treatment Study Group, European Glaucoma Prevention Study Group,
Gordon MO, et al. Validated prediction model for the development of primary open-angle
glaucoma in individuals with ocular hypertension. *Ophthalmology.* 2007;114:10–19.

Treatment of secondary glaucoma is similar to treatment of primary glaucoma, with some exceptions. The underlying cause of the glaucoma should be addressed, if possible. For example, panretinal photocoagulation (PRP) is probably the most vital part of the treatment of neovascular glaucoma and should be done in concert with the appropriate method of IOP reduction. There is currently much interest in the use of intravitreal anti-vascular endothelial growth factor (anti-VEGF) medication as an adjunct to PRP in the treatment of neovascular glaucoma. In uveitic glaucoma, topical, intraocular, and systemic steroids as well as nonsteroidal anti-inflammatory medications are used to treat the inflammatory process. Prostaglandin analogs and parasympathomimetics are generally avoided because of their potential for exacerbating intraocular inflammation.

The efficacy of the therapeutic regimen should be reevaluated periodically. Specifically, a 1-eyed therapeutic trial should be considered to assess the efficacy of new medications; a reverse therapeutic trial can be performed to assess existing regimens. A reverse trial entails discontinuing a medication in only 1 eye and then comparing the effect in the treated versus the untreated eye. This allows assessment of the continued efficacy or side effects of a drug.

Medical Agents

Ocular hypotensive agents are divided into several groups based on chemical structure and pharmacologic action. The groups of agents in common clinical use include

- prostaglandin analogs
- β-adrenergic antagonists (nonselective and selective)
- parasympathomimetic (miotic) agents, including cholinergic and anticholinesterase agents
- carbonic anhydrase inhibitors (oral and topical)
- adrenergic agonists (nonselective and selective α_2-agonists)
- combination medications
- hyperosmotic agents

The actions and adverse effects of the various glaucoma medications are listed in Table 7-1, along with dosage information and other concerns. The reader is referred back to this table throughout the discussions in this chapter. BCSC Section 2, *Fundamentals and Principles of Ophthalmology,* discusses and illustrates the mechanisms of action of these medications in Part V, Ocular Pharmacology.

Netland PA, ed. *Glaucoma Medical Therapy: Principles and Management.* 2nd ed. Ophthalmology Monograph 13. New York: Oxford University Press; 2007.

Table 7-1 Glaucoma Medications

Class/Compound	Brand Name	Strengths	Dosage	Method of Action	IOP Decrease	Side Effects Ocular	Side Effects Systemic	Comments, Including Time to Peak Effect and Washout
Prostaglandin analogs								
Latanoprost	Xalatan	.005%	qd	Increase uveoscleral outflow	25%–32%	Increased pigmentation of iris and lashes, hypertrichosis, blurred vision, keratitis, CME, anterior uveitis, conjunctival hyperemia, reactivation of herpes keratitis	Flulike symptoms, joint/muscle pain, headache	±IOP-lowering effect with miotic Peak: 10–14 hours Washout: 4–6 weeks Maximum IOP-lowering effect may take up to 6 weeks to occur
Travoprost	Travatan	.004%	qd	Same as above	25%–32%	Same as above	Same as above	Same as above
	Travatan Z	.004%	qd	Same as above	25%–32%	Same as above	Same as above	Same as above
Bimatoprost	Lumigan	0.03%	qd	Increase uveoscleral and trabecular outflow	27%–33%	Same as above	Same as above	Same as above
Unoprostone isopropyl	Rescula	0.15%	bid	Increase trabecular outflow	13%–18%	Same as above	Same as above	Peak: unknown Washout: unknown
β-adrenergic antagonists (beta-blockers)								
Nonselective								
Timolol maleate	Timoptic XE	0.25, 0.5%	qd	Decrease aqueous production	20%–30%	Blurring, irritation, corneal anesthesia, punctate keratitis, allergy	Bradycardia, heart block, bronchospasm, lowered blood pressure, decreased libido, CNS depression, mood swings, reduced exercise tolerance	May be less effective if patient on systemic beta-blockers; short-term escape, long-term drift Peak: 2–3 hours Washout: 1 month
	Timoptic	0.25, 0.5%	qd, bid	Same as above				
	Timolol gel	0.5%	qd	Same as above				
Timolol-LA	Istalol	0.5%	qd	Same as above	20%–30%	Same as above	Same as above	Same as above
Timolol hemihydrate	Betimol	0.5%	qd, bid	Same as above	20%–30%	Same as above	Same as above	Less expensive
Levobunolol	Betagan	0.25, 0.5%	qd, bid	Same as above	20%–30%	Same as above	Same as above	Peak: 2–6 hours Report of iritis
Metipranolol	OptiPranolol	0.3%	bid	Same as above	20%–30%	Same as above	Same as above	Peak: 2 hours

Carteolol hydrochloride	Ocupress	1.0%	qd, bid			Intrinsic sympathomimetic	May have less effect on nocturnal pulse, blood pressure Peak: 4 hours Washout: 1 month
Selective							
Betaxolol	Betoptic (S)	0.25%	bid	Same as above	15%–20%	Fewer pulmonary complications	Peak: 2–3 hours Washout: 1 month

Adrenergic agonists

Nonselective

Epinephrine	Epifrin	0.25, 0.5, 1.0, 2.0%	bid	Improve aqueous outflow	15%–20%	Irritation, conjunctival hyperemia (rebound), eyelid retraction, mydriasis, adrenochrome deposits, follicular conjunctivitis (allergy), cystoid macular edema in aphakia, pseudophakia	Hypertension, headache, extra systoles	Peak: variable, initial IOP rise followed by reduction lasting 12–24 hours Washout: 7–14 days Not currently available in the US
Dipivefrin HCL	Propine	0.1%	bid	Same as above	Same as above	Same as above	Prodrug makes systemic effects less likely	Peak/washout: same as epinephrine

α₂-adrenergic agonists

Selective

Apraclonidine HCl	Iopidine	0.5, 1.0%	bid, tid	Decrease aqueous production, decrease episcleral venous pressure	20%–30%	Irritation, ischemia, allergy, eyelid retraction, conjunctival blanching, follicular conjunctivitis, puritis, dermatitis, ocular ache, photopsia, miosis	Hypotension, vasovagal attack, dry mouth and nose, fatigue	Useful in pre- or postlaser or cataract surgery, tachyphylaxis Peak: <1–2 hours Washout: 7–14 days

(Continued)

Table 7-1 (continued)

Class/Compound	Brand Name	Strengths	Dosage	Method of Action	IOP Decrease	Side Effects Ocular	Side Effects Systemic	Comments, Including Time to Peak Effect and Washout
Highly selective								
Brimonidine tartrate 0.2%	Alphagan	0.2%	bid, tid	Decrease aqueous production, increase uveoscleral outflow	20%–30%	Blurring, foreign body sensation, eyelid edema, dryness, less ocular sensitivity/allergy than Iopidine	Headache, fatigue, hypotension, insomnia, depression, syncope, dizziness, anxiety	Primary adrenergic agent in current use, highly α_2 selective Peak: 2 hours Washout: 7–14 days
Brimonidine tartrate in Purite 0.15%	Alphagan P	0.15%	bid, tid	Same as above	Same as above	Same except less allergy than Alphagan	Same except less fatigue and depression than Alphagan	Same as above
Parasympathomimetic (miotic) agents								
Cholinergic agonists (direct acting)								
Pilocarpine HCl	Isopto Carpine	0.2%–10.0%	bid–qid	Increase trabecular outflow	15%–25%	Posterior synechiae, keratitis, miosis, brow ache, cataract growth, angle-closure potential, myopia, retinal tear/detachment, dermatitis, change in retinal sensitivity, color vision changes, epiphora	Increased salivation, increased secretion (gastric), abdominal cramps	Exacerbation of cataract effect, more effective in lighter irides Peak: 1½–2 hours Washout: 48 hours
	Pilocar	0.5, 1.0, 2.0, 3.0, 4.0, 6.0%	bid–qid					
Pilocarpine gel	Pilopine Gel HS	4.0%	qhs	Increase trabecular outflow	15%–25%	Same as above	Same as above	Same as above Peak: 2–3 hours Washout: 48 hours
Carbachol*	Isopto Carbachol	1.5, 3.0%	bid, tid	Same as above	15%–25%	May be useful in patients with pilocarpine sensitivity		Intraoperative carbachol useful to lower IOP

*Also has indirect actions

Anticholinesterase agents (indirect acting)

Echothiophate iodide	Phospholine Iodide	0.125%	qd, bid, qod	Same as above	15%–25%	Intense miosis, iris pigment cyst, myopia, cataract, retinal detachment, angle closure, punctal stenosis, pseudopemphigoid, epiphora	Same as pilocarpine; more gastrointestinal difficulties	Increased inflammation with ocular surgery; may be helpful in aphakia, anesthesia risks (prolonged recovery); useful in eyelid-lash lice, postoperative cataract surgery

Carbonic anhydrase inhibitors

Oral

Acetazolamide	Diamox	62.5, 125, 250 mg	bid–qid	Decrease aqueous production	15%–20%	None	Poor tolerance of carbonated beverages, acidosis, depression, malaise, hirsutism, flatulence, paresthesias, numbness, lethargy, blood dyscrasias, diarrhea, weight loss, renal stones, loss of libido, bone marrow depression, hypokalemia, cramps, anorexia, altered taste, increased serum urate, enuresis	Sulfa allergy, caution to patients susceptible to ketoacidosis, hepatic insufficiency
	Diamox Sequels	500 mg	qd, bid					
Acetazolamide (parenteral)	Diamox	500 mg 5–10 mg/kg	Usually ≤1 qd q6–8 hrs	Same as above	Same as above	Same as above	Same as above	Same as above
Dichlorphenamide	Daranide	50 mg	bid, tid	Same as above	Same as above	Same as above	Same as above	Same as above
Methazolamide	Neptazane	25, 50, 100 mg	bid, tid	Same as above	Same as above	Same as above	Same as above	Same as above

Topical

Dorzolamide	Trusopt	2.0%	bid, tid	Same as above	15%–20%	Induced myopia, blurred vision, stinging, keratitis, conjunctivitis, dermatitis	Less likely to induce systemic effects of CAI, but may occur; bitter taste	Peak: 2–3 hours Washout: 48 hours
Brinzolamide	Azopt	1%	bid, tid	Same as above	Same as above	Less stinging when compared to Trusopt	Same as above	Same as above

(Continued)

Table 7-1 (continued)

Class/Compound	Brand Name	Strengths	Dosage	Method of Action	IOP Decrease	Ocular	Systemic	Comments, Including Time to Peak Effect and Washout
						Side Effects		
Hyperosmotic agents								
Mannitol (parenteral)	Osmitrol	20% soln 50% soln	2 g/kg body wt	Osmotic gradient dehydrates vitreous		IOP rebound, increased aqueous flare	Urinary retention, headache, congestive heart failure, expansion of blood volume, diabetic complications, nausea, vomiting, diarrhea, electrolyte disturbance, renal failure	Caution in heart failure; may precipitate diabetic ketoacidosis; useful in acute increased IOP; isosorbide less nausea, vomiting
Glycerin (oral)		50% soln	4–7 oz	Same as above		Similar to above	Can cause problems in diabetic patients; similar to above	
Fixed combinations								
Timolol/ Dorzolamide	Cosopt (Timoptic/ Trusopt)	0.5%/2%	bid	Decrease aqueous production	25%–30%	Same as nonselective beta-blocker, topical CAI	Same as nonselective beta-blocker, topical CAI	Peak: 2–3 hours Washout: 1 month
Timolol/ Latanoprost	Xalcom	0.5%/0.005%	qd	Same as nonselective beta-blocker and latanoprost	Greater than monotherapy with each individually	Same as nonselective beta-blocker and latanoprost	Same as nonselective beta-blocker and latanoprost	Not currently available in US
Timolol/ Travoprost	DuoTrav	0.5%/0.004%	qd	Same as nonselective beta-blocker and travoprost	Same as above	Same as nonselective beta-blocker and travoprost	Same as nonselective beta-blocker and travoprost	Not currently available in US
	Extravan	0.5%/0.004%	qd					
Timolol/ Bimatoprost	Ganfort	0.5%/0.03%	qd	Same as nonselective beta-blocker and bimatoprost	Same as above	Same as nonselective beta-blocker and bimatoprost	Same as nonselective beta-blocker and bimatoprost	Not currently available in US
Timolol/ Brimonidine tartrate	Combigan	0.5%/0.2%	bid	Same as nonselective beta-blocker and alpha-agonist	Same as above	Same as nonselective beta-blocker and alpha-agonist	Same as nonselective beta-blocker and alpha-agonist	Obtained FDA approval November 2007; the degree of conjunctival hyperemia is less than that with brimonidine alone

Prostaglandin Analogs

Prostaglandin analogs are also referred to as *hypotensive lipids*. Other terms used to categorize this group are *prostamide* (bimatoprost) and *decosanoid* (unoprostone isopropyl). Currently, 4 prostaglandin analogs are approved for clinical use: latanoprost, travoprost, bimatoprost, and unoprostone isopropyl.

All of these drugs work by increasing aqueous outflow. Prostaglandin analogs have a method of action that appears to be both pressure dependent and pressure independent. The exact mechanism by which these drugs increase outflow is not known; however, it has been shown that latanoprost results in increased spaces between the muscle fascicles within the ciliary body, presumably increasing aqueous flow and uveoscleral outflow.

Latanoprost and travoprost are prodrugs that penetrate the cornea and become biologically active after being hydrolyzed by corneal esterase. Both latanoprost and travoprost reduce IOP by 25%–32%. Bimatoprost lowers IOP by 27%–33%; unoprostone is less effective, lowering IOP 13%–18%. Latanoprost, travoprost, and bimatoprost are used once a day, usually at night, and are less effective when used twice daily; unoprostone is used twice daily. Because some patients may respond better to one agent in this class than to another, switching drugs after a trial of 4–6 weeks may prove helpful.

An ocular side effect unique to this class of drugs is the darkening of the iris and periocular skin as a result of an increased number of melanosomes within the melanocytes. The side effect of iris pigmentation is permanent and correlates with baseline iris pigmentation. Blue irides may experience increased pigmentation in 10%–20% of eyes in the initial 18–24 months of therapy, whereas nearly 60% of eyes that are light brown, blue-green, or 2-toned may experience increased pigmentation over the same time period. The long-term sequelae of this side effect are unknown, but there are no data to suggest any additional risk. Other side effects reported in association with the use of a topical prostaglandin analog include conjunctival hyperemia, hypertrichosis (Fig 7-1), trichiasis, distichiasis, hyperpigmentation of the eyelid skin, and hair growth around the eyes. These effects appear to be reversible with drug discontinuation. Exacerbations of underlying herpes keratitis, cystoid macular edema, and uveitis

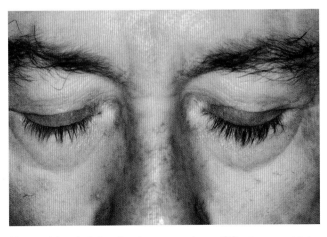

Figure 7-1 Hypertrichosis following latanoprost use OS. *(Courtesy of F. Jane Durcan, MD.)*

have been reported. The latter 2 side effects are more common in eyes with preexisting risk factors for either macular edema or uveitis. Studies to date have demonstrated that the incidence of these side effects varies among these 4 agents. Hyperemia is more common with bimatoprost and travoprost. Because bimatoprost, latanoprost, and travoprost reach peak effect 10–14 hours after administration, bedtime application is recommended to maximize efficacy and decrease patient symptoms related to vascular dilation.

Camras CB, Alm A, Watson P, Stjernschantz J. Latanoprost, a prostaglandin analog, for glaucoma therapy: efficacy and safety after 1 year of treatment in 198 patients. Latanoprost Study Group. *Ophthalmology.* 1996;103:1916–1924.

Higginbotham EJ, Schuman JS, Goldberg I, et al. One-year, randomized study comparing bimatoprost and timolol in glaucoma and ocular hypertension. *Arch Ophthalmol.* 2002;120:1286–1293.

Netland PA, Landry T, Sullivan EK, et al. Travoprost compared with latanoprost and timolol in patients with open-angle glaucoma or ocular hypertension. *Am J Ophthalmol.* 2001;132:472–484.

β-Adrenergic Antagonists

Topical β-adrenergic antagonists lower IOP by inhibiting cyclic adenosine monophosphate (cAMP) production in ciliary epithelium, thereby reducing aqueous humor secretion 20%–50% (2.5 μL/min to 1.9 μL/min), with a corresponding IOP reduction of 20%–30%. The effect of β-adrenergic antagonists, or beta-blockers, on aqueous production occurs within 1 hour of instillation and can be present for up to 4 weeks after discontinuation. Evidence suggests that beta-blockers decrease aqueous production during the day but have much less effect during sleep. As systemic absorption occurs, a contralateral IOP-lowering effect in the untreated eye can also be observed. Most beta-blockers are approved for twice-daily therapy. In many cases, once daily with the nonselective agents is possible. Generally, dosing first thing in the morning is preferred in order to effectively blunt an early-morning pressure rise while minimizing the risk of systemic hypotension during sleep, when aqueous production is diminished. Many nonselective beta-blockers are available in more than 1 concentration. For example, timolol 0.25% is as effective in lowering IOP as timolol 0.5% in many patients.

Beta-blockers are additive in combination with miotics, adrenergic agonists, CAIs (both topical and systemic), and prostaglandin analogs. Combinations of beta-blockers and nonselective adrenergic agonists are only slightly additive, whereas more effect can be expected when beta-blockers are combined with an α_2-adrenergic agonist. The magnitude of additional IOP lowering with prostaglandin analogs remains indeterminate. Approximately 10%–20% of the patients treated with topical beta-blockers fail to respond with significant lowering of the IOP. It should be noted that if a patient is on systemic beta-blocker therapy, the addition of a topical beta-blocker may be significantly less effective. Extended use of beta-blockers may reduce their effectiveness, because the response of beta receptors is affected by constant exposure to an agonist (long-term drift, tachyphylaxis). Similarly, receptor saturation (drug-induced up-regulation of beta receptors) may occur within a few weeks, with loss of effectiveness (short-term escape).

Six topical β-adrenergic antagonists are approved for use for the treatment of glaucoma in the United States: betaxolol, carteolol, levobunolol, metipranolol, timolol maleate, and timolol hemihydrate. All except betaxolol are nonselective β_1 and β_2 antagonists. The activity of β_1 is largely cardiac and that of β_2, largely pulmonary. Because betaxolol is a selective β_1 antagonist, it is safer than the nonselective beta-blockers for use in patients with pulmonary, CNS, or other systemic conditions, but beta-blocker–related adverse effects can still occur. The IOP-lowering effect of betaxolol is less than that of the nonselective β-adrenergic antagonists.

Carteolol demonstrates intrinsic sympathomimetic activity, which means that, while acting as a competitive antagonist, it also causes a slight to moderate activation of receptors. Thus, even though carteolol produces beta-blocking effects, these may be tempered, reducing the effect on cardiovascular and respiratory systems.

Both ocular and systemic adverse effects of β-adrenergic antagonists are listed in Table 7-1. They include bronchospasm, bradycardia, increased heart block, lowered blood pressure, reduced exercise tolerance, and CNS depression. Patients with diabetes may experience reduced glucose tolerance and masking of hypoglycemic signs and symptoms. Abrupt withdrawal of ocular beta-blockers can exacerbate symptoms of hyperthyroidism. Although betaxolol is somewhat less effective than the other β-adrenergic antagonists in lowering IOP, it may be a safer alternative in some patients.

Before the clinician prescribes a beta-blocking agent, it is important to determine whether the patient has ever had asthma, because beta-blockers may induce severe bronchospasm in susceptible patients. The pulse should be measured and the beta-blocker withheld if the pulse rate is slow or if more than first-degree heart block is present. Myasthenia gravis may be aggravated by the use of these drugs. The use of a gel vehicle has been shown to decrease the plasma concentration of beta-blockers compared to the solution modalities.

Other adverse effects of beta-blockers include lethargy, mood changes, depression, altered mentation, light-headedness, syncope, visual disturbance, corneal anesthesia, punctate keratitis, allergy, impotence, reduced libido, and alteration of serum lipids. In children, beta-blockers should be used with caution, because of the relatively high systemic levels achieved. Although topical beta-blockers have been shown to decrease high-density lipoprotein and increase cholesterol levels, there is no evidence that this translates into an actual increase in cardiovascular risk. However, this effect on the plasma lipid profile should be considered, particularly in those patients taking medications that affect plasma lipids. Carteolol may have less effect on serum lipid levels than timolol.

The use of nasolacrimal occlusion or eyelid closure decreases systemic absorption and increases intraocular penetration of medications; nasolacrimal occlusion is particularly important with the use of beta-blockers. For patients who use multiple medications, these procedures may also facilitate a time interval between the instillation of different medications.

Many of the beta-blockers are available as generic agents. Although the generic agents may be less expensive, it is important to realize that in most cases few data are available to prove or disprove equivalent efficacy or similar side effect profiles between branded and generic medications. In addition, because multiple generics are available for a given agent, there is the possibility that differences exist among generic agents—differences that could affect patient care.

Novack GD. Ophthalmic beta blockers since timolol. *Surv Ophthalmol.* 1987;31:307–327.

Van Buskirk EM. Adverse reactions from timolol administration. *Ophthalmology.* 1980;87: 447–450.

Parasympathomimetic Agents

Parasympathomimetic agents, commonly called *miotics,* have been used in the treatment of glaucoma for more than 100 years. They are divided into 2 groups:

- direct-acting cholinergic agonists
- indirect-acting anticholinesterase agents

Direct-acting agents affect the motor end plates in the same way as acetylcholine, which is transmitted at postganglionic parasympathetic junctions, as well as at other autonomic, somatic, and central synapses. Indirect-acting agents inhibit the enzyme acetylcholinesterase, thereby prolonging and enhancing the action of naturally secreted acetylcholine. *Pilocarpine* is the most commonly prescribed direct-acting agent. *Carbachol* has both direct and indirect actions, although its primary mechanism is direct. The only indirect-acting agent still available is *echothiophate iodide* (see Table 7-1), although the availability is limited.

Both direct-acting and indirect-acting agents reduce IOP by causing contraction of the longitudinal ciliary muscle, which pulls the scleral spur to tighten the trabecular meshwork, increasing the outflow of aqueous humor. These agents can reduce the IOP by 15%–25%. The currently accepted indications for miotic therapy include long-term treatment of increased IOP in patients with some filtering angle open and prophylaxis for angle-closure glaucoma prior to iridectomy.

Miotic agents have been associated with numerous ocular side effects. Induced myopia resulting from ciliary muscle contraction is a side effect common to all cholinergic agents. Brow ache may accompany the ciliary spasm, and the miosis interferes with vision in dim light and in patients with lens opacities. They have also been associated with retinal detachment; thus, a peripheral retinal evaluation is suggested before the initiation of therapy. Miotics may be cataractogenic, particularly the indirect-acting agents. In children they may also induce the formation of iris pigment epithelial cysts. In pediatric and adult patients, these agents may cause epiphora by both direct lacrimal stimulation and punctal stenosis. These agents may also cause ocular surface changes resulting in drug-induced pseudopemphigoid.

Other potential ocular side effects include increased bleeding during surgery and increased inflammation and severe fibrinous iridocyclitis postoperatively. Because miotics can break down the blood–aqueous barrier, their use in treating uveitic glaucoma should be limited.

Systemic adverse effects, seen mainly with indirect-acting medications, include diarrhea, abdominal cramps, increased salivation, bronchospasm, and even enuresis. While on indirect-acting agents and for up to 6 weeks after discontinuation, patients should avoid using depolarizing agents such as succinylcholine. Use of miotics may induce a paradoxical angle closure, because contraction of the ciliary muscle leads to forward movement of the lens–iris diaphragm, an increase in the anteroposterior diameter of the lens, and a very miotic pupil. These effects may increase pupillary block.

Although this class of agents effectively lowers IOP, it is often so poorly tolerated because of ocular side effects, that other classes of agents are frequently preferred. In addition, particularly the weaker miotics require frequent instillation, 3 or 4 times daily, further limiting their usefulness. Pilocarpine adsorbed to a polymer gel is administered once daily at bedtime (pilocarpine gel), and induced myopia and miosis are less prominent with the gel than with the drops, but they may still interfere with vision. Pilocarpine is, however, among the most affordable of agents, and the miotics are much better tolerated in eyes that are not phakic. Because of the potential for significant ocular and systemic side effects, indirect-acting parasympathomimetic agents are used less commonly than the direct-acting agents. Indeed, indirect-acting agents are usually reserved for treatment of glaucoma in aphakic and pseudophakic eyes when IOP is not controlled by less toxic agents and in phakic eyes when filtering surgery has failed.

Hoskins HD Jr, Kass MA. Cholinergic drugs. In: Hoskins HD Jr, Kass MA, eds. *Becker-Shaffer's Diagnosis and Therapy of the Glaucomas.* 6th ed. St Louis: Mosby; 1989:420–434.

Carbonic Anhydrase Inhibitors

CAIs decrease aqueous humor formation by direct antagonist activity on ciliary epithelial carbonic anhydrase and perhaps, to a lesser extent only with systemic administration, by production of a generalized acidosis. The enzyme carbonic anhydrase is also present in many other tissues, including corneal endothelium, iris, retinal pigment epithelium, red blood cells, brain, and kidney. More than 90% of the ciliary epithelial enzyme activity must be abolished to decrease aqueous production and lower IOP.

The systemic agents can be given orally, intramuscularly, and intravenously. They are most useful in acute situations (eg, acute angle-closure glaucoma). Oral CAIs begin to act within 1 hour of administration, with maximal effect within 2–4 hours. Sustained-release acetazolamide can reach peak effect within 3–6 hours of administration. For intravenous acetazolamide, the onset of action is within 2 minutes of administration, and peak effect is reached within15 minutes. Because of the side effects of systemic CAIs, however, long-term therapy with these agents should be reserved for patients whose glaucoma cannot be controlled by alternative topical therapy.

Systemic acetazolamide and methazolamide are the oral CAI agents most commonly used; another agent in this group is dichlorphenamide (see Table 7-1). Methazolamide has a longer duration of action and is less bound to serum protein than is acetazolamide. Methazolamide and sustained-release acetazolamide are the best tolerated of the systemic CAIs. Methazolamide is metabolized by the liver, thereby decreasing some of the risk of systemic adverse effects. Acetazolamide is not metabolized and is excreted in urine.

Adverse effects of systemic CAI therapy are usually dose-related. Many patients develop paresthesias of the fingers or toes and complain of lassitude, loss of energy, and anorexia. Weight loss is common. Abdominal discomfort, diarrhea, loss of libido, impotence, and an unpleasant taste in the mouth, as well as severe mental depression, may also occur. There is an increased risk of the formation of calcium oxylate and calcium phosphate renal stones. Because methazolamide has greater hepatic metabolism and causes less acidosis, it may be less likely than acetazolamide to cause renal lithiasis.

CAIs are chemically derived from sulfa drugs, and this may cause allergic reactions and cross reactivity similar to those of sulfa drugs. Aplastic anemia is a rare but potentially fatal idiosyncratic reaction to CAIs. Thrombocytopenia and agranulocytosis can also occur. Although routine complete blood counts have been suggested, they are not predictive of this idiosyncratic reaction and are not routinely recommended. Hypokalemia is a potentially serious complication that is especially likely when oral CAIs are used concurrently with another drug that causes potassium loss (eg, a thiazide diuretic). Serum potassium should be monitored regularly in such patients.

Oral CAIs are potent medications with significant side effects. Therefore, the lowest dose that reduces the IOP to an acceptable range should be used. Methazolamide is often effective in doses as low as 25–50 mg given 2 to 3 times daily. Acetazolamide may be started at 62.5 mg every 6 hours, and higher doses may be used, if tolerated. Sustained-release formulations such as Diamox Sequels may have fewer side effects.

Topical CAI agents are also available for long-term treatment of IOP elevation. Dorzolamide and brinzolamide are sulfonamide derivatives that reduce aqueous formation by direct inhibition of carbonic anhydrase in the ciliary body. They have fewer systemic side effects than the oral agents. Dorzolamide and brinzolamide are currently available for use 3 times daily, although reduction of IOP is only slightly greater when compared to twice-daily therapy. For patients on an adequate oral CAI dose, there is no advantage to also using a topical CAI.

Common adverse effects of topical CAIs include bitter taste, blurred vision, and punctate keratopathy. Ocular surface irritation with dorzolamide may be a result of the drug's relative greater acidity (lower pH) when compared with that of brinzolamide. Eyes with compromised endothelial cell function may also be at risk of corneal decompensation. The brinzolamide suspension may cause more blurring than the dorzolamide solution. Systemic lassitude is a side effect as well.

Fraunfelder FT, Fraunfelder FW, eds. *Drug-Induced Ocular Side Effects*. Boston: Butterworth-Heinemann; 2001.

Strahlman E, Tipping R, Vogel R. A double-masked, randomized 1-year study comparing dorzolamide (Trusopt), timolol, and betaxolol. International Dorzolamide Study Group. *Arch Ophthalmol*. 1995;113:1009–1016.

Adrenergic Agonists

The nonselective adrenergic agonists epinephrine and dipivefrin increase conventional trabecular and uveoscleral outflow. The latter appears to be influenced by epinephrine-induced stimulation of prostaglandin synthesis. Interestingly, epinephrine-related agents may initially increase aqueous production; with long-term use, however, they decrease it. Adding nonselective adrenergic agonists to the administration of beta antagonists usually produces modest additional pressure lowering.

Epinephrine, a mixed alpha and beta agonist, has variable IOP-lowering effect, and many patients become intolerant owing to extraocular reactions.

Dipivefrin is a *prodrug* that is chemically transformed into epinephrine by esterase enzymes in the cornea. Dipivefrin has greater corneal penetration than epinephrine salt, and the activity of this drug before its alteration by the esterase enzymes is relatively low.

Table 7-1 lists potential ocular and systemic side effects of both epinephrine and dipivefrin. Important systemic adverse effects include headache, increased blood pressure, tachycardia, arrhythmia, and nervousness. Epinephrine causes adrenochrome deposits from oxidized metabolites in the conjunctiva, cornea, and lacrimal system, and it may stain soft contact lenses (Fig 7-2). The use of these agents often causes pupillary dilation as a consequence of alpha-agonist action that stimulates norepinephrine receptors, and thus may precipitate or aggravate angle closure in susceptible individuals. Allergic blepharoconjunctivitis occurs in approximately 20% of patients over time. Cystoid macular edema may be precipitated or exacerbated in aphakic and pseudophakic eyes without intact posterior capsules. This maculopathy is usually reversible if recognized early; however, epinephrine or dipivefrin should be used with caution in these eyes. Rebound conjunctival hyperemia is common when these drugs are discontinued. Although this condition is harmless, patients may be disturbed by the appearance and usually need reassurance. Clinically, the nonselective adrenergic agents have been essentially completely replaced with the selective α_2-adrenergic agonists because of their improved efficacy and side effect profiles.

α_2-Adrenergic agonists

Ocular α_1 effects include vasoconstriction, pupillary dilation, and eyelid retraction, whereas ocular α_2 effects are primarily IOP reduction and possible neuroprotection. Apraclonidine and brimonidine are relatively selective α_2 agonists that have been developed for glaucoma therapy. Brimonidine is much more highly selective for the α_2 receptor than is apraclonidine.

Apraclonidine hydrochloride (para-aminoclonidine) is an α_2-adrenergic agonist and a clonidine derivative that prevents the release of norepinephrine at nerve terminals. It

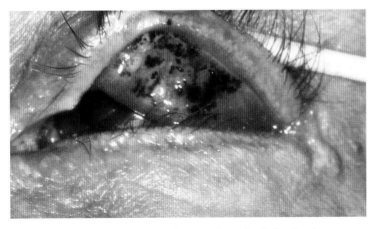

Figure 7-2 Conjunctiva with black adrenochrome deposits following long-term epinephrine use. *(Courtesy of Elizabeth A. Hodapp, MD.)*

decreases aqueous production as well as episcleral venous pressure and improves trabecular outflow. However, its true ocular hypotensive mechanism is not fully understood. When administered preoperatively and postoperatively, the drug is effective in diminishing the acute IOP rise that follows argon laser iridectomy, argon laser trabeculoplasty, Nd:YAG laser capsulotomy, and cataract extraction. Apraclonidine hydrochloride may be effective for the short-term lowering of IOP, but development of topical sensitivity and tachyphylaxis often limits long-term use.

Use of brimonidine tartrate encounters less tachyphylaxis than does apraclonidine, and allergenicity such as follicular conjunctivitis and contact blepharitis-dermatitis (Fig 7-3) is also lower (up to 40% for apraclonidine, less than 15% for brimonidine 0.2%, and less than 10% for brimonidine-Purite 0.15%). Brimonidine-Purite 0.15% has been shown to be as efficacious as brimonidine 0.2% but with a lower incidence of all side effects. It contains a lower concentration without benzalkonium chloride as the preservative at a neutral pH. Cross sensitivity to brimonidine in patients with known hypersensitivity to apraclonidine is minimal. Systemic side effects include dry mouth and lethargy. The use of brimonidine in infants and young children should be avoided because of an increased risk of somnolence, hypotension, seizures, apnea, and serious derangements of neurotransmitters in the CNS, presumably due to increased CNS penetration of the drug. Brimonidine lowers IOP by decreasing aqueous production and increasing uveoscleral outflow. As with beta-blockers, a peripheral mechanism may account for part of the IOP reduction from brimonidine 0.2%, as a 1-week, single-eye treatment trial caused a statistically significant reduction of 1.2 mm Hg in the fellow eye.

Brimonidine's peak IOP reduction is approximately 26% (2 hours postdose). At peak, it is comparable to a nonselective beta-blocker and superior to the selective beta-blocker betaxolol, although at trough (12 hours postdose), the reduction is only 14%–15%, or less effective than the nonselective beta-blockers but comparable to betaxolol during the first 6–12 months of therapy. Though approved for therapy 3 times daily, brimonidine is commonly used twice daily, particularly when used as an adjunctive agent.

Caution is recommended when either apraclonidine or brimonidine is used in patients on a monoamine oxidase inhibitor (MAOI) or tricyclic antidepressant therapy.

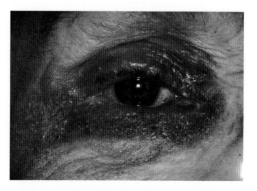

Figure 7-3 Contact blepharitis-dermatitis following alpha-agonist use. *(Courtesy of F. Jane Durcan, MD.)*

Apraclonidine has a much greater affinity for α_1 receptors than does brimonidine and is therefore more likely to produce vasoconstriction in the eye.

Robin AL. Argon laser trabeculoplasty medical therapy to prevent the intraocular pressure rise associated with argon laser trabeculoplasty. *Ophthalmic Surg.* 1991;22:31–37.

Schuman JS, Horwitz B, Choplin NT, David R, Albracht D, Chen K. A 1-year study of brimonidine twice daily in glaucoma and ocular hypertension: a controlled, randomized, multicenter clinical trial. *Arch Ophthalmol.* 1997;115:847–852.

Combined Medications

Medications that are combined and placed in a single bottle have the potential benefits of improved efficacy, convenience, and compliance, as well as reduced cost. Cosopt, the fixed combination of a beta-blocker (timolol maleate 0.5%) and topical CAI (dorzolamide 2%), demonstrates similar efficacy compared with the 2 agents given separately: timolol maleate 0.5% twice daily and Trusopt 2% given 3 times daily. The advantage of this combined therapy may be the convenience and lessened confusion of 1 bottle rather than 2, which may increase the likelihood of greater compliance. However, the twice-daily dosing may create greater exposure to the potential beta-blocker systemic side effects, as beta-blockers alone are generally equally effective when given only once daily. The ocular side effects are the same as for both drugs individually. The indications for this combined medication may be as a substitute for both a beta-blocker and a topical CAI. If Cosopt is used as monotherapy, a monocular trial of timolol should be tried first. If timolol is effective in significantly, but not sufficiently, lowering the IOP, then a monocular trial of dorzolamide should be used with timolol. An alternative trial could involve Cosopt in 1 eye twice daily and timolol in the opposite eye. It is important to prove that the timolol component and the dorzolamide component each have an effect on IOP before the combined medication is chosen, except in emergent situations. Other fixed-combination medications for lowering IOP are approved for use elsewhere in the world. In the United States, new fixed-combination medications are currently undergoing review for approval by the Food and Drug Administration (FDA) (see Table 7-1).

Strohmaier K, Snyder E, DuBiner H, Adamsons I. The efficacy and safety of the dorzolamide-timolol combination versus the concomitant administration of its components. Dorzolamide-Timolol Study Group. *Ophthalmology.* 1998;105:1936–1944.

Hyperosmotic Agents

Hyperosmotic agents are used to control acute episodes of elevated IOP. Common hyperosmotic agents include oral glycerin and intravenous mannitol.

When given systemically, hyperosmotic agents lower the IOP by increasing the blood osmolality, which creates an osmotic gradient between the blood and the vitreous humor, drawing water from the vitreous cavity and reducing IOP. The larger the dose and the more rapid the administration, the greater the reduction in IOP because of the increased gradient. The substance distributed only in extracellular water (eg, mannitol) is more effective than a drug distributed in total body water (eg, urea). When the blood–aqueous barrier is disrupted, the osmotic agent enters the eye faster than when the barrier is intact, thus reducing both the effectiveness of the drug and its duration of action.

Hyperosmotic agents are rarely administered for longer than a few hours because their effects are transient as a result of the rapid reequilibration of the osmotic gradient. They become less effective over time, and a rebound elevation in IOP may occur if the agent penetrates the eye and reverses the osmotic gradient.

Adverse effects of these drugs include headache, mental confusion, backache, acute congestive heart failure, and myocardial infarction. The rapid increase in extracellular volume and cardiac preload caused by hyperosmotic agents may precipitate or aggravate congestive heart failure. Intravenous administration is more likely than oral dosage to cause this problem. In addition, subdural and subarachnoid hemorrhages have been reported after treatment with hyperosmotic agents. Glycerin can produce hyperglycemia or even ketoacidosis in patients with diabetes, because it is metabolized into sugar and ketone bodies. Hypoglycemic agents, as well as oral CAIs, are contraindicated in patients in renal failure or on dialysis.

General Approach to Medical Treatment

Open-Angle Glaucoma

The clinician should tailor therapy for open-angle glaucoma to the individual needs of the patient. As noted previously, a target IOP range is established as a goal. However, the effectiveness of therapy can only be established by careful repeated scrutiny of the patient's optic nerve and visual field status.

Characteristics of the medical agents available for the treatment of glaucoma are summarized in Table 7-1. The clinician making management decisions should keep efficacy and compliance in mind. Treatment is usually initiated with a single topical medication, unless the starting IOP is extremely high, in which case 2 or more medications may be indicated. The selection of the agent for initial medical therapy should be individualized based on the efficacy, safety, and tolerability of the drug and the patient's status and needs. A brief discussion of treatment options with the patient can be effective in determining the optimal choice. Prostaglandin analogs, beta-blockers, α_2-agonists, and topical CAIs are all reasonable choices for first-line therapy. The once-daily prostaglandin analogs are the most effective agents to lower IOP and have the best systemic safety profile. Thus, they are commonly the first class of medications used in most patients. Beta-blockers are the best tolerated in and about the eye. Because of the variability of IOP, it is best (unless the IOP is extremely high) to test the medication in 1 eye until the effectiveness of therapy has been established. At that point, both eyes can be treated.

Patients should be taught how to space their medications, and instructional charts should be given. It may be useful to coordinate the administration of medication with a part of the daily routine such as meals. Patients should be shown how to administer eyedrops properly. Eyedrops to be given at the same time should be separated by at least 5 minutes to prevent washout of the first by the second. Instructions on nasolacrimal occlusion or gentle eyelid closure to reduce the systemic effects from topical eye medications should be given. Teaching the patient to close the eyes for 1–3 full minutes after instillation of the drop helps promote corneal penetration and reduce systemic absorption. An assistive drop device may be considered, especially for patients who live alone or who are unable to successfully instill drops.

If one drug is not adequate to reduce IOP to the estimated desired safe level, the initial agent may be discontinued and another agent tried, preferably as a therapeutic trial in 1 eye. If no single agent controls the pressure, a combination of topical agents should be used. Again, individualizing the choice of agent is helpful for selection of the next best choice. These choices include miotic therapy in nonphakic patients, and, rarely, systemic CAIs may be used for short periods when the clinical situation warrants the risk of adverse effects. Clearly, when the individual requires 3 or more medications, compliance becomes more difficult and the potential for local ocular and systemic side effects increases.

Patients who are intolerant of multiple topical glaucoma agents secondary to local ocular side effects may be experiencing reactions to the preservatives. Benzalkonium chloride (BAK) is the most commonly used agent and is present in nearly all available topical ophthalmic eyedrops. If a reaction is suspected, alternatives include preservative-free timolol maleate (unit dose), brimonidine 0.15% preserved with purite, timolol in gel-forming solution preserved with benzododecinium bromide, and BAK-free travaprost preserved in the bottle with an ionic buffered system. If the level of glaucoma damage permits, it may be beneficial, for rehabilitation of the ocular surface, to stop all topical medications and use nonpreserved artificial tears frequently. The temporary use of oral CAIs may be useful to lower IOP during this period, if clinically warranted.

Patients rarely associate systemic side effects with topical drugs and, consequently, seldom volunteer symptoms. The ophthalmologist must inquire about these symptoms. Communication with the primary care physician is important not only to let the family doctor know the potential side effects of antiglaucoma medication but also to discuss the interactions of any other systemic medications with the glaucoma process. Modification of systemic beta-blocker therapy for hypertension, for example, may affect glaucoma control. Physicians should be aware that compliance may decline as the complexity and expense of the medical regimen increase.

Patients with open-angle glaucoma require careful monitoring. IOP, though important, is only one of the factors to monitor, and optic nerve photographs or drawings and visual fields must be compared periodically to determine the stability of the disease (see Chapter 3). The condition of the patient and the severity of the disease determine how often each of these parameters must be checked. If the cupping or visual field damage shows evidence of progression despite apparent control of acceptable IOP, other diseases should be considered (see the discussion of normal-tension glaucoma in Chapter 4). Other possible explanations include an IOP level too high for the particular patient's optic nerve, IOP that may be spiking at times when the patient is not in the office, thin central corneal thickness, sleep apnea, concomitant angle closure, and poor patient compliance.

Angle-Closure Glaucoma

Medical treatment for acute angle-closure glaucoma is aimed at preparing the patient for laser iridectomy. The goals of medical treatment are to reduce IOP rapidly to prevent further damage to the optic nerve, to clear the cornea, to reduce intraocular inflammation, to allow pupillary constriction, and to prevent formation of posterior and peripheral anterior synechiae (see Chapter 5). Treatment of chronic angle closure is the same as that for POAG, although miotics play a greater role; however, use of miotics may induce a paradoxical increase in IOP if the angle is closed and the trabecular meshwork is nonfunctional.

Use of Glaucoma Medications During Pregnancy or by Nursing Mothers

Unfortunately, there is little definitive information concerning the use of glaucoma medications in pregnant women or nursing mothers. The FDA has designated brimonidine as a class B agent, and all other glaucoma agents are class C. The CAIs have been shown to be teratogenic in rodents, and prostaglandins increase uterine contractility. Thus, although human information is lacking, oral CAIs should not be used by women in their childbearing years or by those who are pregnant. Beta-blockers are concentrated fivefold in breast milk. Because of the effects on infants, beta-blockers, as well as brimonidine, should be avoided in nursing mothers. In general, it is prudent to minimize the use of medications in these patients whenever possible, and the clinician may want to consider laser trabeculoplasty in cases where visual loss is a concern.

Brauner SC, Chen TC, Hutchinson BT, Chang MA, Pasquale LR, Grosskreutz CL. The course of glaucoma during pregnancy: a retrospective case series. *Arch Ophthalmol.* 2006;124(8):1089–1094.

Compliance

Prescribing medications for patients does no good if patients do not use them. The first step in improving compliance is to educate patients. The patient who understands the importance and benefits of treatment is more likely to comply. Education also includes a discussion of treatment alternatives such that the patient can participate in the selection of specific therapies. When patients are aware of the possible side effects, compliance is enhanced. It is also vital to teach patients how to instill medications and confirm that they or someone else will be successful in instilling eyedrops. The next step in enhancing compliance is to design the treatment regimen so that it is as simple as possible. The fewest number of medications, instilled with the least frequency, is optimal. When multiple drugs and doses are needed, coordinate the schedule to daily events and make sure the patient understands the regimen. A written schedule is very helpful.

For patients whose visual function could be aided or enhanced by visual rehabilitation, the American Academy of Ophthalmology (AAO) provides *SmartSight,* a Web site, which is available at http://one.aao.org/SmartSight.

CHAPTER 8

Surgical Therapy for Glaucoma

Surgical treatment for glaucoma is usually undertaken when medical therapy is not appropriate, not tolerated, not effective, or not properly utilized by a particular patient, and the glaucoma remains uncontrolled with either documented progressive damage or a very high risk of further damage. Surgery is usually the primary approach for both congenital glaucoma and pupillary block glaucoma. In patients with primary open-angle glaucoma (POAG), surgery has traditionally been considered when medical therapy has failed. Caution is especially important because of the potential adverse effects of surgery, including bleb-associated problems, cataracts, and infection. Early studies of trabeculectomy as initial therapy for glaucoma, which were performed before the introduction of some contemporary antiglaucoma medications, suggested that trabeculectomy might offer some advantages—better IOP control, reduction in the number of patient visits to the doctor, and possibly better visual field preservation, for example. The results of the Collaborative Initial Glaucoma Treatment Study (CIGTS) confirmed that initial surgical therapy achieves better IOP control than does initial medical therapy. However, this finding did not translate to better visual field stabilization in the average subject because those who received initial surgical treatment had a higher risk of cataract in the longer term. In both groups, there was a low incidence of visual field progression. Based on this study and current practice, most clinicians defer incisional surgery until after an attempt is made to treat with medical therapy.

Lichter PR, Musch DC, Gillespie BW, et al. Interim clinical outcomes in the Collaborative Initial Glaucoma Treatment Study comparing initial treatment randomized to medications or surgery. *Ophthalmology.* 2001;108:1943–1953.

Migdal C, Gregory W, Hitchings R. Long-term functional outcome after early surgery compared with laser and medicine in open-angle glaucoma. *Ophthalmology.* 1994;101:1651–1657.

Musch DC, Gillespie BW, Niziol LM, et al. Cataract extraction in the Collaborative Initial Glaucoma Treatment Study: incidence, risk factors, and the effect of cataract progression and extraction on clinical and quality-of-life outcomes. *Arch Ophthalmol.* 2006;124(12):1694–1700.

When surgery is indicated, the clinical setting must guide the selection of the appropriate procedure. Each of the many possible procedures is appropriate in specific conditions and clinical situations. Many different glaucoma surgical procedures are performed to lower IOP. Among these are trabeculectomy and its variations, nonpenetrating IOP-lowering procedures, implantation of aqueous shunts, angle surgery for congenital and angle-closure glaucoma, and ciliary body ablation. Other procedures, such as iridectomy and gonioplasty, address the problems of aqueous access to the angle. For each condition, it is necessary to understand the indications, contraindications, and preoperative evaluation necessary for surgical planning. Understanding the pathophysiology of the disease, as discussed throughout this volume, is essential to generating an appropriate surgical plan.

Glaucoma surgery can be accomplished with laser or incisional surgical techniques. The discussion in this chapter follows a systematic approach to help the clinician in decision making. Each surgical procedure is described in terms of indications, contraindications, techniques, and complications and other considerations.

Surgery for Open-Angle Glaucoma

Laser Trabeculoplasty

Laser trabeculoplasty (LTP) is a technique whereby laser energy is applied to the trabecular meshwork in discrete spots, usually one half of the circumference of the trabecular meshwork (180°) per treatment. Various modalities of LTP exist, including argon laser trabeculoplasty (ALT), diode laser trabeculoplasty, and selective laser trabeculoplasty (SLT).

Indications

Historically, LTP was indicated when a glaucoma patient who was on maximum tolerated medical therapy and whose angle was open on gonioscopy required lower IOP. Currently, most clinicians still initiate some form of medical therapy before advancing to LTP, but LTP may be considered as an initial or next step in the management of glaucoma. Patients who are intolerant of or noncompliant with initial medical therapy may be candidates for LTP. The question the surgeon and patient must address is when, in the course of glaucoma therapy, it is appropriate to employ LTP.

The Glaucoma Laser Trial (GLT) Research Group conducted a multicenter, randomized clinical trial to assess the efficacy and safety of ALT as an alternative to treatment with topical medication in patients with newly diagnosed, previously untreated POAG. Within the first 2 years of follow-up, ALT as initial therapy appeared to be as effective as medication. However, more than half of the eyes treated initially with laser required the addition of 1 or more medications to control IOP over the course of the study. Further, the medication protocols used in the study no longer resemble the medical regimens commonly employed for the treatment of POAG.

Glaucoma Laser Trial Research Group. The Glaucoma Laser Trial (GLT): 2. Results of argon laser trabeculoplasty versus topical medicines. *Ophthalmology*. 1990;97:1403–1413.

Glaucoma Laser Trial Research Group. The Glaucoma Laser Trial (GLT) and glaucoma laser trial follow-up study: 7. Results. *Am J Ophthalmol*. 1995;120:718–731.

LTP effectively reduces IOP in patients with POAG, pigmentary glaucoma, and exfoliation syndrome. Aphakic and pseudophakic eyes may respond less favorably than phakic eyes. IOP control does not seem to be diminished by subsequent cataract extraction. When effective, LTP is expected to lower IOP 20%–25%. LTP is not effective for treating normal-tension glaucoma and certain types of secondary glaucoma, such as uveitic glaucoma.

Mechanism

Several possible mechanisms of action have been proposed for the increased outflow facility following successful LTP. The treated area of trabecular meshwork may shrink, causing stretching of adjacent areas. Chemical mediators, specifically interleukin-1β and tumor necrosis factor-α, are released from trabecular meshwork cells, increasing outflow facility through induction of specific matrix metalloproteinases. It has been suggested that there is a different mechanism for SLT involving selective effects on pigmented endothelial cells and possible activation of macrophages.

Contraindications

There are few contraindications to LTP for the treatment of POAG when the angle is accessible. LTP is not advised in patients with inflammatory glaucoma, iridocorneal endothelial (ICE) syndrome, neovascular glaucoma, or synechial angle closure, or in patients with developmental glaucoma. LTP can be tried in angle recession, but the underlying tissue alterations may cause it to be ineffective. Another relative contraindication of LTP is the lack of effect in the fellow eye. If the eye has advanced damage and high IOP, LTP is unlikely to achieve the required low target pressure.

Preoperative evaluation

As with all ocular surgery, the preoperative evaluation for LTP should include a detailed medical and ocular history and a comprehensive eye examination. Particular attention must be paid to visual field examination, gonioscopy, and optic nerve evaluation. The angle must be open on gonioscopy. Whereas eyes require some visible pigment in the angle for effective LTP, the degree of pigmentation in the angle will determine the power setting. The more pigmented the trabecular meshwork, the less energy is required for both argon and selective lasers to create the necessary effect.

Technique

In the argon laser procedure, a 50-μm laser beam of 0.1-second duration is focused through a goniolens at the junction of the anterior nonpigmented and the posterior pigmented edge of the trabecular meshwork (Fig 8-1). Application to the posterior trabecular meshwork tends to produce inflammation, pigment dispersion, prolonged elevation of IOP, and peripheral anterior synechiae (PAS). The power setting (300–1000 mW) should be titrated to achieve the desired endpoint: blanching of the trabecular meshwork or production of a tiny bubble. If a large bubble appears, the power is reduced and titrated to achieve the proper effect. As LTP was originally described, laser energy was applied to the entire circumference (360°) of the trabecular meshwork. Evidence suggests that many patients have a satisfactory IOP reduction with less risk of short-term pressure elevation when only one half of the circumference (180°) is treated, using approximately 40–50 applications over 180°.

The procedure with the diode laser is similar; a 75-μm laser beam is focused through a goniolens with a power setting of 600–1000 mW and duration of 0.1 second.

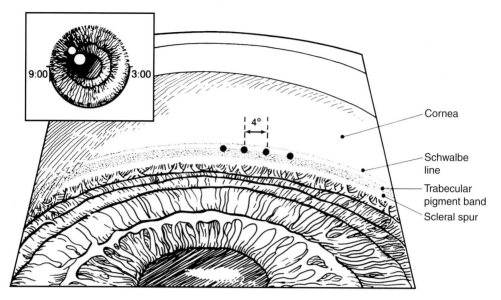

Figure 8-1 Position of argon laser trabeculoplasty treatment in the trabecular meshwork. Inset shows 180° application of laser treatment. *(After Solish AM, Kass MA. Laser trabeculoplasty. In: Waltman SR, Keates RH, Hoyt CS, eds.* Surgery of the Eye. *New York: Churchill Livingstone; 1988:1.)*

Selective laser trabeculoplasty

SLT is an FDA-approved procedure in which the laser targets intracellular melanin. A frequency-doubled (532-nm) Q-switched Nd:YAG laser with a 400-μm spot size is used to deliver 0.4–1.0 mJ of energy for 0.3 ns to perform the procedure. Results suggest that the procedure is safe and effective, with IOP results similar to those achieved with ALT. Preliminary claims also suggest that this procedure may be repeatable, although more recent data question this. Histologic studies have shown less coagulative damage after SLT and fewer structural changes of the trabecular meshwork after SLT compared with ALT. Long-term and re-treatment studies are being conducted to clarify and validate these preliminary claims.

Damji KF, Bovell AM, Hodge WG, et al. Selective laser trabeculoplasty versus argon laser trabeculoplasty: results from a 1-year randomized clinical trial. *Br J Ophthalmol.* 2006;90(12):1490–1494.

Kramer TR, Noecker RJ. Comparison of the morphologic changes after selective laser trabeculoplasty and argon laser trabeculoplasty in human eye bank eyes. *Ophthalmology.* 2001;108:773–779.

Latina MA, Sibayan SA, Shin DH, Noecker RJ, Marcellino G. Q-switched 532-nm Nd:YAG laser trabeculoplasty (selective laser trabeculoplasty): a multicenter, pilot, clinical study. *Ophthalmology.* 1998;105(11):2082–2090.

McIlraith I, Strasfeld M, Colev G, Hutnik CM. Selective laser trabeculoplasty as initial and adjunctive treatment for open-angle glaucoma. *J Glaucoma.* 2006;15(2):125–130.

Weinreb RN, Ruderman J, Juster R, Wilensky JT. Influence of the number of laser burns administered on the early results of argon laser trabeculoplasty. *Am J Ophthalmol.* 1983;95(3):287–292.

Complications

The most significant complication of LTP is a transient rise in IOP, which occurs in approximately 20% of patients. IOP has been reported to reach 50–60 mm Hg, and this transient rise may cause additional damage to the optic nerve. This rise is less common when only 180° of the angle is treated per session.

IOP elevations are of particular concern in patients with advanced cupping. Rises in IOP are usually evident within the first 1–4 hours of treatment, and all patients should be monitored closely for this complication. The adjunctive use of topical apraclonidine 1% or brimonidine 0.2% has been shown to blunt postoperative pressure elevation. Other medications shown to blunt the IOP spikes include beta-blockers, pilocarpine, and carbonic anhydrase inhibitors (CAIs). Hyperosmotic agents and oral CAIs may be helpful in eyes with IOP spikes not responsive to topical medications.

Low-grade iritis may follow LTP. Some surgeons routinely treat with topical anti-inflammatory drugs for 4–7 days; others use them only if inflammation develops. Other complications of LTP include hyphema, the formation of PAS, and the rare persistent elevation of IOP requiring filtering surgery.

Results and long-term follow-up

From 4 to 6 weeks should be allowed before the full effect of the first treatment is evaluated and a decision about additional treatment is made. Approximately 80% of patients with medically uncontrolled open-angle glaucoma experience a drop in IOP for a minimum of 6–12 months following LTP. Longer-term data have shown that 50% of patients with an initial response maintain a significantly lower IOP 3–5 years after treatment. Success at 10 years is approximately 30%. Highest success rates are seen in older patients with POAG and in pseudoexfoliative glaucoma. Eyes with pigmentary glaucoma may show a good initial decrease in IOP, but with continued pigment shedding, this decrease may not be sustained.

Elevation of IOP may recur in some patients after months or even years of control. Additional laser treatment may be helpful in some patients, especially if the entire angle has not been treated previously. Re-treatment of an angle that has been fully treated (approximately 80–100 spots over 360°) has a lower success rate and a higher complication rate than does primary treatment. If initial LTP fails to bring IOP under control, a trabeculectomy should be considered.

Chung PY, Schuman JS, Netland PA, Lloyd-Muhammad RA, Jacobs DS. Five-year results of a randomized, prospective, clinical trial of diode vs argon laser trabeculoplasty for open-angle glaucoma. *Am J Ophthalmol.* 1998;126:185–190.

Mitrev PV, Schuman JS. Lasers in glaucoma management. *Focal Points: Clinical Modules for Ophthalmologists.* San Francisco: American Academy of Ophthalmology; 2001, module 9.

Ritch R, Shields MB, Krupin T, eds. *The Glaucomas.* 2nd ed. St Louis: Mosby; 1996.

Wise JB, Witter SL. Argon laser therapy for open-angle glaucoma: a pilot study. *Arch Ophthalmol.* 1979;97:319–322.

Incisional Surgery for Open-Angle Glaucomas

Incisional surgery is indicated in open-angle glaucoma when IOP cannot be maintained by nonsurgical therapies at a level considered low enough to prevent further pressure-related damage to the optic nerve or visual field loss. The glaucoma may be uncontrolled for various reasons:

- Maximum tolerated medical therapy fails to adequately reduce IOP.
- Glaucomatous optic neuropathy or visual field loss is progressing despite apparent "adequate" reduction of IOP with medical therapy.
- The patient cannot comply with the necessary medical regimen.

Although incisional procedures to lower IOP are traditionally referred to as *filters*, it would be more correct physiologically and anatomically to refer to them as *fistulizing procedures*. In this discussion, the popular term *filter* is used, because it remains in widespread use. The goal of filtering surgery is to create a new pathway (fistula) for the bulk flow of aqueous humor from the anterior chamber through the surgical defect in the sclera into the subconjunctival and sub-Tenon spaces. The filtering procedure most commonly used is the guarded trabeculectomy. Full-thickness procedures have largely fallen into disuse because of both the high complication rate and the introduction of antifibrotic agents in particular.

Indications

Incisional surgery is indicated for the treatment of glaucoma when a patient whose optic nerve function is failing or is likely to fail is already on the maximum tolerated medical therapy and is not likely to achieve a sufficient IOP reduction with laser treatment.

This statement raises several important considerations. The presence of glaucoma with a high probability of optic nerve damage is a clear indication. With the potential complications of glaucoma surgery, however, it is not reasonable to perform a trabeculectomy in an eye with ocular hypertension and a low risk of developing damage. In less clear-cut situations—for example, when 1 eye has sustained significant damage and the IOP is high in the fellow eye despite maximum tolerated medical therapy—some surgeons will recommend surgery prior to unequivocal detection of damage.

The maximum tolerated medical therapy can be confirmed only when therapy is advanced beyond the tolerated level and patient intolerance is documented. This is clearly unnecessary and frustrating for both physician and patient. An alternative concept is *core therapy*, in which treatment consists of those medications likely to work well in combination. If a patient does not have a satisfactory IOP response, the physician may make a few alterations, but it is likely that further medical intervention will simply delay indicated surgery. Although a large number of drugs are available for use in this setting, IOP response diminishes each time a drug is added. Also, determining the maximum tolerated level does not require the use of every class of IOP-lowering medication.

Failure of medical therapy may be the result of poor patient compliance with therapy, in itself a relative indication for surgery. Some patients may use their medications only shortly before an office visit. Thus, there may be progression despite apparent acceptable IOP. It is difficult to elicit an accurate history in this situation. When poor patient compliance is suspected, it may be appropriate to move to surgery sooner, as further changes in medical therapy are unlikely to improve IOP control.

Although the hallmark of glaucoma is progressive optic nerve damage, it is actually relatively uncommon to make a surgical decision based on the detection of progressive change in the optic nerve or retinal nerve fiber layer. The main clinical indications for surgery are progression of visual field damage and uncontrolled IOP, even though multiple field examinations may be required to determine with certainty that a damaged field has become more damaged. Many decisions to operate are based on a clinical judgment that the IOP is too high considering the stage of the disease. Thus, whereas an IOP of 25 mm Hg is not an indication for surgery in an eye with ocular hypertension, surgery may be indicated to lower this IOP in the setting of advanced glaucomatous optic neuropathy. It is not always necessary to perform LTP before proceeding to trabeculectomy. Certain conditions tend not to respond well to LTP. Eyes with very high IOP and advanced optic nerve damage are unlikely to achieve substantial and sufficient IOP lowering with LTP.

Weinreb RN, Mills RP, eds. *Glaucoma Surgery: Principles and Techniques.* 2nd ed. Ophthalmology Monograph 4. San Francisco: American Academy of Ophthalmology; 1998:20.

Contraindications

Relative contraindications for glaucoma filtering surgery can be ocular or systemic. A blind eye should not be considered for incisional surgery. Ciliary body ablation is a better alternative for lowering IOP in such eyes if necessary for pain control, although even this procedure is not without risk. The risk of sympathetic ophthalmia should always be kept in mind when any procedure on a blind eye or an eye with poor visual potential is considered. Conditions that predispose to trabeculectomy failure such as active anterior segment neovascularization (rubeosis iridis) or active iritis are relative contraindications. The underlying problem should be addressed first, or a surgical alternative such as aqueous shunt implantation should be considered. It may be extremely difficult to perform a successful trabeculectomy in an eye that has sustained extensive conjunctival injury (eg, after retinal detachment surgery or chemical trauma) or that has an extremely thin sclera from extensive prior surgery or necrotizing scleritis, and in such cases the likelihood of success is also reduced because of an increased risk of scarring.

Filtering surgery is less successful in younger or aphakic/pseudophakic patients. A lower success rate is also found in patients with certain types of secondary glaucomas (eg, uveitic or neovascular) or in those who have had previously failed filtration procedures. Black patients have a higher failure rate with filtering surgery.

Preoperative evaluation

Before contemplating a surgical procedure, the ophthalmologist must consider factors such as the patient's general health, presumed life expectancy, and status of the fellow eye. The patient must be medically stable for an invasive ocular procedure under local anesthesia. Preoperative evaluation should determine and document factors that may affect surgical planning, as well as those that determine the structural and functional status of the eye.

Control of preoperative inflammation with corticosteroids helps reduce postoperative iritis and scarring of the filtering bleb. In the rare instances when they are used, anticholinesterase agents should be discontinued if possible and replaced temporarily by alternative medications at least 3–6 weeks before surgery to reduce bleeding and iridocyclitis. Systemic CAIs should be discontinued postoperatively and topical CAIs used in the fellow eye, if needed.

In preparation for surgery, IOP should be reduced as closely as possible to normal levels so that the risk of expulsive choroidal hemorrhage is minimized. Antiplatelet medications should be discontinued, and systemic hypertension should be controlled.

Patients should be informed of the purpose and expectations of surgery: to arrest or delay progressive visual loss caused by their glaucoma. Patients should understand that glaucoma surgery alone rarely improves vision and that they may still need to use glaucoma medications postoperatively; that surgery may fail completely; that they could lose vision as a result of surgery; and that glaucoma may progress despite successful surgery.

It is important to note that a patient with far advanced visual field loss or field loss that is impinging on fixation is at risk of loss of central acuity following a surgical procedure. The most common cause of loss of visual acuity after trabeculectomy is cataract. Hypotony maculopathy and cystoid macular edema may also cause vision loss. Loss of central visual field in the absence of other explanations ("wipeout") may occur, but rarely. Advanced age, preoperative visual field with macular splitting, and early postoperative hypotony are risk factors for wipeout. Early, undetected, postoperative elevation of IOP may also be associated with wipeout. Bleb infections and endophthalmitis may occur long after filtering surgery and may also cause vision loss.

Costa VP, Smith M, Spaeth GL, Gandham S, Markovitz B. Loss of visual acuity after trabeculectomy. *Ophthalmology*. 1993;100:599–612.

Greenfield DS. Dysfunctional glaucoma filtration blebs. *Focal Points: Clinical Modules for Ophthalmologists*. San Francisco: American Academy of Ophthalmology; 2002, module 4.

Trabeculectomy technique

Knowledge of both the internal and external anatomy of the limbal area is essential for successful incisional surgery. Trabeculectomy is a guarded partial-thickness filtering procedure performed by removal of a block of peripheral corneal tissue beneath a scleral flap. The scleral flap provides resistance and limits the outflow of aqueous, thereby reducing the complications associated with early hypotony such as flat anterior chamber, cataract, serous and hemorrhagic choroidal effusion, macular edema, and optic nerve edema.

Because of the lower incidence of postoperative complications, trabeculectomy is the most commonly performed filtering operation. The use of antifibrotic agents such as mitomycin C and 5-fluorouracil, along with releasable sutures or laser suture lysis, enhances the longevity of guarded procedures, offers lower IOPs, and avoids some of the complications associated with full-thickness procedures.

Successful trabeculectomy involves reduction of IOP and avoidance or management of complications. Unlike cataract surgery, the success of trabeculectomy often depends on appropriate and timely postoperative intervention to influence the functioning of the filter. Complete healing of the epithelial and conjunctival wound with incomplete healing of the scleral wound is the goal of this procedure.

A trabeculectomy can be broken down into several basic steps:

- *Exposure:* A corneal or limbal traction suture can rotate the globe down, providing excellent exposure of the superior sulcus and limbus, which can be very helpful for a limbus-based conjunctival flap (Fig 8-2). A superior rectus bridle suture has the same effect but is more likely to cause postoperative ptosis and subconjunctival hemorrhage. The speculum should be adjusted to keep pressure off the globe.

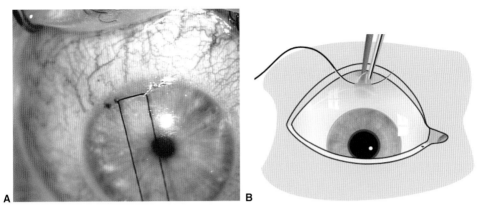

Figure 8-2 Exposure for trabeculectomy: a corneal traction suture **(A)** or superior rectus bridle suture **(B)** is inserted. *(Part A courtesy of Keith Barton; part B courtesy of Alan Lacey. Both parts reproduced with permission of Moorfields Eye Hospital.)*

- *Conjunctival wound:* Traditionally, the trabeculectomy has been positioned at 12 o'clock or in either superior quadrant, depending on surgeon preference. There is evidence that with the use of antiproliferative agents, the trabeculectomy bleb should be positioned at 12 o'clock to reduce the risk of bleb exposure and dysesthesia. A fornix-based or limbus-based conjunctival flap can be used (Figs 8-3, 8-4). Each technique has advantages and disadvantages. The fornix-based flap is easier to fashion but requires very careful suturing to achieve a watertight closure at the end of the procedure. The advantage of a fornix-based conjunctival flap is the creation of a subconjunctival scar anterior to the scleral flap, thereby encouraging posterior aqueous flow and a more posterior drainage bleb. The limbus-based conjunctival flap is technically more challenging, but it permits a secure closure well away from the limbus. The incision should be positioned 8–10 mm posterior to the limbus, and care should be taken to avoid the tendon of the superior rectus muscle. The advantage of a limbus-based flap is a lower risk of leakage; the disadvantage is the creation of a subconjunctival scar posterior to the scleral flap, impeding posterior flow of aqueous and encouraging bleb formation closer to the limbus.
- *Scleral flap:* The exact size and shape of the scleral flap does not seem critical. Rather, it is the relationship of the flap to the underlying sclerostomy that provides resistance to outflow. Although flap design will vary by surgeon preference, a common technique involves creating a 3- to 4-mm triangular, trapezoidal, or rectangular flap (Fig 8-5). If a fornix-based conjunctival flap is used, it is best to avoid dissecting the flap anteriorly into clear cornea, since anterior flap dissection facilitates early wound leakage. In a strict sense, the term *trabeculectomy* is inaccurate, because the procedure usually involves a peripheral posterior keratectomy rather than removal of trabecular meshwork. There is no advantage in extending the block posteriorly into sclera, and the risk of bleeding from iris root and ciliary body is greater.
- *Paracentesis* (Fig 8-6): To enable the surgeon to control the anterior chamber, a paracentesis should be performed. This allows instillation of balanced salt solution (BSS) or viscoelastic and intraoperative testing of the patency of the

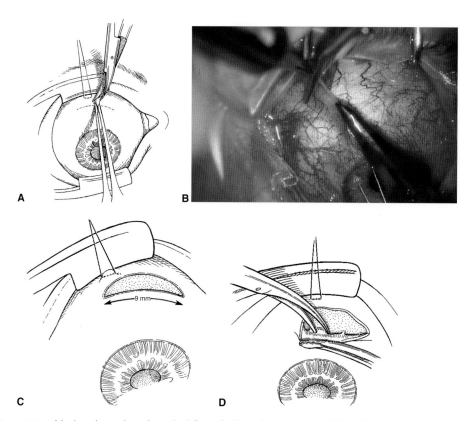

Figure 8-3 Limbus-based conjunctival flap. **A,** Drawing shows initial incision through conjunctiva and Tenon's capsule. **B,** Clinical photograph corresponding to *A* shows the initial incision for the creation of a limbus-based conjunctival flap. **C,** Completion of conjunctiva–Tenon's incision 8–10 mm posterior to limbus. **D,** Anterior dissection of conjunctiva–Tenon's flap with excision of Tenon's episcleral fibrous adhesions. *(Parts A, C, and D modified with permission from Weinreb RN, Mills RP, eds.* Glaucoma Surgery: Principles and Techniques. *2nd ed. Ophthalmology Monograph 4. San Francisco: American Academy of Ophthalmology; 1998:29–31. Part B courtesy of Robert D. Fechtner, MD.)*

filtration site. BSS is instilled through the paracentesis, and sutures are added to the scleral flap until flow is minimal. When a postoperative flat chamber occurs, the paracentesis already in place is used to re-form the chamber. Using the existing paracentesis is much safer than trying to create a paracentesis in an eye with a flat chamber.

- *Sclerostomy:* The sclerostomy is commonly created with the use of a punch, although a block may also be cut with the use of a fine blade (Fig 8-7). Aqueous drainage is generally not restricted by the size of the sclerostomy. A very small hole can drain more aqueous than is required to control IOP. However, the sclerostomy must be large enough to avoid occlusion by iris, but small enough so that it is overlapped on all sides by scleral flap. More overlap, a thicker flap, and tighter sutures are generally associated with less flow, and the converse is also true.

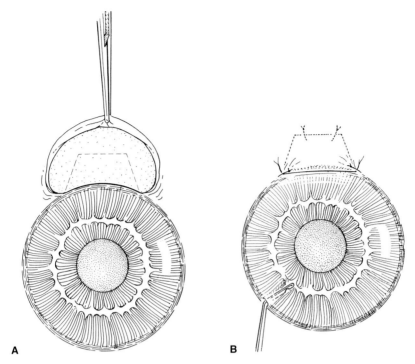

A   **B**

Figure 8-4   Fornix-based conjunctival flap (alternative to limbus-based flap). **A,** Drawing shows initial incision through conjunctiva and the insertion of Tenon's capsule. The arc length of the initial incision is approximately 6–7 mm. The tissue adjacent to the incision is undermined with blunt scissors before the scleral flap is prepared. **B,** The flap is closed either at both ends with interrupted sutures or with a running mattress suture. *(Modified with permission from Weinreb RN, Mills RP, eds.* Glaucoma Surgery: Principles and Techniques. *2nd ed. Ophthalmology Monograph 4. San Francisco: American Academy of Ophthalmology; 1998:43.)*

- *Iridectomy:* An iridectomy is performed to reduce the risk of iris occluding the sclerostomy, especially in phakic eyes, and to prevent pupillary block (see Fig 8-7D). Care should be taken to avoid amputation of ciliary processes or disruption of the zonular fibers or hyaloid face.
- *Closure of scleral flap:* With the advent of laser suture lysis and releasable sutures, many surgeons close the flap tightly, thereby minimizing postoperative anterior chamber shallowing. After a few days or weeks, these techniques may be used to release and promote flow. It is important to test the scleral flap integrity before closing the conjunctiva. When mitomycin C is used, suture tension and suture numbers should be adjusted until almost no spontaneous flow can be seen. To ensure that the trabeculectomy will still function after suture adjustment, the surgeon can test the flow. It should be possible to induce flow by gentle depression of the posterior scleral lip (Fig 8-8).

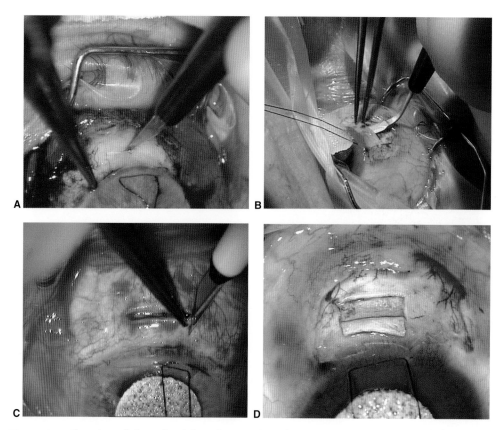

Figure 8-5   Creation of the scleral flap. Preparation of split-thickness scleral flap 4 mm wide and 2–2.5 mm from front to back. **A,** Posterior margin is dissected with a fine blade. **B,** A crescent knife is used to dissect a partial-thickness scleral tunnel. **C,** The sides of the tunnel are opened to create a flap. **D,** The final appearance. *(Courtesy of Keith Barton. Reproduced with permission of Moorfields Eye Hospital.)*

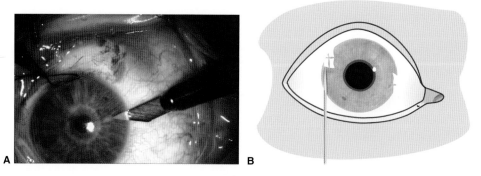

Figure 8-6   A paracentesis is created through clear cornea. This may be radial **(A)** or oblique **(B).** *(Part A courtesy of Keith Barton; part B courtesy of Alan Lacey. Both parts reproduced with permission of Moorfields Eye Hospital.)*

Figure 8-7 The surgeon can create a sclerostomy by **(A)** inserting a punch under the scleral flap; **(B)** snaring the posterior lip of the anterior chamber entry site; and **(C)** removing a punch (0.75–1 mm) of peripheral posterior cornea. A peripheral iridectomy is then made (shown here in an albino eye) with the use of iridectomy scissors **(D)**. *(Clinical photographs courtesy of Keith Barton; drawing courtesy of Alan Lacey. All parts reproduced with permission of Moorfields Eye Hospital.)*

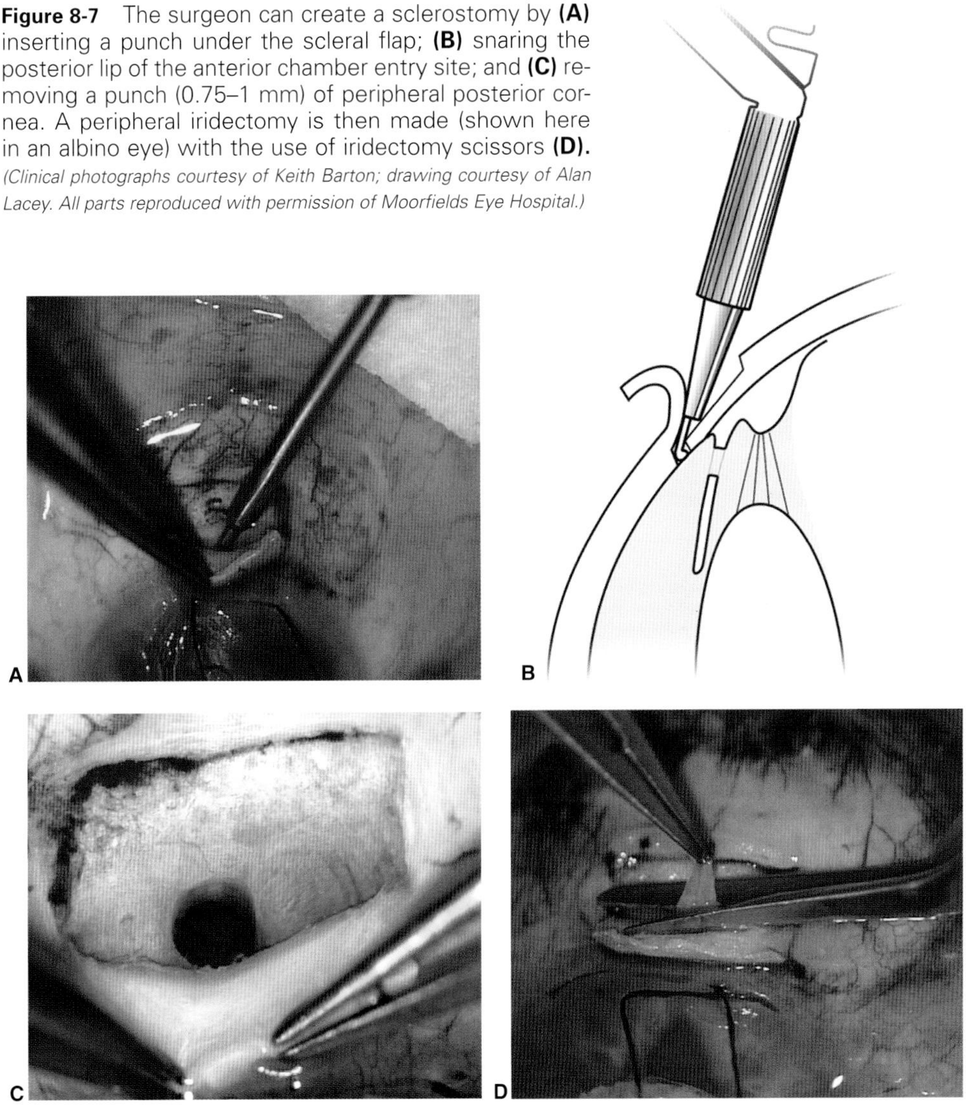

- *Flow adjustment:* Before closing the conjunctiva, the surgeon may adjust the flow around the flap by placing additional sutures or removing sutures. When mitomycin C is used, adjustment of suture numbers and tension to prevent postoperative anterior chamber shallowing may not be sufficient to prevent postoperative hypotony; thus, it is important to reduce flow to a minimum prior to conjunctival closure.
- *Closure of conjunctiva:* Many techniques have been developed for conjunctival closure (Fig 8-9). For a fornix-based flap, conjunctiva is secured at the limbus. For a limbus-based flap, conjunctiva and Tenon's capsule are closed separately or in a single layer.

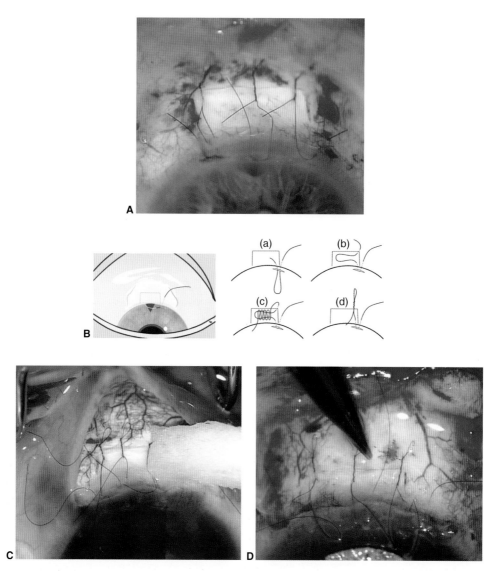

Figure 8-8 In a mitomycin C (MMC) trabeculectomy, the scleral flap is closed relatively tightly so that spontaneous drainage is minimal. Closure may be performed with the use of releasable sutures **(A, B)** that can be removed later at the slit lamp in order to increase flow, or with interrupted sutures that may be removed by laser later. **B** demonstrates the order in which each movement is made. In both cases, the surgeon should check the flow at the end of scleral closure using a sponge **(C)** or fluorescein **(D)**. *(Clinical photographs courtesy of Keith Barton; drawing courtesy of Alan Lacey. All parts reproduced with permission of Moorfields Eye Hospital.)*

Antifibrotic agents

The application of antifibrotic agents such as 5-fluorouracil (5-FU) and mitomycin C (MMC) results in greater success and lower IOP following trabeculectomy; however, the rate of serious postoperative complications may increase, and these agents must not be used indiscriminantly. Antifibrotic agents should be used with caution in primary trabeculectomies on young patients with myopia because of an increased risk of hypotony maculopathy.

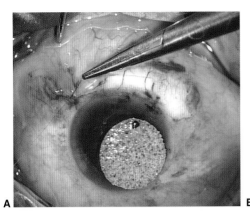

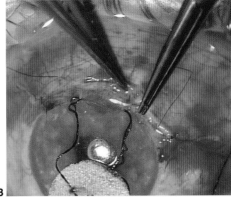

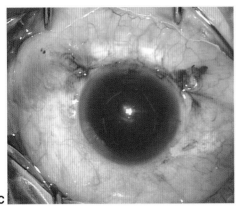

Figure 8-9 Conjunctival closure. Careful conjunctival closure is essential to prevent aqueous leakage, especially when a fornix-based conjunctival flap is used. Closing each extremity of the incision tightly with a purse-string suture **(A)** stretches the limbal edge of the conjunctiva, facilitating tight closure at the limbus. One or more conjunctival mattress sutures **(B)** prevent conjunctival recession. When the integrity of the conjunctival closure is in doubt, it can be tested with injection of viscoelastic under the conjunctiva to demonstrate that the bleb inflates without leakage **(C)**. *(Courtesy of Keith Barton. Reproduced with permission of Moorfields Eye Hospital.)*

The pyrimidine analog 5-FU inhibits fibroblast proliferation and has proven useful in reducing scarring after filtering surgery. The agent undergoes intracellular conversion to the active deoxynucleotide 5-fluoro-2′-deoxyuridine 5′-monophosphate (FdUMP), which interferes with DNA synthesis through its action on thymidylate synthetase.

Although it was originally advocated for high-risk groups such as patients with aphakic or pseudophakic eyes, neovascular glaucoma, or a history of failed operations, this agent is now used on a routine basis by many surgeons. 5-FU (50 mg/mL on a surgical sponge) may be used intraoperatively in a fashion similar to that described next for mitomycin C. Regimens for postoperative administration vary according to the observed healing response. Individual doses of 5–10 mg in 0.1–0.5 cc can be injected. The total dose can be titrated to the observed healing response and corneal toxicity. Complications such as corneal epithelial defects commonly occur and require discontinuation of 5-FU injections. The site of injection can be varied from 180° away to the upper fornix adjacent to the bleb. 5-FU is highly alkaline, and injection close to the scleral flap should be avoided so that the risk of intraocular exposure is reduced.

Mitomycin C is a naturally occurring antibiotic-antineoplastic compound that is derived from *Streptomyces caespitosus*. It acts as an alkylating agent after enzyme activation resulting in DNA cross-linking. MMC is a potent antifibrotic agent. It is most commonly administered intraoperatively by placement of a surgical sponge soaked in MMC within the subconjunctival space in contact with sclera at the planned trabeculectomy site. Concentrations in current usage are typically between 0.1 and 0.5 mg/mL with a duration of application from 0.5 to 5 minutes. Most surgeons use the higher concentrations for shorter durations and vice versa. Few data are available to compare regimens, and most surgeons increase concentration or duration based on risk factors for trabeculectomy failure. MMC is toxic and highly mutagenic. Intracameral exposure must therefore be avoided.

Flap management

Techniques allowing tighter initial wound closure of the scleral flap help prevent early postoperative hypotony. The use of releasable flap sutures or the placement of additional sutures that can be cut postoperatively to facilitate outflow following trabeculectomy are 2 of these techniques. In laser suture lysis (LSL), the conjunctiva is compressed with either a Zeiss goniolens or a lens designed for suture lysis (such as a Hoskins, Ritch, Mandelkorn, or Blumenthal lens), and the argon laser (set at 300–600 mW at a duration of 0.02–0.1 seconds with a spot size of 50–100 μm) can usually lyse the selected nylon suture with one application. It is important to avoid creating a full-thickness conjunctival burn. Shorter duration of laser energy and avoidance of pigment or blood are helpful. Most surgeons wait at least 48 hours before performing LSL. Filtration is best enhanced if lysis or suture release is completed within 2 weeks or before the occurrence of flap fibrosis. This period may be lengthened to several months when antifibrotic agents have been used.

Postoperative considerations in filtering surgery

The success of glaucoma surgery depends on careful postoperative management. Topical corticosteroids are typically administered intensively (at least 4 times daily) initially and tapered as the clinical course dictates. Topical antibiotics, cycloplegic agents (atropine), or mydriatics (phenylephrine) may also be used. Topical corticosteroids should be tapered according to the degree of conjunctival hyperemia, which may continue for 2 months or more, rather than in response to the visible anterior chamber reaction, which usually resolves more quickly. Long-term use of prophylactic antibiotics is generally not recommended. Trabeculectomies require intensive early postoperative care, and frequent office visits (once weekly or more) are necessary in the first postoperative month. During this period, it is common for bleb massage to be performed, 5-FU injections to be given, or sutures to be lysed or removed. Conversely, if hypotony occurs, it will not go undiagnosed for a prolonged period.

Complications of filtering surgery

Early and late complications of filtering surgery are listed in Table 8-1. Bleb-related complications may occur early (within 3 months of surgery) or late (after 3 months postoperatively). Early complications include wound leakage and hypotony, shallow or flat anterior chamber, and serous or hemorrhagic ciliochoroidal effusions. Late complications include bleb-related endophthalmitis, bleb leakage, ocular hypotony and associated maculopathy or choroidal hemorrhage, bleb failure, overhanging blebs, painful blebs, ptosis, or eyelid retraction. The filtering bleb can leak, produce dellen, or expand so as to interfere with eyelid function or extend onto the cornea and interfere with vision or cause irritation. Blebs may also encapsulate or fibrose, causing an increased IOP. Filtering blebs are dy-

Table 8-1 Complications of Filtering Surgery

Early Complications	Late Complications
Infection	Leakage or failure of the filtering bleb
Hypotony	Cataract
Shallow or flat anterior chamber	Blebitis
Aqueous misdirection	Endophthalmitis/bleb infection
Hyphema	Symptomatic bleb (dysesthetic bleb)
Formation or acceleration of cataract	Bleb migration
Transient IOP elevation	Hypotony
Cystoid macular edema	Ptosis
Hypotony maculopathy	Eyelid retraction
Choroidal effusion	
Suprachoroidal hemorrhage	
Persistent uveitis	
Dellen formation	
Loss of vision	

namic. They evolve over time and must be monitored. All patients must be informed of the warning signs of endophthalmitis and instructed to seek ophthalmic care immediately should they develop a red eye or other signs of infection.

Late-onset bleb-related endophthalmitis is a potentially devastating complication of filtering surgery. The incidence of postoperative endophthalmitis associated with glaucoma surgery with or without antifibrosis drugs has been reported to range from 0.06% to 13.2%. Risk factors for bleb-related endophthalmitis include blepharitis or conjunctivitis, ocular trauma, nasolacrimal duct obstruction, contact lens use, chronic bleb leak, male gender, and young age. Trabeculectomy performed at the inferior limbus is associated with a high risk of bleb-related endophthalmitis compared with trabeculectomy at the superior limbus. Use of adjunctive antifibrosis drugs such as 5-FU or MMC has been associated with increased risk of bleb-related endophthalmitis, perhaps because these blebs are often thin-walled and avascular. Patients may present with blebitis or with blebitis and endophthalmitis (Fig 8-10).

Hypotony after filtering surgery is usually due to overfiltration through the scleral flap. Bleb leakage may also occur as a manifestation of overfiltration, but the leakage itself may not be the main cause of the hypotony. Aqueous leakage from a filtering bleb may occur as an early or late complication of surgery. Early-onset bleb leaks are usually related to wound closure. The techniques of choroidal drainage and anterior chamber re-formation should be familiar to any surgeon who performs filtering surgery, because this operation carries a risk of flat chamber as a result of overdrainage and secondary choroidal detachment. Suprachoroidal fluid is drained through one or more posterior sclerotomies, as the chamber is deepened through a paracentesis. Late-onset leaks occur more frequently after full-thickness filters such as posterior lip sclerectomy or after use of antifibrosis drugs. Untreated bleb leaks may lead to vision-threatening complications, including shallowing of the anterior chamber, PAS formation, cataract, corneal decompensation, choroidal effusion, suprachoroidal hemorrhage, endophthalmitis, and hypotony maculopathy. Clinical manifestations of hypotony maculopathy include decreased vision, hypotony, optic nerve and retinal edema, and radial folds of the macula.

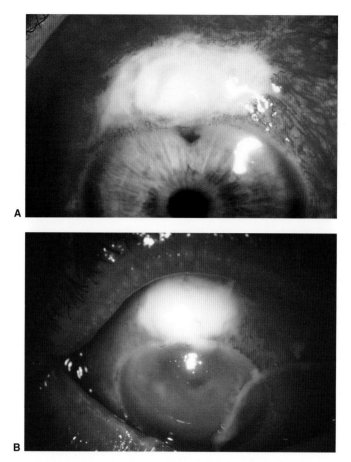

Figure 8-10 Bleb-related infection. Patients may present with blebitis, which is characterized by mucopurulent infiltrate within the bleb, localized conjunctival hyperemia, and minimal intraocular inflammation **(A)**. Bleb-related endophthalmitis **(B)** is characterized by diffuse bulbar conjunctival hyperemia, purulent material within the bleb, and anterior chamber cellular reaction, and sometimes by hypopyon formation and marked vitritis. Location of the bleb at the inferior limbus is associated with a high risk of bleb-related infection. *(Part A courtesy of Richard K. Parrish; part B courtesy of Keith Barton. Part B is reproduced with permission of Moorfields Eye Hospital.)*

Failure of the bleb may occur following filtering surgery. Eyes with failing blebs may have reduced bleb height, increased bleb-wall thickness, vascularization of the bleb, loss of conjunctival microcysts, and increased IOP. Risk factors for bleb failure include anterior segment neovascularization, black race, aphakia, prior failed filtering procedures, uveitis, prior cataract surgery, and young age. Initial management of failing blebs often includes use of antiglaucoma medications and digital massage. In eyes that do not respond to this initial therapy, transconjunctival needle revision may restore aqueous flow.

The use of contact lenses with a filtering bleb presents special problems. Contact lenses may be difficult to fit in the presence of a filtering bleb, or the lens may ride against the bleb, causing discomfort and increasing the risk of infection. Several options can be considered for the patient who has high myopia, needs a trabeculectomy, and prefers not to wear spectacles. Refractive surgery options include photorefractive keratectomy (PRK), laser in situ keratomileusis (LASIK), or intracorneal ring segments prior to trabeculectomy. Clear lens extraction (either before or after or combined with trabeculectomy) is controversial. In some circumstances, hard or soft contact lens use under close supervision may be considered after trabeculectomy. Contact lens use is more often feasible in patients after aqueous shunt implantation than after trabeculectomy. When an initial filtering procedure is not adequate to control the glaucoma and resumption of medical therapy is not successful, revision of original surgery, repeat filtering surgery at a new site, or aqueous shunt implantation and possibly cyclodestructive procedures may be indicated.

Budenz DL, Hoffman K, Zacchei A. Glaucoma filtering bleb dysesthesia. *Am J Ophthalmol.* 2001;131(5):626–630.

Camras CB. Diagnosis and management of complications of glaucoma filtering surgery. *Focal Points: Clinical Modules for Ophthalmologists.* San Francisco: American Academy of Ophthalmology; 1994, module 3.

Greenfield DS. Dysfunctional glaucoma filtration blebs. *Focal Points: Clinical Modules for Ophthalmologists.* San Francisco: American Academy of Ophthalmology; 2002, module 4.

Haynes WL, Alward WL. Control of intraocular pressure after trabeculectomy. *Surv Ophthalmol.* 1999;43:345–355.

Full-Thickness Sclerectomy

Full-thickness filtering operations were formerly performed by removal of a block of limbal tissue with a punch, trephine, laser, or cautery. Full-thickness filtering procedures were associated with a high risk of hypotony and endophthalmitis, and they no longer have a role in clinical practice.

Combined Cataract and Filtering Surgery

Both cataract and glaucoma are conditions that show increasing prevalence with aging. It is not surprising that many patients with glaucoma eventually develop cataracts either naturally or as a result of the effects of glaucoma therapy.

Indications

Cataract surgery is usually combined with trabeculectomy in the following situations:

- cataract requiring extraction in a glaucoma patient who has advanced cupping and visual field loss
- cataract requiring extraction in a glaucoma patient who requires medications to control IOP but who tolerates medical therapy poorly
- cataract requiring extraction in a glaucoma patient who requires multiple medications to control IOP

The success rate of combined surgery in terms of IOP control is reduced. Thus, in uncontrolled glaucoma, combined surgery is usually performed only in specific circumstances, such as primary angle-closure glaucoma uncontrollable either with medications or after laser iridectomy when cataract surgery alone is unlikely to provide successful IOP control and trabeculectomy alone would be hazardous. The precise number of medications representing "multiple medications" varies depending on the surgeon and the individual patient. Many surgeons perform trabeculectomy with cataract surgery when the IOP is stable but the patient is using 2 to 3 IOP-lowering medications. The goal in these cases is to avoid perioperative problems with elevated IOP and to achieve a long-term reduction in the number of medications required. However, many surgeons would perform cataract surgery alone in a patient who has controlled IOP using 1 medication, with mild to moderate cupping and little or no visual field loss.

Relative contraindications

Combined cataract and filtering surgery should be avoided in the following situations, in which glaucoma surgery alone is preferred:

- glaucoma that requires a very low target IOP
- advanced glaucoma with uncontrolled IOP and immediate need for successful reduction of IOP

Considerations

A combined procedure may prevent a postoperative rise in IOP. Combined procedures are generally less effective than filtering procedures alone in controlling IOP over time, although combined procedures using small-incision phacoemulsification techniques with an antifibrotic agent appear to have better success rates than trabeculectomy combined with extracapsular cataract surgery. For patients in whom glaucoma is the greatest immediate threat to vision, filtering surgery alone is usually performed first. The postoperative discontinuation of miotics, if used, is often enough to increase visual acuity so that cataract extraction and IOL implantation may be delayed.

Several clinical challenges are common in patients with coexisting cataract and glaucoma. Medical therapy for glaucoma may create chronic miosis, and the surgeon must deal with a small pupil. Patients with exfoliation syndrome often have fragile zonular support of the lens, and vitreous loss is therefore more common in such complicated eyes. As with all surgery, the risks, benefits, and alternatives should be discussed with the patient.

Technique

Several surgical approaches to coexisting cataract and glaucoma are now in use, and a debate has continued since the development of successful small-incision clear corneal cataract extraction. Single-site combined surgery with phacoemulsification had been the commonly accepted approach when a scleral tunnel technique was used. Two-site surgery with a clear corneal cataract extraction and a standard trabeculectomy has gained in popularity. Long-term control of IOP is better with combined glaucoma and cataract operations compared with cataract surgery alone. For patients who have IOP controlled medically, clear corneal cataract surgery alone may be the appropriate choice. As no violation of conjunctiva or sclera occurs, there is little reason to perform an incidental trabeculectomy. Rather, standard trabeculectomy can be performed when dictated by independent indications. Although little evidence exists to compare long-term outcomes with these different approaches, it makes sense for the surgeon to perform his or her best cataract procedure, because the primary indication for surgery is the presence of cataract.

Balyeat HD. Cataract surgery in the glaucoma patient. Part 1: A cataract surgeon's perspective. *Focal Points: Clinical Modules for Ophthalmologists.* San Francisco: American Academy of Ophthalmology; 1998, module 3.

Friedman DS, Jampel HD, Lubomski LH, et al. Surgical strategies for coexisting glaucoma and cataract: an evidence-based update. *Ophthalmology.* 2002;109:1902–1913.

Jampel HD, Friedman DS, Lubomski LH, et al. Effect of technique on intraocular pressure after combined cataract and glaucoma surgery: an evidence-based review. *Ophthalmology.* 2002;109:2215–2224.

Skuta GL. Cataract surgery in the glaucoma patient. Part 2: A glaucoma surgeon's perspective. *Focal Points: Clinical Modules for Ophthalmologists.* San Francisco: American Academy of Ophthalmology; 1998, module 4.

Weinreb RN, Mills RP, eds. *Glaucoma Surgery: Principles and Techniques.* 2nd ed. Ophthalmology Monograph 4. San Francisco: American Academy of Ophthalmology; 1998:65–85.

Surgery for Angle-Closure Glaucoma

The first clinical decision point following the diagnosis of angle-closure glaucoma is to distinguish between angle closure based on a pupillary block mechanism and angle closure based on another mechanism. Laser iridectomy is the procedure of choice to relieve pupillary block, but this is of no use in an eye with complete synechial closure as a result of neovascularization or chronic inflammation. It is sometimes necessary, however, to perform the iridectomy as much for diagnostic purposes as for therapeutic ones. For example, the diagnosis of plateau iris can be definitely confirmed only when a patent iridectomy fails to change peripheral iris configuration and relieve angle closure.

The treatment of pupillary block glaucoma, whether primary or secondary, is a laser or an incisional iridectomy. These procedures provide an alternate route for aqueous trapped in the posterior chamber to enter the anterior chamber, which allows the iris to recede from its occlusion of the trabecular meshwork (Fig 8-11). Laser surgery has become the preferred method in almost all cases. Both the argon laser and the Nd:YAG laser are effective, but the Nd:YAG laser has become the more popular instrument used. Cataract extraction is also effective as therapy for angle closure secondary to pupillary block. Following the successful resolution of pupillary block, IOP may return to normal or may remain elevated. At this point, the indications for surgery become similar to those for POAG, except for possible surgical goniosynechialysis. Pupillary block associated with aphakia or an anterior chamber intraocular lens usually requires a surgical iridectomy, because vitreous easily occludes laser iridectomies. When cataract surgery results in aphakia or anterior chamber intraocular lens placement, a surgical iridectomy should be performed at 12 o'clock at the time of the cataract surgery.

For eyes with secondary angle closure not caused by pupillary block, an attempt should be made to identify and treat underlying conditions. For example, an eye with rubeosis iridis from diabetic retinopathy should have retinal ablation prior to glaucoma surgery. In early cases, the IOP elevation may be reversible. Even in the presence of complete

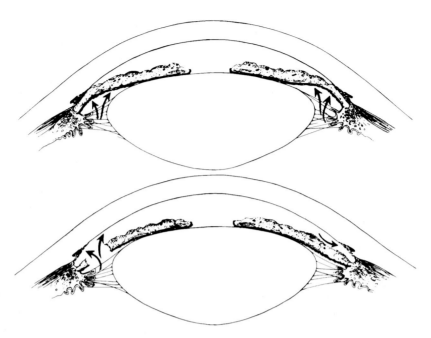

Figure 8-11 Angle-closure glaucoma. Laser or surgical iridectomy breaks the pupillary block and results in opening of the entire peripheral angle if no permanent peripheral anterior synechiae are present. *(Reproduced and modified with permission from Kolker AE, Hetherington J, eds.* Becker-Shaffer's Diagnosis and Therapy of the Glaucomas. *5th ed. St Louis: Mosby; 1983.)*

synechial angle closure from rubeosis, neovascularization may regress following retinal ablation, allowing subsequent successful filtering surgery.

Laser Iridectomy

Indications

The indications for iridectomy include the presence of pupillary block and the need to determine the presence of pupillary block. Laser iridectomy is also indicated to prevent pupillary block in an eye considered at risk, as determined by gonioscopic evaluation or because of an angle-closure attack in the fellow eye.

Contraindications

An eye with active rubeosis iridis may bleed following laser iridectomy. The risk of bleeding is also increased in a patient taking systemic anticoagulants, including aspirin. The argon laser may be more appropriate than the Nd:YAG should laser iridectomy be performed in such an individual. Although laser iridectomy is not helpful for angle closure not caused by a pupillary block mechanism, it is sometimes necessary to perform the laser iridectomy to ensure that pupillary block is not present.

Preoperative considerations

In the setting of acute angle closure, it is often difficult to perform laser iridectomy because of the cloudy cornea, shallow chamber, and engorged iris. The clinician should attempt to break the attack medically and then proceed to surgery. Corneal edema may be improved prior to laser by pretreatment with topical glycerin. It is easiest to penetrate the iris in a crypt. The surgeon should take care to keep the iridectomy peripheral and covered by eyelid, if possible, to avoid monocular diplopia. Pretreatment with pilocarpine may be helpful by stretching and thinning the iris. Pretreatment with apraclonidine can help blunt IOP spikes.

Technique

The argon laser may be used to produce an iridectomy in most eyes, but very dark and very light irides present technical difficulties. Using a condensing contact lens, the typical initial laser settings are 0.02–0.1 second of duration, 50-μm spot size, and 800–1000 mW of power. There are a number of variations in technique, and iris color dictates which technique is chosen. Complications include localized lens opacity, acute rise in IOP (which may damage the optic nerve), transient or persistent iritis, early closure of the iridectomy, posterior synechiae, and corneal and retinal burns.

The Q-switched Nd:YAG laser generally requires fewer pulses and less energy than an argon laser to create a patent iridectomy and has become the preferred technique for most eyes. Also, the effectiveness of this laser is not affected by iris color, and the iridectomy created by this laser does not close as often over the long term as one created by argon laser. With a condensing contact lens, the typical initial laser setting is 2–8 mJ. Potential complications include corneal burns, disruption of the anterior lens capsule or corneal endothelium, bleeding (usually transient), postoperative IOP spike, inflammation, and delayed closure of the iridectomy. To prevent damage to the lens, the surgeon must use caution with the Q-switched Nd:YAG laser in performing further enlargement of the opening once patency is established. The location should be as peripheral as possible, at the point where the distance between the iris and lens is greatest.

Postoperative care

Bleeding may occur from the iridectomy site, particularly with the Nd:YAG laser. Often, compression of the eye with the laser lens will tamponade the vessel, thereby slowing bleeding until coagulation can occur. In rare cases when this does not work, it may be helpful to use the argon laser to coagulate the vessel. Postoperative pressure spikes may occur, as with LTP, and they are treated as described in the section on LTP. Inflammation is treated as necessary with topical corticosteroids.

Murphy PH, Trope GE. Monocular blurring: a complication of YAG laser iridotomy. *Ophthalmology.* 1991;98:1539–1542.

Ritch R, Shields MB, Krupin T, eds. *The Glaucomas.* 2nd ed. St Louis: Mosby; 1996.

Shields MB. *Textbook of Glaucoma.* 4th ed. Philadelphia: Williams & Wilkins; 2000.

Laser Gonioplasty, or Peripheral Iridoplasty

Indications

Gonioplasty, or iridoplasty, is a technique to deepen the angle. It is occasionally useful in angle-closure glaucoma resulting from plateau iris. Stromal burns are created with the argon laser in the peripheral iris to cause contraction and flattening. It is difficult to diagnose plateau iris unless an iridectomy has been created and the angle configuration has not changed and, therefore, remains occludable.

Contraindications

The contraindications are the same as those for laser iridectomy.

Preoperative considerations

An angle that is closed from plateau iris will not open with creation of a laser iridectomy, because the underlying mechanism is not pupillary block. This is often a difficult condition to diagnose accurately.

Technique

Typical laser settings are 0.1–0.5 second duration, 200- to 500-μm spot size, and 200–500 mW of power. This procedure can be used to open the angle temporarily, in anticipation of a more definitive laser or incisional iridectomy, or in other types of angle closure such as plateau iris syndrome and nanophthalmos. Argon laser gonioplasty may be useful to treat synechial angle closure, in patients with angle closure of months' to even years' duration (laser goniosynechialysis). A gonioscopy lens with a diameter smaller than the corneal diameter may be used, allowing simultaneous compression gonioscopy if necessary. A spot size of 100–200 μm is used, but otherwise the settings are the same as for gonioplasty.

Wand M. Argon laser gonioplasty for synechial angle closure. *Arch Ophthalmol.* 1992;110: 363–367.

Incisional Surgery for Angle Closure

Peripheral iridectomy

Surgical iridectomy may be required if a patent iridectomy cannot be achieved with a laser. Such situations include a cloudy cornea, a flat anterior chamber, and insufficient patient cooperation.

Cataract extraction

When pupillary block is associated with a visually significant cataract, lens extraction might be considered as a primary procedure. However, laser iridectomy may stop an acute attack of pupillary block, so that cataract surgery may be performed more safely at a later time.

Chamber deepening and goniosynechialysis

When PAS develop in cases of angle-closure glaucoma, iridectomy alone may not relieve the glaucoma adequately. Chamber deepening through a paracentesis with intraoperative gonioscopy may break PAS of relatively recent onset. A viscoelastic agent and/or an iris or cyclodialysis spatula may be useful, in a procedure known as *goniosynechialysis,* to break synechiae.

Campbell DG, Vela A. Modern goniosynechialysis for the treatment of synechial angle-closure glaucoma. *Ophthalmology.* 1984;91:1052–1060.

Shingleton BJ, Chang MA, Bellows AR, Thomas JV. Surgical goniosynechialysis for angle-closure glaucoma. *Ophthalmology.* 1990;97:551–556.

Other Procedures to Lower IOP

Incisional and nonincisional procedures to control IOP include aqueous shunt implantation, ciliary body ablation, cyclodialysis, and viscocanalostomy and other nonpenetrating procedures.

Aqueous Shunt Implantation

Many different types of devices have been developed that aid filtration by shunting aqueous to a site away from limbus, such as the equatorial subconjunctival space (Table 8-2). Aqueous shunts, or glaucoma drainage devices, in current use generally have a tube placed into the anterior chamber, in the ciliary sulcus, or through the pars plana into the vitreous cavity. Aqueous flows out through the device to an extraocular reservoir, which is placed in the equatorial region on the sclera (Fig 8-12). Aqueous shunts can be broadly categorized as nonvalved devices, which have no flow restrictor, or valved devices, which have a flow restrictor. The most popular nonvalved devices are the Molteno (Molteno Ophthalmic Ltd, Dunedin, New Zealand) and Baerveldt (Advanced Medical Optics, Inc, Santa Ana, CA) designs. The most widely used valved device is the Ahmed (New World Medical, Inc, Rancho Cucamonga, CA). The size of the plate varies and can influence IOP control and complications postoperatively. The anterior chamber tube shunt to an encircling band (ACTSEB) described by Schocket used an encircling element intended for

Table 8-2 Aqueous Shunts

	Molteno		Baerveldt		Ahmed	
	Single plate	Double plate	250	350	Single plate	Double plate
Surface area	135 mm²	270 mm²	250 mm²	350 mm²	184 mm²	364 mm²
Height profile	2.16 mm	2.16 mm	0.84 mm	0.84 mm	1.90 mm	1.90 mm
Plate material	Polypropylene	Polypropylene	Silicone	Silicone	Polypropylene or silicone	
Flow resistor	No	No	No	No	Yes	Yes

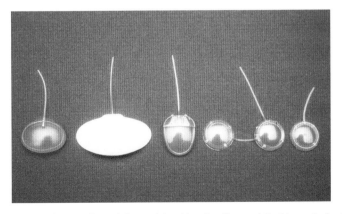

Figure 8-12 Aqueous shunts, from left to right: Krupin, Baerveldt, Ahmed, double-plate Molteno, single-plate Molteno.

scleral buckling with tubing attached to the encircling band. A variation on the ACTSEB can be used on eyes with a previously placed scleral buckle.

Weinreb RN, Mills RP, eds. *Glaucoma Surgery: Principles and Techniques.* 2nd ed. Ophthalmology Monograph 4. San Francisco: American Academy of Ophthalmology; 1998:65–85.

Indications

The devices mentioned and other, similar types of implants are generally reserved for difficult glaucoma cases in which conventional filtering surgery has failed or is likely to fail. One form of "failure" may be the inability of the patient to be a suitable candidate for trabeculectomy. An aqueous shunt should be considered in the following clinical settings:

- *Failed trabeculectomy with antifibrotics:* It may be appropriate to perform a repeat trabeculectomy in some clinical situations. However, when the factors that precipitated the initial failure cannot be modified, or when it is not technically possible to repeat the trabeculectomy, an aqueous shunt may be the procedure of choice.

- *Active uveitis:* Although few randomized, prospective data are available comparing trabeculectomy with antifibrotics to aqueous shunts in the setting of active uveitis, the success of trabeculectomy in the setting of active inflammation is disappointingly low. In certain types of uveitis, for example, young patients with juvenile idiopathic arthritis, the success rate of trabeculectomy is low, and aqueous shunt implantation is often the primary surgical treatment.

- *Neovascular glaucoma:* Eyes with neovascular glaucoma (NVG) are at a high risk of trabeculectomy failure. In one prospective study, the 5-year success rate of trabeculectomy with 5-FU in NVG was 28%. When possible, retinal ablation is performed prior to glaucoma surgery in cases of NVG. When the IOP mandates urgent surgery, or when the NVG does not respond to retinal ablation, an aqueous shunt is indicated. The management of NVG is likely to change with the use of monoclonal antibodies to vascular endothelial growth factor.

- *Inadequate conjunctiva:* In patients who have undergone severe trauma or extensive surgery (eg, retinal detachment surgery), trabeculectomy success is reduced because these patients' eyes have excessive conjunctival scarring. An aqueous shunt can be placed, even in the presence of a scleral buckle. When vitrectomy has been performed, the tube can be placed through the pars plana.

- *Aphakia:* Aphakic eyes have a poor prognosis for the success of conventional filtering surgery even when MMC is used. Many surgeons use aqueous shunt implantation as a primary procedure in uncontrolled aphakic glaucoma.

Other factors should be considered when a patient is evaluated for possible aqueous shunt surgery:

- *Poor candidate for trabeculectomy:* In addition to the clinical settings just described, lack of an intact blood–aqueous barrier is a relative indication for an aqueous shunt.

- *Potential for improved visual acuity:* It may not be appropriate to perform incisional surgery, which requires a prolonged convalescence, in an eye with little potential for useful vision. However, when the potential for useful vision remains, it is worth the risks and potentially complicated postoperative course of aqueous shunt surgery.
- *Need for lower IOP:* After a failed trabeculectomy, medical therapy should be resumed. If IOP is not controlled, additional surgery must be considered.

Contraindications

Aqueous shunt surgery may have a complicated postoperative course. Thus, it is relatively contraindicated in patients unable to comply with self-care in the postoperative period. Borderline corneal endothelial function is a relative contraindication for anterior chamber placement of a shunt.

Preoperative considerations

Preoperative evaluation should be similar to that for trabeculectomy. During the ophthalmic examination, the clinician should note the motility examination, the status of the conjunctiva, the health of the sclera at the anticipated shunt and external reservoir sites, the location of PAS near possible shunt insertion sites, and the location of vitreous in the eye.

Techniques

Although aqueous shunts differ in design, the basic techniques for implantation are similar. The superotemporal quadrant is preferred over the superonasal quadrant, because surgical access is more easily achieved in the former. For the valved devices, the shunt must be primed before implantation. The extraocular plate or valve mechanism is sutured between the vertical and horizontal rectus muscles posterior to the muscle insertions. The tube portion of the shunt is then routed either anteriorly to enter the chamber angle, or through the pars plana for posterior implantation in eyes that have had a vitrectomy. Typically, the shunt is covered with tissue such as sclera, pericardium, or cornea to help prevent erosion. Dura has also been used in the past but should now be avoided because of the potential risk of prion transmission.

For the nonvalved devices, there are a number of techniques to restrict flow in the early postoperative period, such as stenting the tube lumen or ligating the tube with a suture. Restricting flow is not necessary with devices that contain a flow restrictor, although hypotony and a flat chamber can still sometimes occur with them. Doses of antifibrotic agents similar to those used in trabeculectomy do not appear to improve the success of glaucoma aqueous shunt surgery. For devices with 2 plates, the second plate and its interconnecting tube may be placed either over or under the superior rectus muscle; the distal plate is attached to the sclera in a manner similar to that in which the proximal plate is attached.

A confounding cause of hypotony can be leakage of aqueous around the outside of the shunt at the anterior chamber entry site. In general, shunts should be introduced into the anterior chamber via a needle incision that is no larger than the diameter of the shunt (23 gauge for most shunts). When the patient's eye has thin sclera or when the shunt is introduced through partial-thickness sclera, a tighter entry site (eg, 25 gauge) may be required.

Postoperative management

The IOP in the early postoperative period can be variable. In nonvalved devices in which the tube has been occluded, early IOP spikes are best managed medically. After sufficient time has passed for a capsule to form around the extraocular reservoir, the occluding suture is released for the nonvalved devices. Topical corticosteroids, antibiotics, and cycloplegics are used as with trabeculectomy. Elevation of the IOP occurs around 2–8 weeks postoperatively, which probably represents encapsulation around the extraocular reservoir. Aqueous suppression can control the IOP, and this elevation usually improves or resolves spontaneously within 1–6 months.

Complications

Success rates have been encouraging, but the implant procedures share many of the complications associated with conventional filtering surgery. Unique problems related to the shunts and plates also arise. Early overfiltration in an eye with the shunt in the anterior chamber results in a flat chamber and shunt–cornea touch. This shunt–cornea touch can compromise the cornea. Even when no touch occurs, however, an area of corneal decompensation can appear near the shunt. Eyes must be monitored for late complications such as shunt erosion or plate migration. Motility disturbances may also occur. Shunt obstruction, plate migration, or shunt erosion may require surgical revision. Table 8-3 lists several common complications, along with methods for avoiding or managing them.

Gedde SJ, Herndon LW, Brandt JD, Budenz DL, Feuer WJ, Schiffman JC. Surgical complications in the Tube Versus Trabeculectomy Study during the first year of follow-up. *Am J Ophthalmol.* 2007;143(1):23–31.

Gedde SJ, Schiffman JC, Feuer WJ, Herndon LW, Brandt JD, Budenz DL. Treatment outcomes in the Tube Versus Trabeculectomy Study after one year of follow-up. *Am J Ophthalmol.* 2007;143(1):9–22.

Sidoti PA, Heuer DK. Aqueous shunting procedures. *Focal Points: Clinical Modules for Ophthalmologists.* San Francisco: American Academy of Ophthalmology; 2002, module 3.

Wilson MR, Mendis U, Paliwal A, Haynatzka V. Long-term follow-up of primary glaucoma surgery with Ahmed glaucoma valve implant versus trabeculectomy. *Am J Ophthalmol.* 2003;136:464–470.

Ciliary Body Ablation Procedures

Several surgical procedures reduce aqueous secretion by destroying a portion of the ciliary body. The secretory activity of ciliary body epithelium can be inhibited by treatment with cyclocryotherapy and thermal lasers such as continuous-wave Nd:YAG, argon, and diode (Fig 8-13).

Indications

Ciliary ablation is indicated to lower IOP in eyes that have poor visual potential or that are poor candidates for incisional surgery. Incisional surgery for blind eyes should be avoided, if possible, because of the small risk of sympathetic ophthalmia. Diode laser cyclophotocoagulation (CPC) is often the treatment of choice for IOP-lowering in painful blind eyes or in eyes unlikely to respond to other modes of therapy. Interventions such as retro-

Table 8-3 Aqueous Shunt Surgery Complications and Prevention/Management Options

Complication	Prevention/Management
Shunt–cornea touch	Avoid by making the anterior chamber insertion parallel with the iris plane and using a shunt occlusion technique to avoid a flat chamber. Pars plana and ciliary sulcus insertion avoid this complication.
Flat chamber and hypotony	Flat chamber and hypotony caused by overfiltration are best avoided by the use of a valved device, an occlusion technique, or viscoelastic agents. Aqueous leakage around the shunt at the anterior chamber entry site is another important cause of hypotony. Avoid by ensuring that the entry site is watertight around the shunt. A flat chamber with shunt–cornea touch and serous choroidal detachment should be managed by early re-formation of the anterior chamber and correction of the overdrainage. To correct overdrainage, use shunt occlusion techniques or correct entry site problems by resiting the shunt if necessary. Viscoelastic can help maintain the chamber. A flat chamber resulting from a complication such as suprachoroidal hemorrhage must be managed based on the clinical setting.
Shunt occlusion	Avoid by beveling the shunt away from uveal tissue (iris) or vitreous. A generous vitrectomy should be performed if needed. Although it is possible to use Nd:YAG laser to clear an occlusion, surgical intervention is often required.
Plate migration	Avoid by securing plate tightly to sclera with nonabsorbable sutures. If the plate migrates, the intraocular tube may become longer or retract. Plate migration toward the limbus requires repositioning of the plate in the equatorial subconjunctival space. Plate migration away from the limbus is rarely significant enough to warrant repositioning but may require a tube-extender if the tube retracts from the anterior chamber.
Valve malfunction	Test valves for patency before insertion of the shunt. Several techniques have been described to unclog a valve.
Shunt exposure or erosion	Repair shunt exposure by removing any protruding sutures that have precipitated the erosion, securing tube tightly to sclera, covering shunt with reinforcing material (eg, sclera, cornea, or pericardium), and mobilizing conjunctiva. Donor sclera must be adequately covered with conjunctiva, or further erosion may occur. If adequate conjunctiva is not available, conjunctival autograft or amniotic membrane may be used. Exposure increases the risk of endophthalmitis. In some settings, the shunt should be removed if adequate coverage cannot be achieved.

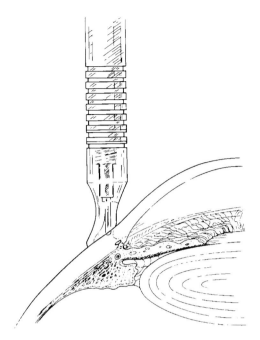

Figure 8-13 Cyclophotocoagulation. The diode laser handpiece attachment from one manufacturer is shown. After the edge of the probe is aligned with the limbus, approximately 17–19 applications are placed 270° around the limbus, with a power of 1.5–2 W and a duration of approximately 2 seconds. *(Reproduced with permission from Weinreb RN, Mills RP, eds.* Glaucoma Surgery: Principles and Techniques. *2nd ed. Ophthalmology Monograph 4. San Francisco: American Academy of Ophthalmology; 1998:165.)*

bulbar alcohol injection, retrobulbar chlorpromazine injection, or enucleation are rarely performed now because of improved CPC techniques.

Contraindications

Ciliary ablation is relatively contraindicated in eyes with good vision because of the risk of loss of visual acuity.

Preoperative evaluation

This step is the same as for incisional glaucoma surgery.

Methods and considerations

Cyclocryotherapy and Nd:YAG laser CPC are rarely performed, having been largely replaced by transscleral diode laser CPC, which is better tolerated, causing less pain and inflammation. Also, even though there is a degree of unpredictability with diode laser CPC, this method is considerably more predictable than its predecessors in its effect.

An *endoscopic laser delivery system* has been advocated for use with cataract surgery or in pediatric, pseudophakic, or aphakic eyes. Use of the argon laser aimed at the ciliary processes through a goniolens is possible in a small percentage of patients.

Postoperative management

Pain following these procedures may be substantial, and patients should be provided with adequate analgesics, including narcotics, during the immediate postoperative period.

Complications

Each of these procedures may result in prolonged hypotony, pain, inflammation, cystoid macular edema, hemorrhage, and even phthisis bulbi. Sympathetic ophthalmia is a rare but serious complication.

Pastor SA, Singh K, Lee DA, et al. Cyclophotocoagulation: a report by the American Academy of Ophthalmology. *Ophthalmology*. 2001;108:2130–2138.

Cyclodialysis

Cyclodialysis creates a direct communication between the anterior chamber and the suprachoroidal space. It can occur traumatically or surgically. Surgical cyclodialysis is now rarely performed, but in the past may have been helpful in aphakic patients who did not respond to filtering surgery. In this procedure, a spatula is passed from the suprachoroidal space into the anterior chamber through a small scleral incision approximately 4 mm posterior to the limbus. Many complications can occur after the procedure, including bleeding, inflammation, and Descemet's detachment. Profound hypotony, or an equally significant rise in IOP should the cleft close, may also occur.

Nonpenetrating Glaucoma Surgery

Although the most widely accepted IOP-lowering incisional surgeries involve creating a direct communication between the anterior chamber and the subconjunctival space, nonpenetrating surgery has also been proposed. Nonpenetrating glaucoma procedures were initially described in the early 1970s. The goal was to achieve IOP lowering while avoiding some of the complications of standard trabeculectomy.

Recently, interest in nonpenetrating surgery has been revived. Several variations all involve a deep sclerectomy. These include deep sclerectomy with or without a collagen implant and *viscocanalostomy,* which is augmentation of the deep sclerectomy with injection of viscoelastic into Schlemm's canal. Both deep sclerectomy and viscocanalostomy involve creation of a superficial scleral flap and a deeper scleral dissection underneath to leave behind only a thin layer of sclera and Descemet's membrane.

Currently, few long-term prospective, randomized data compare these new procedures with trabeculectomy. In theory, nonpenetrating surgery may avoid some of the complications associated with penetrating filtering surgery. However, the procedures are technically challenging, and initial results suggest that IOP reduction may be less than with trabeculectomy.

Netland PA, Ophthalmic Technology Assessment Committee, Glaucoma Panel, American Academy of Ophthalmology. Nonpenetrating glaucoma surgery. *Ophthalmology*. 2001;108:416–421.

Sarodia U, Shaarawy T, Barton K. Nonpenetrating glaucoma surgery: a critical evaluation. *Curr Opin Ophthalmol*. 2007;18(2):152–158.

Primary Congenital Glaucoma

For those glaucomas occurring within the first few years of life, initial surgical therapy is generally more effective than medical treatment. Goniotomy and trabeculotomy are the preferred procedures in primary congenital glaucoma. Goniotomy is possible only in an eye with a relatively clear cornea, whereas trabeculotomy can be performed whether the cornea is clear or cloudy. A standard trabeculotomy performed superiorly can be converted to trabeculectomy if needed. Published success rates are similar for trabeculotomy and goniotomy in eyes with clear corneas.

For an eye that has failed one of these procedures, debate continues whether the next procedure should be trabeculectomy with an antifibrotic agent or an aqueous shunt. CPC is another procedure that can be considered in intractable cases. These procedures in infants are probably best performed by clinicians experienced in the surgical treatment of childhood glaucomas. See also BCSC Section 6, *Pediatric Ophthalmology and Strabismus.*

Goniotomy and Trabeculotomy

Indications

The presence of childhood glaucoma is an indication for surgery. The selection of procedure will, in part, depend on the training and experience of the surgeon.

Contraindications

Contraindications to surgery include an infant with unstable health, an infant with multiple anomalies with poor prognosis, and a grossly disorganized eye.

Preoperative evaluation

Thorough examination in the office is not always possible. Sometimes a bottle feeding will distract a young infant enough to allow tonometry and dilated examination. When this is not possible, examination under anesthesia is necessary. Surgery can be performed at the same or at a subsequent session. It is best not to dilate the eye expected to have angle surgery in order to better protect the lens during the procedure. BCSC Section 6, *Pediatric Ophthalmology and Strabismus,* includes a section on examination techniques and tips written by pediatric ophthalmologists.

Technique

Most surgeons fill the anterior chamber with viscoelastic to prevent collapse and to tamponade bleeding. A disadvantage of viscoelastic use is that a postoperative IOP spike may occur if not all of the viscoelastic material is removed from the eye. With a *goniotomy,* a needle-knife is passed across the anterior chamber, and a superficial incision is made in the anterior aspect of the trabecular meshwork under gonioscopic control (Fig 8-14). A clear cornea is necessary to provide an adequate view of the chamber angle.

In a *trabeculotomy,* a fine wirelike instrument (trabeculotome) is inserted into Schlemm's canal from an external incision and then rotated into the anterior chamber, tearing the trabecular meshwork (Fig 8-15). Schlemm's canal is more easily identified if a partial-thickness scleral flap is first elevated, similar to what occurs in a trabeculectomy. A

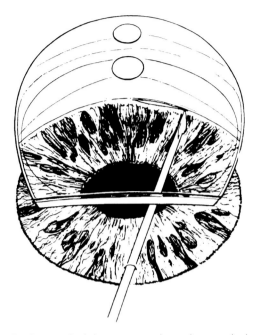

Figure 8-14 Goniotomy incision as seen through a surgical contact lens.

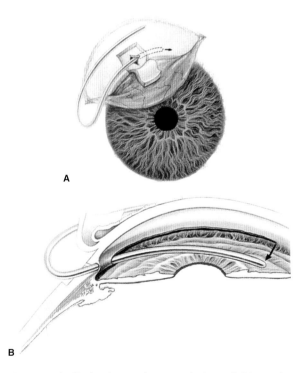

A

B

Figure 8-15 Trabeculotomy. **A,** Probe is gently passed along Schlemm's canal with little resistance for 6–10 mm. **B,** By rotating the probe internally *(arrow),* the surgeon ruptures the
trabeculum, and the probe appears in the anterior chamber with minimum bleeding. *(Reproduced
and modified with permission from Kolker AE, Hetherington J, eds.* Becker-Shaffer's Diagnosis and Therapy of the Glaucomas. *5th ed. St Louis: Mosby; 1983.)*

gradual cutdown can then be made so that the canal can be clearly identified. Alternative techniques have been developed in which a suture, usually 6-0 polypropylene (Prolene), is threaded through Schlemm's canal and the end is retrieved. The 2 ends of the suture are then pulled, and the suture ruptures the trabecular meshwork and passes into the anterior chamber. The suture is then removed. This process may be performed over 180° or 360° of the angle. Trabeculotomy is particularly useful if the cornea is too cloudy to allow adequate visualization for goniotomy. However, the abnormal angle anatomy associated with congenital glaucomas sometimes precludes localization of Schlemm's canal.

Complications

Complications of both of these operations include hyphema, infection, lens damage, and uveitis. Descemet's membrane may be stripped during trabeculotomy. General anesthesia may cause serious complications in children, and bilateral procedures are indicated in some children because of anesthetic risks. There is a long-term risk of amblyopia, and the child must be followed closely over time. IOP elevation may recur at any time.

Beck AD, Lynch MG. Pediatric glaucoma. *Focal Points: Clinical Modules for Ophthalmologists.* San Francisco: American Academy of Ophthalmology; 1997, module 5.

Basic Texts

Glaucoma

Anderson DR, Patella VM. *Automated Static Perimetry*. 2nd ed. St Louis: Mosby; 1999.

Drance SM, Anderson DR, eds. *Automatic Perimetry in Glaucoma: A Practical Guide*. Orlando, FL: Grune & Stratton; 1985.

Epstein DL, Allingham RR, Schuman JS, eds. *Chandler and Grant's Glaucoma*. 4th ed. Baltimore: Williams & Wilkins; 1997.

Harrington DO, Drake MV. *The Visual Fields: A Textbook and Atlas of Clinical Perimetry*. 6th ed. St Louis: Mosby; 1989.

Hart WM Jr, ed. *Adler's Physiology of the Eye: Clinical Application*. 9th ed. St Louis: Mosby; 1992.

Minckler DS, Van Buskirk EM, eds. Glaucoma. In: Wright KW, ed. *Color Atlas of Ophthalmic Surgery*. Philadelphia: Lippincott; 1992.

Ritch R, Shields MB, Krupin T, eds. *The Glaucomas*. 2nd ed. St Louis: Mosby; 1996.

Shields MB. *Textbook of Glaucoma*. 4th ed. Baltimore: Williams & Wilkins; 1998.

Stamper RL, Lieberman MF, Drake MV, eds. *Becker-Shaffer's Diagnosis and Therapy of the Glaucomas*. 7th ed. St Louis: Mosby; 1999.

Tasman WS, Jaeger EA, eds. *Duane's Ophthalmology*. Philadelphia: Lippincott; 2007.

Thomas JV, Belcher CD III, Simmons RJ, eds. *Glaucoma Surgery*. St Louis: Mosby; 1992.

Zimmerman TJ, Kooner KS, Sharir M, Fechtner RD. *Textbook of Ocular Pharmacology*. Philadelphia: Lippincott; 1997.

Related Academy Materials

Focal Points: Clinical Modules for Ophthalmologists

Individual modules are available in pdf format at aao.org/focalpointsarchive. Print modules are available only through an annual subscription.

Campagna JA. Traumatic hyphema: current strategies (Module 10, 2007).

Giaconi JA, Coleman AL. Evidence-based medicine in glaucoma: clinical trials update (Module 3, 2008).

Greenfield DS. Dysfunctional glaucoma filtration blebs (Module 4, 2002).

Hawkins AS, Edward DP. Cyclodestruction as a treatment for glaucoma (Module 10, 2004).

Johnson CA, Spry PG. Advances in automated perimetry (Module 10, 2002).

Mikelberg FS. Normal-tension glaucoma: the next generation of glaucoma management (Module 12, 2000).

Mitrev PV, Schuman JS. Lasers in glaucoma management (Module 9, 2001).

Moster MR, Azuara-Blanco A. Techniques of glaucoma filtration surgery (Module 6, 2000).

Salinas-Van Orman E, Bashford KP, Craven ER. Nerve fiber layer, macula, and optic disc imaging in glaucoma (Module 8, 2006).

Savage JA. Gonioscopy in the management of glaucoma (Module 3, 2006).

Sheth BP. Drugs and pregnancy (Module 7, 2007).

Sidoti PA, Heuer DK. Aqueous shunting procedures (Module 3, 2002).

Wilson RM, Brandt JD. Update on glaucoma clinical trials (Module 9, 2003).

Print Publications

Arnold AC, ed. *Basic Principles of Ophthalmic Surgery* (2006).

Netland PA, ed. *Glaucoma Medical Therapy: Principles and Management.* 2nd ed. (Ophthalmology Monograph 13, 2007).

Rockwood EJ, ed. *ProVision: Preferred Responses in Ophthalmology.* Series 4. Self-Assessment Program. 2-vol set (2007).

Walsh TJ, ed. *Visual Fields: Examination and Interpretation.* 2nd ed. (Ophthalmology Monograph 3, 1996; reviewed for currency 2000).

Weinreb RN, Mills RP, eds. *Glaucoma Surgery: Principles and Techniques.* 2nd ed. (Ophthalmology Monograph 4, 1998; reviewed for currency 2001).

Wilson FM II, ed. *Practical Ophthalmology: A Manual for Beginning Residents.* 5th ed. (2005).

Online Materials

American Academy of Ophthalmology. Ophthalmic News and Education Network: Clinical Education Case Web site; http://www.aao.org/education/products/cases/index.cfm

American Academy of Ophthalmology. Ophthalmic News and Education Network: Clinical Education Course Web site; http://www.aao.org/education/products/courses/index.cfm

Basic and Clinical Science Course (Sections 1–13); http://www.aao.org/education/bcsc_online.cfm

Maintenance of Certification Exam Study Kit, Glaucoma, version 2.0 (2007); http://www.aao.org/moc

Rockwood EJ, ed. *ProVision: Preferred Responses in Ophthalmology.* Series 4. Self-Assessment Program. 2-vol set (2007); http://one.aao.org/CE/EducationalContent/Provision.aspx

Specialty Clinical Updates: Glaucoma, Vol 1 (2003); http://www.aao.org/education/products/scu/index.cfm

CDs/DVDs

Basic and Clinical Science Course (Sections 1–13) (CD-ROM; 2008).

Budenz DL, Brandt JD, Fellman RL, et al. *LEO Clinical Update Course: Glaucoma* (DVD; 2006).

Front Row View: Video Collections of Eye Surgery. Series 1 (DVD; 2006).

Front Row View: Video Collections of Eye Surgery. Series 2 (DVD; 2007).

Preferred Practice Patterns

Preferred Practice Patterns are available at http://one.aao.org/CE/PracticeGuidelines/PPP.aspx.

Preferred Practice Patterns Committee, Glaucoma Panel. *Open-Angle Glaucoma Suspect* (2005).

Preferred Practice Patterns Committee, Glaucoma Panel. *Primary Angle Closure* (2005).

Preferred Practice Patterns Committee, Glaucoma Panel. *Primary Open-Angle Glaucoma* (2005).

Ophthalmic Technology Assessments

Ophthalmic Technology Assessments are available at http://one.aao.org/CE/Practice Guidelines/Ophthalmic.aspx and are published in the Academy's journal, *Ophthalmology.* Individual reprints may be ordered at http://www.aao.org/store.

Ophthalmic Technology Assessment Committee. *Aqueous Shunts in Glaucoma* (2008).

Ophthalmic Technology Assessment Committee. *Automated Perimetry* (2002).

Ophthalmic Technology Assessment Committee. *Corneal Thickness Measurement in the Management of Primary Open-Angle Glaucoma* (2007).

Ophthalmic Technology Assessment Committee. *Cyclophotocoagulation* (2001; reviewed for currency 2006).

Ophthalmic Technology Assessment Committee. *Laser Peripheral Iridotomy for Pupillary-Block Glaucoma* (1994; reviewed for currency 2003).

Ophthalmic Technology Assessment Committee. *Nonpenetrating Glaucoma Surgery* (2001; reviewed for currency 2006).

Ophthalmic Technology Assessment Committee. *Optic Nerve Head and Retinal Nerve Fiber Layer Analysis* (2007).

Complementary Therapy Assessments

Complementary Therapy Assessments are available at http://one.aao.org/CE/Practice Guidelines/Therapy.aspx.

Complementary Therapy Glaucoma Task Force. *Marijuana in the Treatment of Glaucoma* (2003).

To order any of these materials, please order online at www.aao.org/store, or call the Academy's Customer Service toll-free number 866-561-8558 in the U.S. If outside the U.S., call 415-561-8540 between 8:00 AM and 5:00 PM PST.

Study Questions

Although a concerted effort has been made to avoid ambiguity and redundancy in these questions, the authors recognize that differences of opinion may occur regarding the "best" answer. The discussions are provided to demonstrate the rationale used to derive the answer. They may also be helpful in confirming that your approach to the problem was correct or, if necessary, in fixing the principle in your memory.

1. In eyes without glaucoma, the average normal corneal thickness is
   a. 520 μm
   b. 540 μm
   c. 560 μm
   d. 580 μm
   e. 600 μm

2. In AGIS, the Advanced Glaucoma Intervention Study, patients had significantly better outcomes if their intraocular pressure (IOP) was controlled
   a. below 18 mm Hg at all visits
   b. below 18 mm Hg at 50% of visits
   c. below 14 mm Hg at all visits
   d. below 14 mm Hg at 50% of visits

3. In the CNTGS, Collaborative Normal-Tension Glaucoma Study, progression was reduced by nearly threefold by a reduction in IOP of
   a. 20%
   b. 30%
   c. 40%
   d. 50%

4. A feature *not* associated with exfoliation syndrome is
   a. spontaneous lens dislocation
   b. earlier cataract formation
   c. higher incidence of vitreous loss during cataract surgery
   d. volatile IOPs
   e. deeper anterior chamber angles

5. In pigmentary dispersion syndrome with elevated IOP,
   a. laser iridotomy may help deepen the chamber
   b. laser trabeculoplasty requires greater energy settings
   c. African-American ancestry is more common
   d. myopic nerves may make detection of early glaucomatous change more difficult
   e. the risk of hypotony maculopathy after filtering surgery with antimetabolites is reduced

6. All of the following statements about aqueous humor are true *except*
   a. Aqueous humor is formed at a rate of approximately 2–3 μL/min.
   b. There is a 1% turnover in aqueous volume each minute.
   c. Normal aqueous humor has a high protein content.
   d. As aqueous humor flows from the posterior chamber through the pupil and into the anterior chamber, its composition is altered.

7. Patients with primary angle closure usually have
   a. short axial length
   b. an anterior chamber depth <2.1 mm
   c. increased anterior curvature of the lens
   d. small cornea diameter and radius of curvature
   e. all of the above

8. Screening for glaucoma based solely on IOP >21 mm Hg
   a. may miss up to half of the people with glaucoma in the screened population
   b. is a good strategy because glaucomatous damage is caused exclusively by pressures that are higher than 21 mm Hg
   c. is effective because IOPs in a population have a Gaussian distribution
   d. is effective because a clear line exists between safe and unsafe IOP

9. The preferred therapy for primary congenital glaucoma is
   a. topical beta-blockers
   b. topical brimonidine
   c. trabeculotomy or goniotomy
   d. oral acetazolamide

10. Sturge-Weber syndrome
    a. is usually bilateral
    b. is always inherited in an autosomal dominant pattern
    c. is more common in males
    d. is rarely associated with glaucoma
    e. may be associated with glaucoma in infants

11. Goldmann tonometry
    a. is not affected by alteration in scleral rigidity
    b. is unaffected by laser in situ keratomileusis (LASIK)
    c. may give an artificially high IOP measurement with increased central corneal thickness
    d. may give pressure measurements taken over a corneal scar that are falsely low

12. Elevated episcleral venous pressure may be associated with all the following *except*
    a. Sturge-Weber syndrome
    b. facial cutaneous angiomas, such as nevus flammeus
    c. foreshortening of the conjunctival fornices
    d. thyroid-associated orbitopathy
    e. dilation of episcleral vessels

13. Automated perimetry
    a. requires the pupil diameter to be at least 5 mm to obtain reliable results
    b. often employs "staircase" strategies to estimate the threshold sensitivity at individual locations
    c. is useful for the detection of glaucomatous vision loss but not for assessing progression of loss
    d. prevents lens rim artifacts, which are common with manual perimetry

14. With regard to neurofibromatosis:
    a. It may be associated with glaucoma.
    b. Anterior segment abnormalities and angle closure may develop.
    c. Plexiform neuromas may produce S-shaped upper eyelid deformities.
    d. Plexiform neuromas are a hallmark of the type 1 variant of neurofibromatosis.
    e. All of the above are true.

15. With regard to anterior chamber angle pigmentation, all of the following are true *except*
    a. Pigmentation commonly increases with age.
    b. Decreased pigmentation is common following ocular trauma with hyphemas.
    c. Both exfoliation syndrome and pigment dispersion syndrome have increased angle pigmentation.
    d. the Sampaolesi line is a scalloped line of pigment deposition anterior to the Schwalbe line.
    e. Pigmentation of the angle is dynamic and changes over time.

16. Which of the following systemic disorders is *not* typically associated with glaucoma?
    a. tuberous asclerosis
    b. juvenile xanthogranuloma
    c. ocular dermal melanocytosis
    d. Fuchs endothelial dystrophy
    e. Bourneville syndrome

17. The anterior optic nerve
    a. has a diameter of approximately 1.5 mm
    b. is commonly divided into 4 regions (nerve fiber layer, prelaminar, laminar, and retro-laminar)
    c. receives its blood supply from both the central retinal artery and the posterior ciliary arteries
    d. is composed primarily of retinal ganglion cell axons, vascular tissues, glial tissues, and extracellular matrix
    e. all of the above

18. The prevalence of glaucoma is
    a. equal in blacks and whites
    b. 2 times more common in whites than in blacks
    c. 8 to 10 times more common in whites than in blacks
    d. 3 to 4 times higher in blacks than in whites
    e. 2 times higher in blacks than in whites

19. The inheritance pattern of the 8 primary loci for adult-onset glaucoma is mainly
    a. autosomal recessive
    b. autosomal dominant
    c. sex-linked
    d. none of the above

20. The percentage of primary congenital glaucoma that is now known to have a definite genetic component is
    a. 1%
    b. 10%
    c. 25%
    d. 50%
    e. 75%

21. Which of the following is *least* compelling as a risk factor for primary open-angle glaucoma (POAG)?
    a. IOP
    b. age
    c. race
    d. diabetes mellitus
    e. family history

22. The gene known to be associated with aniridia is
    a. *CYP1B1*
    b. *PITX2*
    c. *FOXC1*
    d. *PAX6*
    e. *LMX1B*

23. Which of the following is *not true* regarding the gene known to cause *GLC1A*-associated glaucoma?
    a. It involves an abnormality of the TIGR/myocilin protein.
    b. It is associated with juvenile open-angle glaucoma.
    c. It is associated with adult open-angle glaucoma.
    d. It is found on chromosome 1.
    e. It is associated with a single, specific mutation.

24. Anterior chamber depth
    a. is less in women than in men
    b. increases with increasing age
    c. is increased by hyperopia
    d. is decreased in very high myopia
    e. rarely correlates with anterior chamber volume

25. Long-term (10-year) success after laser trabeculoplasty is achieved in what percentage of patients?
    a. 90%
    b. 70%
    c. 50%
    d. 30%
    e. none

26. Incisional surgery for glaucoma may be required in all of the following situations *except*
    a. Maximal tolerated medical therapy fails to adequately reduce IOP.
    b. The patient is treated with multiple glaucoma medications and has had an adverse reaction to a glaucoma medication.
    c. Medical therapy necessary to control IOP is not well tolerated or places the patient at unacceptable risk.
    d. Glaucomatous optic neuropathy or visual field loss is progressing despite apparently "adequate" reduction of IOP with medical therapy.
    e. The patient cannot comply with the necessary medical regimen.

27. A single intraoperative application of mitomycin C has been associated with an increased risk of
    a. hypotony
    b. bleb hyperemia
    c. bleb leaks and infections
    d. all of the above
    e. a and c only

28. Aqueous shunts are indicated for all of the following conditions or situations *except*
    a. elevated IOP despite maximal medical therapy
    b. a failed trabeculectomy
    c. conjunctival scarring
    d. poor prognosis for success of trabeculectomy
    e. iridocorneal endothelial (ICE) syndrome

29. Complications of cyclophotocoagulation include
    a. hypotony
    b. vision loss
    c. phthisis bulbi
    d. all of the above
    e. a and b only

30. All of the following statements regarding Goldmann applanation tonometry are true *except*
    a. The diameter of the applanated area is 3.06 mm.
    b. The tear film creates surface tension that increases the force of applanation.
    c. The cornea tends to resist deformation, which tends to balance out the surface tension effect of the tear film.
    d. The IOP tends to be overestimated in eyes with low scleral rigidity.

31. Each of the following conditions may produce nerve fiber bundle visual field defects similar to those seen in glaucoma *except*
    a. chronic papilledema
    b. optic disc drusen
    c. AION (anterior ischemic optic neuropathy)
    d. occipital infarction
    e. branch retinal artery occlusion

32. All of the following are histologic changes in glaucoma *except*
    a. posterior bowing of the lamina cribrosa
    b. thinning of the retinal nerve fiber layer
    c. loss of the outer nuclear layer of the retina
    d. loss of ganglion cells in the retina
    e. peripapillary atrophy

33. The ICE syndrome includes all of the following *except*
    a. Chandler syndrome
    b. Axenfeld-Rieger syndrome
    c. iris nevus syndrome
    d. essential iris atrophy

34. All of the following are true of ciliary block glaucoma, or malignant glaucoma, *except*
    a. It responds to aqueous suppressants and hyperosmotic medical management in approximately 50% of cases.
    b. It results from posterior misdirection of aqueous into the vitreous cavity.
    c. It occurs only after incisional surgery and never following laser treatment.
    d. It occurs most commonly in eyes with a history of angle-closure glaucoma.
    e. It may occur in aphakic or pseudophakic eyes.

35. Which of the following causes of developmental glaucoma does *not* involve trabeculodysgenesis as a part of its pathophysiology?
    a. Sturge-Weber
    b. homocystinuria
    c. aniridia
    d. Peters anomaly

36. Which of the following beta-blockers demonstrates the relative selectivity in the manner described?
    a. betaxolol: relatively selective for β_2-receptors
    b. timolol: relatively selective for β_1-receptors
    c. levobunolol: relatively selective for β_2-receptors
    d. betaxolol: relatively selective for β_1-receptors
    e. levobunolol: relatively selective for β_1-receptors

37. All of the following statements concerning pilocarpine are true *except*
    a. By relaxing tension on the zonular fibers, it may cause narrowing of the anterior chamber.
    b. It is a direct cholinergic agonist.
    c. It reduces IOP by increasing aqueous flow.
    d. It inhibits acetylcholinesterase.
    e. It is relatively contraindicated in the treatment of uveitic glaucoma.

38. The secondary angle-closure glaucoma in which peripheral anterior synechiae (PAS) extend anterior to the Schwalbe line is
    a. Axenfeld-Rieger syndrome
    b. neovascular glaucoma
    c. ICE syndrome
    d. Fuchs heterochromic iridocyclitis

39. The condition in which iris neovascularization is *not* associated with PAS and secondary angle closure is
    a. Fuchs heterochromic iridocyclitis
    b. ocular ischemic syndrome
    c. central retinal vein occlusion
    d. chronic retinal detachment

40. An 80-year-old white man presents with poor vision in his right eye with sudden onset of pain and conjunctival hyperemia. The examination reveals an IOP of 45 mm Hg with a prominent cell and flare reaction without keratic precipitates, a dense cataract, and an open anterior chamber angle. The most likely diagnosis is
    a. phacolytic glaucoma
    b. phacoantigenic glaucoma
    c. ICE syndrome
    d. Fuchs heterochromic iridocyclitis

41. The most common cause of glaucoma in which elevated IOP and optic nerve damage are present in only one eye is
    a. Sturge-Weber syndrome
    b. blunt trauma
    c. pseudoexfoliation syndrome
    d. Axenfeld-Rieger syndrome

42. Chandler syndrome is
    a. part of the ICE syndrome
    b. associated with stretch holes in the iris
    c. associated with secondary angle closure and elevated IOP
    d. also known as *essential iris atrophy*
    e. a and c
    f. b and d

43. Failure of trabeculectomy with loss of IOP control
    a. most commonly results from endophthalmitis
    b. almost always is a sequela of bleb encapsulation
    c. is most frequently the result of episcleral scarring
    d. is commonly associated with choroidal effusions

44. In the Ocular Hypertension Treatment Study (OHTS), patients with ocular hypertension were randomized to medical therapy or observation. Which of the following is *true*?
    a. The IOP-lowering target of 20% was achieved in almost all patients with a single medication at 5 years of follow-up.
    b. The conversion rate to glaucoma was identical in the two groups.
    c. The most common finding among the patients who converted to glaucoma was an optic nerve hemorrhage.
    d. IOP lowering in the treated group was approximately 22.5%.

Answers

1. **b.** Average corneal thickness, determined by optical and ultrasonic pachymetry, is approximately 530–545 μm in eyes without glaucoma.

2. **a.** AGIS found that patients with IOP consistently less than 18 mm Hg and an average IOP of 12.2 mm Hg had significantly better outcomes than patients with greater IOP fluctuations and higher average IOP.

3. **b.** In CNTGS, the target set was a 30% reduction of IOP.

4. **e.** Patients with exfoliation syndrome tend to have narrow anterior chamber angles.

5. **d.** Patients with pigmentary dispersion syndrome are usually myopic with increased pigmentation of the trabecular meshwork. As a result, they require less energy with laser trabeculoplasty and have a higher incidence of hypotony maculopathy. Laser peripheral iridectomy may flatten the peripheral iris contour but will not deepen the anterior chamber in this condition.

6. **c.** Aqueous humor is essentially protein free (1/200 to 1/500 of the protein found in plasma), which allows for optical clarity.

7. **e.** Each of the statements is correct.

8. **a.** Pooled data from large epidemiologic studies indicate that the mean IOP is approximately 16 mm Hg, with a standard deviation of 3 mm Hg. IOP, however, has a non-Gaussian distribution with a skew toward higher pressures, especially in individuals older than 40 years. For the population as a whole, no clear line exists between safe and unsafe IOP. Screening for glaucoma based solely on IOP >21 mm Hg may miss up to half of the people with glaucoma in the screened population.

9. **c.** Medications have limited long-term value for primary congenital glaucoma in most cases, and the preferred therapy is surgical. The initial procedures of choice are goniotomy or trabeculotomy if the cornea is clear, and trabeculotomy ab externo if the cornea is hazy. Brimonidine should not be used in infants, and topical beta-blockers should be used cautiously.

10. **e.** Sturge-Weber syndrome is usually a unilateral condition. There is no race or gender predilection, and no inheritance pattern has been established. Glaucoma occurs in 30%–70% of children with this syndrome. When glaucoma is seen in infants with this syndrome, it is thought to be due to congenital anterior chamber anomalies (similar to congenital glaucoma).

11. **c.** Increased central corneal thickness may give an artificially high IOP, and decreased central corneal thickness may give an artificially low IOP. IOP measured after PRK and laser in situ keratomileusis (LASIK) may be reduced because of changes in the corneal thickness induced by these procedures. Pressure measurements taken over a corneal scar will be falsely high secondary to increased corneal rigidity.

12. **c.** Foreshortening of the conjunctival fornices does not affect episcleral venous pressure.

13. **b.** Automated perimetry uses a variety of "staircase" strategies to estimate the threshold sensitivity. The strategy chosen will affect the speed and reproducibility of the visual field produced.

14. **e.** Each of the statements about neurofibromatosis is correct.

15. **b.** Ocular trauma with hyphemas usually will increase anterior chamber angle pigmentation.

16. **d.** Fuchs endothelial dystrophy is an ocular disorder that can, in very rare situations, cause a secondary angle-closure glaucoma.

17. **e.** Each of the statements is correct.

18. **d.** The prevalence of glaucoma in the black population is estimated to be 3 to 4 times higher than that in the white population.

19. **b.** The majority of the 8 described POAG loci appear to be inherited in an autosomal dominant pattern.

20. **e.** It is surprising that the 3 genes identified for primary congenital glaucoma are estimated to account for 75% of all known forms of the disease.

21. **d.** The data are the least compelling for diabetes mellitus being a risk factor for high-pressure POAG.

22. **d.** *CYP1B1* is responsible for primary congenital glaucoma. *PITX2* is associated with Rieger syndrome. *FOXC1* is associated with iridogoniodysgenesis, and *LMX1B* is associated with nail-patella syndrome.

23. **e.** More than 40 mutations are known for *GLC1A*.

24. **a.** Anterior chamber depth decreases with increasing age and correlates with anterior chamber volume. Anterior chamber depth tends to be reduced in hyperopia and increased with myopia.

25. **d.** Although initial success rates are high after laser trabeculoplasty, the success rate declines over time to approximately 50% after 3–5 years and 30% after 10 years.

26. **b.** Many patients require more than one glaucoma medication to control their disease. Adverse reactions may occur with any glaucoma medication. These reactions resolve when the medication is discontinued. Usually an alternate medication or laser trabeculoplasty can be used to successfully treat the patient.

27. **e.** Use of mitomycin C during filtering surgery has been associated with persistent ocular hypotony, bleb leaks, and infections. The blebs are often less vascular than the surrounding tissues that are not treated with mitomycin C.

28. **a.** The usual primary glaucoma surgery is trabeculectomy. If patients have failed prior trabeculectomy, have inadequate conjunctiva (eg, due to extensive prior ocular surgery), or have a poor prognosis for successful trabeculectomy (eg, active uveitis, neovascular glaucoma, ICE syndrome), they may be candidates for aqueous shunt surgery.

29. **d.** Cyclophotocoagulation may be associated with vision loss, hypotony, pain, inflammation, cystoid macular edema, hemorrhage, and even phthisis bulbi. Sympathetic ophthalmia is a rare but serious complication.

30. **d.** The IOP in eyes with low scleral rigidity may be underestimated with applanation tonometry, although this effect is more pronounced when techniques of indentation tonometry are used.

31. **d.** All of the choices except occipital infarction may produce nerve fiber bundle defects that can mimic the visual field loss seen in glaucoma. Occipital infarction would typically produce a homonymous hemianopia.

32. **c.** Loss of the outer nuclear layer is not observed in glaucoma. Glaucoma results in loss of ganglion cells and their axons, which make up the retinal nerve fiber layer.

33. **b.** Iris nevus syndrome, Chandler syndrome, and essential iris atrophy are 3 clinical variants of the ICE syndrome that have been described. Axenfeld-Rieger syndrome is a disorder of the iris stroma that may have other associated ocular and systemic abnormalities.

34. **c.** Ciliary block, or malignant, glaucoma is characterized by a shallow anterior chamber with elevated IOP as a result of posterior misdirection of aqueous. It occurs most commonly following intraocular surgery in eyes with a history of angle-closure glaucoma, but it may also follow laser iridectomy or other procedures. It has been reported in aphakic and pseudophakic eyes as well as phakic eyes.

35. **b.** Trabeculodysgenesis is probably the most common pathophysiologic mechanism behind the entire category of developmental glaucomas. It has never been reported in homocystinuria.

36. **d.** Because of its relative β_1 selectivity, betaxolol has fewer pulmonary side effects. Timolol and levobunolol are nonselective beta-blockers.

37. **d.** An indirect cholinergic agonist would inhibit cholinesterase. Pilocarpine is a direct-acting cholinergic agonist.

38. **c.** In the ICE syndrome, the characteristic abnormal corneal endothelium allows for the PAS to extend anterior to the Schwalbe line. Neovascular glaucoma and Fuchs heterochromic iridocyclitis have a normal corneal endothelium. In Axenfeld-Rieger syndrome, the Schwalbe line is displaced anteriorly; however, the PAS are limited to this anterior displacement.

39. **a.** Fine neovascularization of the iris and anterior chamber angle occurs in Fuchs heterochromic iridocyclitis, but it is not associated with angle closure and PAS formation. The other three conditions can cause iris neovascularization associated with PAS and secondary angle-closure glaucoma.

40. **a.** This is the classic presentation of a patient with phacolytic glaucoma. Without keratic precipitates, both phacoantigenic glaucoma and Fuchs heterochromic iridocyclitis are unlikely. Fuchs heterochromic iridocyclitis is associated with cataract formation, primarily posterior subcapsular cataracts, but it tends to present in a much younger patient. ICE syndrome occurs in younger patients and causes a secondary angle-closure glaucoma.

41. **b.** Blunt trauma resulting in angle damage and decreased outflow facility may lead to IOP elevation even decades after the trauma occurred.

42. **e.** Chandler syndrome is part of the ICE syndrome and commonly presents with corneal edema.

43. **c.** Subconjunctival and episcleral fibrosis and scarring are the most common reasons for bleb failure. Most bleb encapsulations spontaneously resolve, and endophthalmitis is relatively uncommon.

44. **d.** Although all patients who were treated initially received 1 medication and the target IOP lowering was 20%, approximately 50% required at least 2 medications to maintain the target at 5 years. The average IOP lowering was 22.5%, and the treated group had significantly lower conversion rates to glaucoma.

Index

(*f* = figure; *t* = table)

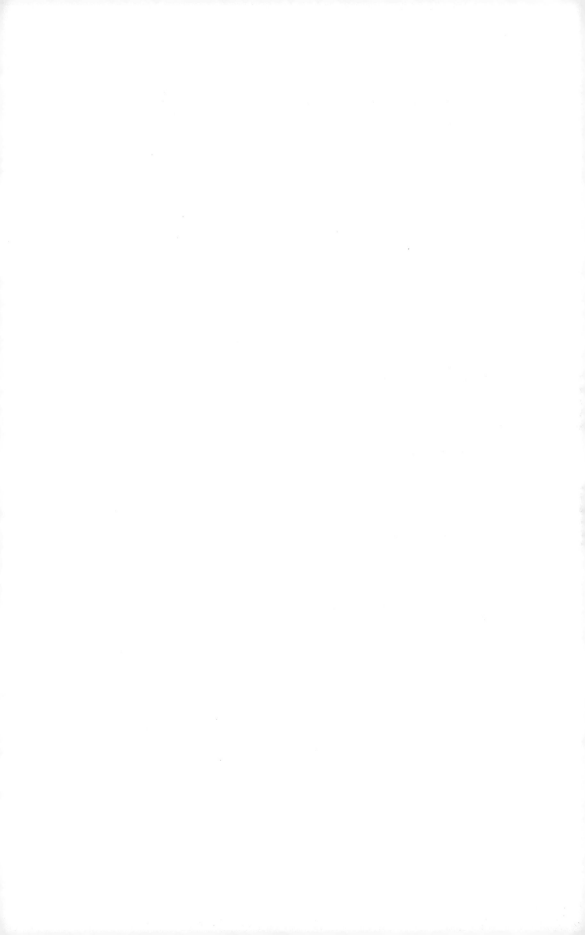